Neural Plasticity and Disorders of the Nervous System

Neural Plasticity and Disorders of the Nervous System provides comprehensive coverage of the pathophysiology of neurological disorders emphasizing those disorders where expression of plasticity is evident. Including the basis for the expression of neural plasticity; how reorganization of the nervous system can cause hyperactivity in sensory systems producing central neuropathic pain, tinnitus and paresthesia; the role of little-known non-classical pathways in pain and sensory disorders and their subcortical connections; hyper- and hypoactivity of motor systems after injury, and the role of spinal reflexes and internal processing in the spinal cord. Phantom symptoms and disorders of nerves and associated disorders are discussed, along with disorders that can be cured by microvascular decompression operations. A detailed and comprehensive description of the organization of pain circuits and sensory and motor nervous systems is also included. *Neural Plasticity and Disorders of the Nervous System* is aimed at students and graduates of neuroscience and medicine.

DR. AAGE R. MØLLER is Professor and holder of the M. F. Jonsson Chair at the University of Texas at Dallas, School of Behavioral and Brain Sciences and Callier Center for Communication Disorders. He teaches neuroscience, disorders of neurological disorders and the physiological and anatomical basis for intraoperative neurophysiologic monitoring.

Neural Plasticity and Disorders of the Nervous System

AAGE R. MØLLER

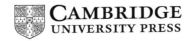
CAMBRIDGE
UNIVERSITY PRESS

CAMBRIDGE UNIVERSITY PRESS
Cambridge, New York, Melbourne, Madrid, Cape Town, Singapore, São Paulo

Cambridge University Press
The Edinburgh Building, Cambridge CB2 2RU, UK

Published in the United States of America by Cambridge University Press, New York

www.cambridge.org
Information on this title: www.cambridge.org/9780521846677

© A. Møller 2006

First published 2006

Printed in the United Kingdom at the University Press, Cambridge

A catalog record for this publication is available from the British Library

ISBN-13 978-0-521-84667-7 hardback
ISBN-10 0-521-84667-6 hardback

Contents

Acknowledgements

I have had valuable help from many individuals in writing this book. I want especially to thank Mark Steckert, MD, Ph.D., Keith Tansey, MD, Ph.D., Carl Noe, MD, and Margareta B. Møller, MD, D. Med.Sci., for their valuable comments on earlier versions of the manuscript. Steve Lomber, Ph.D., and Tres Thompson, Ph.D., also provided valuable comments on earlier versions of the manuscript.

Many of my students at the University of Texas at Dallas School of Behavioral and Brain Sciences have provided valuable feedback and comments. I want to thank Hilda Dorsett for preparing most of the artwork for the book, and Renee Workings and Erik Lakes for help with editing the manuscript.

I also want to thank Martin Griffiths, Editor, and Jayne Aldhouse, Production Manager, Cambridge University Press, for their excellent work on the book.

I would not have been able to write this book without the support of the School of Behavioral and Brain Sciences at the University of Texas at Dallas.

Last but not least I also want to thank my wife, Margareta B. Møller, for her patience with my absorption in this book and for her encouragement during my writing of it.

Dallas, June 2004
Aage R. Møller, Ph.D. (D. Med.Sci)

Abbreviations

5-HT	Serotonin
AI	Primary auditory cortex
ABR	Auditory brainstem responses
ALS	Amyotrophic lateral sclerosis
AMPA	Amino-3-hydroxy-5-methyl-4-isoxazolepropionic acid
AP	Action potential
BDNF	Brain derived neurotrophic factor
BK	Bradykinin
BPPV	Benign paroxysmal positional vertigo
CCK	Cholecystokinin
CGRP	Calcitonin gene-related peptide,
CM	Centromedian (nucleus of thalamus)
CMAP	Compound muscle action potentials
CMT-I	Charcot-Marie-Tooth
CN	Cranial nerve
CNS	Central nervous system
CPG	Central pattern generator
CRPS I	Complex regional pain syndrome type I
CRPS II	Complex regional pain syndrome type II
DBS	Deep brain (electrical) stimulation
DLPT	Dorsolateral pontomesencephalic tegmentum
DPV	Disabling positional vertigo
DREZ	Dorsal root entry zone
DRG	Dorsal root ganglia
EMG	Electromyography
EP	Epinephrine

EPSP	Excitatory post synaptic potentials
FRA	Flexor reflex afferents
GABA	Gamma aminobutyric acid
GAD	Glutamic acid decarboxylase
GBS	Guillain-Barre syndrome
Gly	Glycine
GPe	Globus pallidus external part
GPi	Globus pallidus internal part
GPN	Glossopharyngeal neuralgia
H+	Proton
HD	Huntington's disease
HFS	Hemifacial spasm
HMSN-I	Hereditary motor sensory neuropathies
HTM	High threshold mechanoreceptors
IASP	International Association for the Study of Pain
IC	Inferior colliculus
ICC	Central nucleus of the IC
IPS	Intraparietal sulcus
LGN	Lateral geniculate nucleus
LGP	Lateral segment of pallidus
LTM	Low threshold mechanoreceptors
LTR	Local twitch response
MGB	Medial geniculate body
MGP	Medial segment of globus pallidus
MI	Primary motor cortex
MLF	Medial longitudinal fasciculus
MLR	Middle latency responses
MPTP	Methylphenyltetrahydropyridine
MS	Multiple sclerosis
MSA	Multiple system atrophy
MVD	Microvascular decompression
NA	Noradrenaline (Norepinephrine)
NE	Norepinephrine
NIHL	Noise induced hearing loss
NMDA	N-methyl-D-aspartate
NST	Nucleus of the solitary tract
PAG	Periaqueductal gray
PD	Parkinson's disease
PF	Prefrontal (cortex)
PMA	Premotor (cortical) areas

PTS	Permanent threshold shift
RBD	Rapid eye movement sleep behavior disorder
REM	Rapid eye movement (sleep)
REZ	Root entry (exit) zone
RPC	Reticularis pontis caudalis
RSD	Reflex sympathetic dystrophy
RVM	Rostral ventromedial medulla
SC	Superior colliculus
SCI	Spinal cord injuries
SDR	Selective dorsal root rhizotomy
SG	Sympathetic ganglion
SI	Primary somatosensory cortex
SII	Secondary somatosensory cortex
SMA	Supplementary motor areas
SMP	Sympathetic maintained pain
SNc	Substantia nigra pars compacta
SNr	Substantia nigra pars reticulata
SOC	Superior olivary complex
SP	Substance P
SSRI	Selective serotonin re-uptake inhibitor
STN	Subthalamic nucleus
STT	Spinothalamic tract
TENS	Transdermal electric nerve stimulation
TGN	Trigeminal neuralgia
TIA	Transient ischemic attack
TMJ	Temporomandibular joint
TRT	Tinnitus retraining therapy
TTS	Temporary threshold shift
V1	Primary visual cortex (striate cortex)
V2–5	Extrastriate visual cortices
VB	Ventrobasal nuclei (of thalamus)
Vim	Ventral intermediary nucleus (of the thalamus)
VLL	Ventral nucleus of the lateral lemniscus
VLo	Ventralis lateralis pars oralis
VMpo	Ventromedial posterior oralis (nuclei of thalamus)
VOR	Vestibular ocular reflex
VPI	Ventral posterior inferior (nuclei of thalamus)
VPL	Ventral posterior lateral (nuclei of thalamus)
VPM	Ventral medial (thalamic) nucleus
WBS	Williams-Beuren syndrome
WDR	Wide dynamic range (neurons)

Introduction

Historically, the search for the cause of a disorder of the nervous system has been focused on finding morphological or chemical abnormalities, while symptoms and signs of many disorders of the nervous system can be caused by changes in function other than those that are not directly caused by morphological or chemical abnormalities.

It is well known that activation of neural plasticity is an effective means for treating disorders of the nervous system, but it is less recognized that expression of neural plasticity can also cause symptoms and signs of disorders of the nervous system, and such facts have received less attention than morphological abnormalities.

The focus on morphological changes rather than functional changes for diagnosis and treatment, and for describing the pathology of disorders of the nervous system, is natural: morphological abnormalities (pathologies) are easy to visualize but it is difficult to determine the cause of functional changes. The focus on easily observable factors such as morphological changes is most aptly illustrated through the story about the drunken man who looks for his lost keys under the streetlight – not because this was the place he lost his keys, but because there was better light there.

In a similar way, the focus on genetically related disorders has been on a person's genetic makeup, but genetics alone do not determine whether a person develops the disease in question. For example, a genetic disease can manifest itself in only one of two identical twins, despite the fact that the other twin has exactly the same genetic makeup. Furthermore, when, for example, animals (mice) that are genetically identical are exposed to noise that produces hearing loss, all animals do not achieve exactly the same degree of hearing loss or acquire the same degree of age-related hearing loss, although the variations are smaller in animals that are heavily inbred. Obviously, genetics does not tell the whole story – whether or not a gene is inactivated or activated is important, but it has only recently received noticeable attention. Again, the reason for the focus on genetics is that it is so clearly observable.

There is thus considerable evidence that several factors contribute to the symptoms and signs of most disorders of the nervous system and, in fact, few disorders are caused by a single factor or a single event. Some diseases only manifest themselves when several factors are present, while each factor alone will not cause noticeable signs or symptoms. In other disorders of the nervous system, different factors add to the symptoms and signs, and some disorders manifest only after a sequence of events has occurred before any symptoms of disease become apparent. The search for the cause of a disorder is therefore often counterproductive but patients often demand to get to know what has caused their disease. It is even difficult to get physicians to accept that a specific disease is caused by several different factors interacting in complex ways.

The focus on so-called objective tests, which mainly detect gross morphological abnormalities, has been a distraction in searching for accurate diagnoses and treatments for many disorders of the nervous system.

The fact that induction of neural plasticity can reverse or correct certain pathologic conditions of the nervous system means that induction of neural plasticity is a valuable addition to the medical arsenal of treatments. Directing treatment towards correcting the abnormal function that causes the symptoms and signs of a disease is more beneficial to the patient, than attempts to treat the abnormal test results. This requires a thorough knowledge of not only the normal physiology that makes up a given system, but also its pathophysiology – a topic that is sparsely taught in medical schools.

Increase in understanding of how functional changes in the nervous system can cause symptoms and signs of diseases has already led to more efficient treatments, with fewer side effects, and it seems likely that we have just seen the beginning of a development that focuses on functional changes in the nervous system as a cause of symptoms and signs of disease. Fully utilization of these advancements in diagnosis and treatment of disorders of the nervous system will lead to better treatment of many disorders of the nervous system. More focus on understanding of the pathophysiology of neurological disorders and greater focus on the role of functional changes in disorders of the nervous system would benefit diagnosis and treatment of many diseases. To accomplish that, the concept of multi causes of neurological disorders must be communicated to individuals who are involved in diagnosis and treatment of neurological disorders.

Our understanding of the pathology of neurological disorders has been achieved through the use of many different approaches and studies of patients with different diseases and using different morphological, chemical and physiological methods have contributed to our understanding of the pathophysiology of many disorders of the nervous system. Postmortem studies of tissue samples and morphology have been important in gaining understanding of pathologies of the nervous system. These different approaches have often produced different research results and researchers with different backgrounds often arrive at different results. The same is the case in diagnosis of disorders of the nervous system where physicians of different specialties use different methods to arrive at different diagnoses and thus instate different treatments. It is almost like the old story about the six blind men and the elephant.

They all came to different results from their examination. "A wall!" "A snake!" "A spear!" "A tree!" "A fan!" "A rope!" They told the prince: "We are sorry. But we cannot agree on what an elephant is like. We each touched the same animal. But to each of us the animal is completely different." The prince spoke gently, "The elephant is a very large animal. Its side is like a wall. Its trunk is like a snake. Its tusks are like spears. Its legs are like trees. Its ears are like fans. And its tail is like a rope. So you are all right. But you are all wrong, too. For each of you touched only one part of the animal. To know what an elephant is really like, you must put all those parts together."

We can all agree that the nervous system is very large and its disorders are quite complex. We need to put all the information we have together in order to most effectively understand it. Therefore, this book discusses neurological disorders from several angles, one being specifically the role of functional changes and accompanied by the role of neural plasticity in causing symptoms and signs of diseases of the nervous system.

Proper evaluation of neurological disorders requires a thorough knowledge of not only the anatomy and physiology of the nervous system, but also an understanding of pathophysiology and the role of contributing factors such as neural plasticity.

Functional changes may cause symptoms that cannot be explained from the observed morphological changes but such symptoms are often ignored because of lack of "hard diagnostic evidence" such as imaging and chemical abnormalities. This means that however important such sophisticated imaging methods are in determining the anatomical location of many lesions they have also contributed to incorrect diagnoses. Imaging methods do not detect changes that occur on the cellular level, such as sprouting or elimination of axons or dendrites, nor do they detect changes in synaptic efficacy or threshold. Slightly injured nerves or fiber tracts do not appear different from normal nerves or fiber tracts, yet such changes may cause dramatic symptoms such as severe pain, tinnitus or motor disturbances that alters the life of a patient.

When attempting to diagnose disorders such as trauma to the spinal cord and the cerebrum it is important to recognize the immense complexity of these systems with many interconnected subsystems. For example spasticity that is a result of spinal cord injury cannot be explained by the simple deficits from severed pathways or destroyed gray matter. Symptoms and signs such as spasm and tremor have complex causes because of the complicated and interrelated neural processing that normally occurs in the many parts of the motor systems. Knowledge about the normal function of motor systems and the pathophysiology related to various injuries can benefit treatment and diagnosis, which is a prerequisite for successful treatment. In a similar way, hyperactive disorders such as pain and severe tinnitus have complex causes that require a thorough understanding of not only the anatomy and physiology of the systems involved but also of the mechanisms of neural plasticity.

This book focuses on the pathophysiology of disorders of the nervous system with an emphasis on the role of neural plasticity in creating symptoms and signs. It provides up-to-date knowledge and understanding of the pathophysiology of disorders of the nervous system in a way that can be directly applied to diagnosis and treatment of disorders of the nervous system.

Other factors that are important in evaluation of symptoms and signs of disorders of the nervous system are the stability of an individual's nervous system and its inherent reserves or redundancy.

The fact that the symptoms and signs of two individuals with the same disorder may differ has been an obstacle in diagnosis and treatment of disorders of the nervous system. Biological systems and especially the human central nervous system are extremely complex systems and the nervous systems in different individuals have different degrees of instability and different amounts of reserves. Even two systems that normally function in exactly the same way can have different degrees of stability, and such differences may only manifest when an insult to the nervous system occurs. That neither one of the two individuals had signs of malfunction before that event may be explained by the fact that the instability in itself does not affect the normal function of the system. A particular event may not affect the function of a system that has a high degree of stability, but the same event may cause a major change in the function of the system that had a lower degree of stability. There are many examples of situations where the degree of stability determines the reaction to an external event.

Age-related changes affect different individuals differently and that may also be explained by differences in inherent stability of their nervous system and by the amount of reserves that individuals possess. These reserves decrease with age and changes such as the known change in the balance between inhibition and excitation change the inherent stability of the nervous system. How much insult is needed to cause symptoms depends on these factors and because it is not known beforehand what the limits of stability or redundancy are, the effect of an insult cannot be predicted.

Think of a rod with a flat end placed on a table. It will remain upright until the table shakes a certain amount. How much must the table shake in order that the rod will tumble? It depends on the size of the surface and some random factors. The size of the supporting surface does not affect the rod as long as the table does not shake. If the size of the supporting surface changes nothing happens until the table shakes.

Drugs and surgical operations have been the main means for treatment of disorders of the nervous system. Promotion of expression of neural plasticity for the purpose of correcting abnormal function, and for compensating for lost functions, have not been fully utilized in treatment of neurological disorders, and its capacity has been grossly underestimated. There are many disorders that can benefit from similar kinds of intervention; perhaps the clearest example of the efficiency of inducing expression of neural plasticity is the use of TENS in the treatment of certain forms of pain, but there are many other disorders that can benefit from similar kinds of intervention. Inducing neural plasticity is also effective for treating such disorders as tinnitus, as well as some vestibular disorders. Plastic reorganization of the nervous system after injuries and strokes can promote the regaining of lost functions. Currently, physical therapy is the most used method to promote expression of neural plasticity, but more advanced and directed methods such as electrical stimulation of the cerebral cortex have recently been shown to enhance rehabilitation after strokes. Even some of the symptoms and signs of disorders that are caused by morphological changes can often be ameliorated by inducing neural plasticity that is aimed at shifting function to other parts of the central nervous system. Typically, treatments that make use of expression of neural plasticity have few if any side effects, but use of these methods requires knowledge about anatomy and physiology of the nervous system and, specifically, about neural plasticity.

The understanding of neural plasticity is expanding rapidly, both from studies in animals and studies in humans, to the benefit of diagnosis and treatment of disorders of the nervous system. The results of these studies need to be applied to the treatment of patients. This book is intended to assist in that endeavor by providing pivotal and up-to-date information about the pathophysiology of key disorders of the nervous system. The book provides an in-depth discussion of the role of neural plasticity in disorders of the nervous system. The first chapter discusses the basis for neural plasticity and the following five chapters discuss disorders of nerves, sensory systems and motor systems. Pain and cranial nerves and vestibular disorders (neurotology) are covered in two separate chapters. The role of neural plasticity in causing symptoms and signs such as phantom sensations, cross-modal interaction, spasm and spasticity is also discussed in these chapters. There is a chapter that focuses upon the anatomical and physiological basis for pain that is caused by stimulation of nociceptors, and pain in which neural plasticity is involved is described. The book additionally provides the anatomical and physiological basis for understanding the role of neural plasticity in diseases of the nervous system, and the basis for its use to treat specific disorders. The pathophysiology of neurological disorders is discussed and the different chapters also cover the applicable normal anatomy and physiology of the systems in question.

Anatomical and physiological basis for neural plasticity

Introduction

The nervous system is plastic and expression of neural plasticity can compensate for losses and adapt to changing demands, but the induced changes in the function of the nervous system can also cause symptoms and signs of disease. In fact, such functional change causes or contributes to the symptoms of many disorders of the nervous system. This chapter provides an overview of the mechanisms involved in expression of neural plasticity in general, its role in compensating for deficits and adapting to changing demands, and in creating signs and symptoms of disease. The mechanisms involved in expression of neural plasticity and the physiological and anatomical basis for expression of neural plasticity are discussed.

In the following chapters of this book, we will discuss the pathophysiology of neurological disorders and the role of expression of neural plasticity. In these chapters we will discuss the different symptoms and signs that are caused by expression of neural plasticity while this chapter will provide an overview of the role of expression of neural plasticity and the physiological and anatomical basis for expression of neural plasticity.

1.1   Advantages to the organism from neural plasticity

The beneficial effects of expression of neural plasticity can be divided into three main groups:

    a.   Necessary for normal postnatal development.
    b.   It makes the nervous system adapt to changing demands.

> c.   It can compensate for loss of function and reorganize the nervous system to replace lost functions.

1.1.1   Postnatal development

Perhaps the greatest advantage to humans from neural plasticity is the postnatal development of skills and adaptation to different tasks. The fact that the nervous system of humans, unlike many animal species, are born immature is an advantage because it allows the organization and function of the nervous system to be controlled according to needs and by input from the environment [47].

Such environmental regulation of nervous system development is critical for establishing of normal functions including that of sensory functions. The classical studies of ocular dominance by Wiesel [124, 126] clearly demonstrated the importance of (visual) input for normal development and effectively showed that the effect of closing one eye produced different results from that of closing both eyes. These findings have been confirmed and extended in many later studies [57, 100, 101, 124, 127] that have confirmed that adequate stimulation is necessary for the normal physiological and anatomical development of the nervous system.

> The study by Wiesel and Hubel [124] in cats was one of the first studies that clearly showed the existence of critical periods during which development was guided through sensory input and that adequate sensory input was necessary for the development of normal sensory functions. Wiesel and Hubel also found that the deficits from early visual deprivation were largely preserved and only little recovery occurred after opening the eyes of the animals [126]. Additionally, they found that monocular and binocular deprivation had a different effect on the morphology and function of cells in the lateral geniculate nucleus (LGN) and the primary visual cortex. While few cells in the primary visual (striate) cortex could be activated from the monocular deprived eye many cells could be activated from binocular deprived eyes although the response of many of the cells was not normal [127]. This was an unexpected finding and it illustrates the complexity of the expression of neural plasticity from early deprivation of input. It means that the effect of deprivation of input to one eye depends on the input to the other eye. Bilateral morphological abnormalities were found in the LGN but there were no observed morphological changes in the cerebral cortex.

Most studies on the role of neural plasticity in postnatal development have been performed in animals but more recently studies with humans have been possible through the introduction of auditory prostheses (cochlear implants), which allows the effect of input to the auditory system at different ages to be studied after such input has been established through cochlear implants [52, 106, 113]. Operations for strabismus have yielded similar opportunities [88].

These studies in humans have confirmed the characteristics known from animal experiments that appropriate sensory input is necessary for normal development of the (sensory) nervous system. The existence of critical periods in human studies has also been confirmed [58, 61, 98, 107, 137], which means that the sensory stimulation that occurs before a certain time in the life of children is more effective in changing the functions of the nervous system than input that occurs later in life. Thus cochlear implants that are applied early in life serve better than those implanted in older individuals, confirming that neural plasticity is more pronounced in the young individual than the older organism [61, 107, 137].

The normal postnatal development of the nervous system is a programmed expression of neural plasticity that can be affected by external events such as change in demands and sensory input, and internally by intellectual activity. Deprivation of sensory input causes detectable changes in the function of neurons in the cerebral sensory cortex as shown in the auditory system in studies of congenitally deaf cats. Postnatal deprivation of auditory sensory input causes neural degeneration of the cerebral cortex in a layer specific manner and it can be at least partly restored by electrical stimulation of the auditory nerve in the cochlea (using devices that are similar to the cochlear implants that are used in humans as auditory prostheses) [58] and animals can learn to make use of the input from the electrical stimulation of the auditory nerve [52]. The best results are obtained when such stimulation is provided early in life, thus another example of the existence of a critical period for re-organization of the cortex [57].

The auditory system is organized according to the frequency of sounds and such frequency maps exist throughout the auditory system including the various auditory areas of cerebral cortices (see [79]). It is assumed that these maps are the result of the frequency selectivity of the basilar membrane of the cochlea causing excitation of the sensory cells in accordance with the frequency of sounds. It is assumed that the resulting tonotopic organization of the nervous system together with the frequency tuning of individual nerve cells is important for proper processing of auditory information. Since sounds through cochlear implants do not activate the same groups of nerve cells as the same sounds would do in the normal cochlea, cochlear implants do not generate the same frequency maps as the normal cochlea. If the frequency maps are important for discrimination of sounds such as speech sounds, the nervous system must therefore reorganize after implantation of cochlear implants to achieve a mapping of the CNS that is in accordance with the activation that the cochlear implants provide. It is not known if the normal frequency maps are created in response to sound stimulation during postnatal development, or are independent of sound stimulation. (Deaf animals that have been deprived of stimulation of the auditory nerve have only a rudimentary cochleotopic organization in brainstem nuclei [38] and in the auditory cortex according to some studies [36, 38].) The adaptation to cochlear implants may therefore be different in individuals who were born deaf and those with hearing experience.

Studies of the auditory system have shown that apoptosis, formation of new connections or elimination of connections [16] and changes of synaptic efficacy are all parts of normal postnatal development of the CNS [102]. Some of these changes are programmed (caused by genetic guidance), and some are caused by expression of neural plasticity evoked by sensory input [56, 100].

Little is known about the role of neural plasticity in development of motor skills. Walking, for example, may be programmed in the spinal cord (locomotory control pattern generator, see Chapter 5), but dexterity and other manual skills that require training must involve expression of neural plasticity for adaptation to demands.

The development of facial expressions from the mass movement of the face seen in young children may be a sign of postnatal organization that involves severing of connections within the facial motonuclei where synapses that connect different populations of facial motoneurons in young individuals have not yet become unmasked (compare that with development of synkinesis of face muscles after facial nerve injuries and in hemifacial spasm, pp. 333, 334).

The enhanced capacity for neural plasticity in children also can make the CNS in children more vulnerable to injuries and many pediatric neurological disorders are related to the high degree of plasticity of the developing brain [48]. Impaired plasticity may lead to symptoms and signs of various kinds where cognitive impairments play important roles. Excessive plasticity may lead to maladaptation of various kinds. These matters are extremely complex and the expression of abnormalities depends on many factors such as genetics, epigenetics and environmental factors of various kinds and have not until recently attracted much attention.

Errors in the normal postnatal development may cause more or less severe abnormalities. Failure to block synapses and inadequate pruning of the nervous system may play a role in developmental disorders of many different kinds such as schizophrenia and autism [67, 84]. Similar errors may cause disorders that can manifest later in life such as neurodegenerative disorders such as Alzheimer's and Huntington's diseases. Whether apoptosis is entirely genetically controlled or, more likely, controlled by a combination of environmental and internal factors, has been debated, especially as regards disorders such as autism [67]. There are critical periods regarding vulnerability to insults from environmental factors that can interfere with normal postnatal development [98] as there are critical periods regarding the necessity of sensory input for normal postnatal development [57, 100, 125].

> It was early recognized that input to a cell during early postnatal development is important for adequate generation of proteins in the cell [10]. More recent studies in the avian auditory system have shown that changes in auditory receptors cause changes in neurons in the auditory brainstem [8] and alter protein synthesis in these neurons [100, 108]. Rapid changes in protein synthesis, ribosome and ribosomal RNA has been demonstrated in chick cochlear nucleus [100, 108] after ablation of the cochlea. The hypothesis that synaptic input to these neurons is important in regulating their protein synthesis and metabolism was supported by the finding that administering of Tetrodotoxin (TTX) neurotoxin causes similar changes as ablation of the cochlea and changes in protein synthesis seem to be the earliest cellular sign of reduced input to nerve cells [40]. Also protease activity is beginning to become recognized as an important factor in regulating the activity of nerve cells [17, 116] (see p. 21).

1.1.2   Adaptation to changing demands

That the ability to re-organize is greater in the immature nervous system than in the mature nervous system that was first demonstrated in the classical studies by Wiesel and Hubel [124, 125], has been confirmed in later studies of other sensory systems. The existence of similar "critical periods" where the nervous system can most easily be molded by input to the organism was shown in studies in cats [52, 57]. Other studies, performed in the chicken, have shown that the transition of the critical period where the organization of the cochlear nucleus is most sensitive to removal of the cochlea is sharp [100]. (Some investigators have called this form of neural plasticity "environmental regulation of nervous system development" [100], whereas other investigators have used the term neural plasticity.)

The mature nervous system was earlier regarded as being relatively stable, except for changes that are related to aging. The demonstration of the "kindling phenomenon" (in rats) by Goddard [34] was one of the first published reports that indicates that the function of the adult nervous system can be changed by external factors (electrical stimulation of the amygdala). Later, many studies have brought evidence that the function of the mature nervous system can be changed within wide limits through expression of neural plasticity [42, 46, 54, 72, 96, 99, 105, 111, 112, 119, 121].

While the expression of neural plasticity that is prominent in childhood can proceed throughout the entire life, the ability of the nervous system to change its function after the critical postnatal period decreases with age. For example, while individuals who lose vestibular function at a young age can recover totally relatively quickly, older individuals take longer time to recover and the recovery is not complete. This is an example of adaptation to changing demands that occurs through changes in function and re-routing of neural information. Such switching of functions takes a considerably longer time with increasing age and it becomes incomplete if the injury occurs after a certain age of the individual, again indicating that the young organism is more flexible than the mature organism. Above the age of 60 years, recovery from loss of vestibular function is incomplete (see Chapter 6). This means expression of neural plasticity that is necessary for switching the functions that are normally provided by the vestibular system (such as control of posture) to other systems (such as proprioceptive systems) decreases with age. The ability to recover other functions such as language recovery is much less age related.

An example of how changes in demand can alter the organization of the nervous system was described in individuals who made extensive use of one or more fingers [26]. Also Braille users develop observable changes in the organization of their somatosensory cortex [110]. Even the simplest of the components of the motor system, the monosynaptic stretch reflex, is highly plastic and the size of the stretch response can increase and decrease as a result of behavioral manipulations (such as presentation of reward) [131].

All these forms of plastic changes require active external processes in order to be expressed. Even maintaining skill and functions requires actions ("use it or lose it") and appropriate use of motor skills and sensory input is important for achieving optimal neural functions.

1.1.3   Compensation for damage and injury

A typical example of expression of neural plasticity that is to the benefit to the organism is the recovery after ischemic strokes, which initiates expression of neural plasticity that causes re-organization of the nervous system to make other parts of the CNS take over some of the functions that were lost from the destruction of neural tissue. For example, injury to cortical areas elicits a sequence of self-repair mechanisms, including redirection of tasks to other cortical areas, and reorganization of these remote areas. This injury-induced reorganization includes the enlargement of the cortical areas representative of the (new/redirected) body structure involved, and it may provide the neural substrate for adaptation and recovery of motor behavior after injury [29].

Injuries to sensory organs, sensory nerves or CNS structures elicit expression of neural plasticity. For example, injury to sensory cells such as cochlear hair cells causes morphological changes in the afferent nerve fibers, a process in which neurotrophic factors are involved [2].

Individuals who adapt to artificial limbs likewise rely on expression of neural plasticity to induce proper changes in the proprioceptive and motor systems. This process is more complex than expression of neural plasticity that affects a single system because visual and somatosensory inputs cooperatively play important roles in adapting to amputations.

These changes occur spontaneously in response to injury (including amputations) and it has been known for a long time that training can facilitate the shift of processing from damaged parts of the CNS to other functional parts. Training is the best known method for rehabilitation that can facilitate expression of neural plasticity but additional methods are under development such as electrical stimulation of the cerebral cortex [91].

1.1.4   *Other beneficial effects of expression of neural plasticity*

Not all beneficial effects of neural plasticity have been fully explored. For example, the finding that sound stimulation can slow age-related hearing loss [117, 130] might be caused by expression of neural plasticity. The same may be the case for the "toughening" of ears regarding susceptibility to noise induced hearing loss [1, 15, 73]. The use of electrical stimulation of the cerebral cortex to enhance the effect of training is another recent finding of a beneficial effect of expression of neural plasticity [21].

1.2   Disadvantages to the organism from neural plasticity

The involvement of neural plasticity in creating symptoms of disease has been most extensively studied in connection with pain [18, 54, 69, 71, 94, 95, 121, 133–136] (pain is discussed in Chapter 4); but the symptoms and signs of other disorders such as tinnitus, spasm and synkinesis have also been related to expression of neural plasticity. Research regarding pain has produced most of our knowledge about expression of neural plasticity that causes symptoms and signs of diseases but evidence of the implication of neural plasticity in other symptoms and signs is emerging.

The extensive parallel processing in pain circuits including connections with autonomic and limbic systems can be a substrate for many kinds of plastic changes that can affect routing and processing of nociceptive input [93, 95]. The neural circuits that are involved in generation of the activity that is perceived as pain without stimulation of nociceptors (central neuropathic pain) are incompletely known but are likely to be even more complex than those circuits that are processing information from nociceptors (Chapter 4). Attempts by the organism to compensate for loss of sensory input through expression of neural plasticity involve increasing the sensitivity of neural systems, but this compensation can cause hyperactive symptoms such as tinnitus, central neuropathic pain and exaggerated muscle activity.

There are several reasons why it is difficult to diagnose disorders that are caused by expression of neural plasticity. One reason is related to the fact that anatomical location of the physiological abnormality that causes the symptoms is often different from the anatomical location to which the symptoms are referred.

Phantom sensations are the clearest demonstration of symptoms caused by physiological abnormalities, the anatomical location of which is different from that to which the abnormal sensations (pain, tingling or tinnitus) are referred [4, 13, 45, 70]. The phantom limb syndrome experienced by amputees, and tinnitus that occurs despite a severed auditory nerve, are clear symptoms that have a central origin but are referred to a peripheral origin (the amputated limb or the ear). Paresthesia (tingling) and central neuropathic pain are other examples of phantom sensations. The abnormal neural activity that causes tinnitus in individuals with severed auditory nerve is generated somewhere in the central nervous system, despite the fact that the patient feels that the abnormal activity ("ringing" sensation) comes from the ear [78].

Changes in processing of sensory input, such as distortion of sounds, or sounds appearing louder than normal, cross modal interaction [13, 75] and altered temporal summation, are common signs of expression of neural plasticity in the auditory system [32]. Altered temporal integration also occurs in connection with neuropathic pain [77]. In that way, tinnitus and neuropathic pain have many similarities [76]. Sensitization is another sign of altered processing that is best known from pain where both peripheral and central sensitization can cause hypersensitivity [6, 115] (see Chapter 4) but it probably also plays a role in other hyperactive disorders such as tinnitus (see Chapter 3) as well as some movement disorders (see Chapters 5 and 6). The wind-up phenomenon [39, 115] is a sign of sensitization (see p. 209). Hyperacusis and hyperpathia are other examples of hypersensitivity that are caused by altered processing in the CNS brought about by expression of neural plasticity.

Incorrect redirection of information after injuries can cause synkinesis,[1] which is another example of unwanted manifestation of expression of neural plasticity. Allodynia[2] that often is present together with neuropathic pain is

---

[1] Synkinesis: Voluntary contraction of muscles is accompanied by involuntary contractions of other muscles.

[2] Allodynia: Pain sensation from normally innocuous stimulation (touch) of the skin.

another example of abnormal routing of information that occurs as a result of expression of neural plasticity. Cross-modal interactions that occur in sensory systems in connection with disorders such as tinnitus may be caused by abnormal involvement of non-classical ascending sensory pathways [82], thereby providing subcortical connections to the amygdala. Activation of non-classical sensory pathways is an example of redirection of sensory information to the dorsal portion of the thalamus providing a subcortical route to limbic structures (see Chapter 3).

Changes in the function of the central nervous system caused by expression of neural plasticity may cause increased tonus of muscles and increased reflexes. These changes in function may be nature's way of compensating for lost motor function but too much increase of reflex response can give pathologic signs such as spasticity and hyper-reflexes. In a similar way, expression of neural plasticity triggered by hearing loss may increase the sensitivity of the ear and certain parts of the auditory nervous system as a compensation for loss of sensitivity but overcompensation may cause some forms of tinnitus (see Chapter 3). Expression of neural plasticity is also involved in disorders of the balance systems (dizziness, vertigo, see Chapter 6).

Movement disorders such as spasticity and paresis and paralysis that occur in connection with spinal cord injuries are often regarded to be caused by morphologic damage to neural structures while many of the symptoms in fact are related to functional changes that may be induced by misdirected expression of neural plasticity. The beneficial effect of physical therapy and training in disorders of motor systems may result from reversal of functional changes that were induced by expression of neural plasticity.

1.3   Promoters of neural plasticity

Both external and internal events may cause expression of neural plasticity. Deprivation of input is perhaps the strongest promoter of plastic changes in sensory systems, but insults such as trauma, inflammation and compression or irritation to sensory nerves are also frequent causes of expression of neural plasticity. Novel sensory stimulations, and overstimulation, may also promote expression of neural plasticity and it may affect the balance between inhibition and excitation. Injuries to the CNS such as from strokes and trauma also cause expression of neural plasticity. Age-related morphological and chemical changes may also promote expression of neural plasticity.

Different kinds of insult to the nervous system and novel activation of one part of the nervous system can cause changes in the function of remote parts of the nervous system. For example, forebrain structures can influence more caudal structures of the brain. Change in input from large myelinated axons, sprouting within the dorsal horn [134] and loss of inhibitory neurons through apoptosis [7] are additional examples of changes in function of remote parts of the nervous system. Therefore, nerves and their nuclei and other parts of the CNS to which they relate must be regarded as an integrated system where abnormalities in one part can affect the function of other parts. Receptors, nerves and nuclei of sensory systems should be viewed as integrated systems with regard to being involved in symptoms and signs of disorders. For motor systems, muscles, motor nerves and the spinal cord (and cranial motonuclei) should be regarded as integrated systems where all components together may be involved in causing expression of neural plasticity. However, our knowledge about the role of neural plasticity in creating symptoms and signs of disease is limited and expression of plasticity often occurs without any known cause.

Many studies have shown that plastic changes in the function of specific parts of the CNS can be induced by novel stimulation [50] or overstimulation [85, 86, 96, 114].

It is commonly experienced that the beneficial effect of deep brain stimulation that is used to inactivate specific structures in the basal ganglia or the thalamus for treatment of movement disorders or pain decreases with time. This reduced efficacy over time may be a result of expression of neural plasticity because the stimulation is regarded as a novel stimulation. The expression of neural plasticity then tends to reverse the effect of treatment.

> Signs that deprivation of sensory input may cause reorganization of neural structures comes from animal experiments that have shown that the auditory [42, 96, 99, 111, 112] as well as the somatosensory sensory cortex [46, 50, 72, 119] may reorganize when specific areas have been deprived of input. It has been shown that regions of the cerebral cortex that are adjacent to the areas that are deprived of input expand to occupy the deprived cortical areas [46, 72].
>
> One of the first demonstrations of neural plasticity evoked by novel stimulation was that of Goddard who showed that repeated electrical stimulation of the amygdala nuclei in rats changed the function of these nuclei in such a way that the electrical stimulation began to evoke seizure activity after 4–6 weeks' electrical stimulation [34]. Goddard named this phenomenon "kindling". The kindling phenomenon has later been demonstrated in many other parts of the CNS [118] and even in motonuclei (the facial nucleus) [74] [105].

Various forms of treatment may induce expression of neural plasticity. Physical training is an effective means to promote neural plasticity that can compensate for loss of function and reduce the symptoms associated with injuries to the nervous system. Neural plasticity may also be promoted by means of artificial (electrical) stimulation of CNS structures. Recently electrical stimulation of the auditory cerebral cortex has found use in treatment of tinnitus [20] and for enhancing the beneficial effect of training in stroke patients [91].

There are thus many forms of neural plasticity and many factors can elicit expression of neural plasticity. It is often not known which of these factors are involved in the expression of plasticity that cause symptoms and signs of disease and which cause the changes that are beneficial to the organism, or if the same factors may cause expression of both forms of plasticity.

1.4   Basis for neural plasticity

Plastic changes in the nervous system can occur in four main ways:

1. By (functional) changes in synaptic efficacy, the extreme of which is unmasking of dormant synapses, or masking of efficient synapses.
2. By reducing or modifying protein synthesis and proteinase activity in nerve cells.
3. By creation of new anatomical connections (sprouting of axons and dendrites) or elimination of existing connections or by altering synapses morphologically.
4. By elimination of nerve cells (apoptosis).

Many morphological connections are not functional because the synapses with which they make contact to a target cell are ineffective (not conducting), or because the input is not able to exceed the threshold of the target neuron due to insufficient temporal integration. Such unused connections are a form of redundancy of the nervous system that can be utilized when required such as in response to change in demand or after injuries.

Expression of neural plasticity can cause reorganization of the nervous system to different extents, and it may affect connections between cells in specific structures of the CNS such as parts of the cerebral cortex and it may change the processing of information and re-direct neural information.

Redirection of information can cause neural activity that is elicited by sensory stimulation to reach brain regions that are not normally involved in such processing, or it may cause information to bypass certain populations of neurons that are normally activated. For example, re-routing can cause sensory information to reach the limbic system through a subcortical route via dorsal thalamic nuclei thus bypassing the processing that normally occurs in the cerebral cortices before the information reaches limbic structures. Similar change in the routing of information may cause information to bypass the primary sensory cortices and reach secondary and association cortices directly.

Expression of neural plasticity may alter the excitability of neurons or shift the relationship between excitation and inhibition and thereby cause hypoexcitability or (more often) cause hyperexcitability. Plastic changes in the function of the CNS may occur at different rates (long-term or short-term changes). Expression of neural plasticity that causes symptoms and signs of disease that occur over a long time period tend to become stable and long lasting. Such changes may be caused by formation or elimination of synapses or by modification of their size and efficacy, or by local sprouting of axons and dendrites.

Neural plasticity has many similarities with learning. Some of the earliest hypotheses regarding neural plasticity in fact concerned learning [37]. Neural plasticity has been associated with long-term potentiation (LTP), which has been studied extensively in the hippocampus [65].

1.4.1   Functional changes

Whether or not input to a cell will activate the cell so that an action potential is generated in the cell's axon depends on

1. the input to cells
2. presynaptic activation
3. efficacy of synapses
4. sensitization
5. the availability of neural transmitters
6. protein synthesis and protease activity
7. the balance between inhibition and excitation and the threshold of the cell (resting membrane potential).

Input

Change in the input can functionally open or close synapses. Thus, a change from sustained activity to burst activity, which is often seen in slightly injured nerves (Chapter 2), may cause activation of target neurons that are normally not activated by (normal) sustained activity (Fig. 1.1). This is because temporal summation of the EPSP of several incoming impulses is necessary to generate an excitatory postsynaptic potential (EPSP) that can exceed the neuron's threshold. Assuming that the neuron in question functions according to the "integrate-and-fire" model the decay of the EPSP prevents sufficient summation of input when the intervals between incoming impulses are large. Impulses with short interval such as occur in burst activity may generate EPSPs of sufficient amplitude to reach the threshold of a target neuron that normally was not activated by sustained activity (Fig. 1.1). This would have the same effect as other forms of unmasking of the synapses in question.

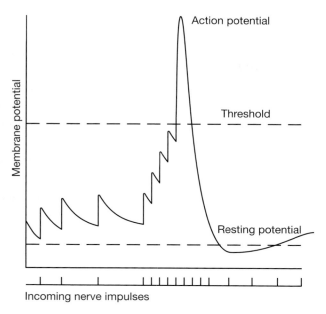

Fig. 1.1 Hypothetical description of the effect of burst activity on excitation of a cell.

This also explains why artificial (electrical) stimulation of high frequency is more effective in activating cells than low frequency stimulation and it may activate cells that are unresponsive to low frequency stimulation.

Presynaptic activation

The degree of expression of neural plasticity depends on the presynaptic activation [5, 109] and the efficacy of a synapse is dependent on how it has been activated earlier (activity dependent synaptic plasticity; long-term potentiation (LPT), long-term depression (LTD)). Some synapses become more efficient after having been activated. Different kinds of drugs can manipulate synaptic efficacy. Some of the anatomical and physiological basis for activity-induced neural plasticity is expressed in Hebb's principle [37] although that hypothesis originally regarded learning. Hebb's principle states that neurons that are activated together establish morphological connections [37]. This means that formation of new connections occurs because of increased neural activity. This has often been referred to as "Neurons that fire together, wire together" [5, 109]. In addition the efficacy of a synapse increases when presynaptic and postsynaptic inputs occur at the same time (synchronized). Activity-dependent synaptic plasticity (Hebbian plasticity) involves postsynaptic activity-controlled regulation of membrane ionic channels [64].

The finding that changes occur in many nuclei after alteration of auditory input (deprivation [31, 32] or overstimulation [114]) including the cerebral cortex [25, 50] implies that such experience-dependent plasticity (Hebbian plasticity) is anatomically more widespread than earlier believed. Jenkins and co-workers (1990) [46] showed that stimulation of the somatosensory system could change the way that body parts were represented on the somatosensory cortex. Studies in the rat have shown widespread changes in the molecular composition and cellular morphology throughout the brainstem after modifications of auditory input [41]. This naturally has implications for the treatment of hearing deficits through artificial stimulation (cochlear and brainstem implants) but these findings also have general importance in understanding of the effects of novel stimulation (or absence of stimulation).

Neurons depend on their innervation to maintain their integrity in both adult and young animals [2, 100] and motoneurons depend on the integrity of their (efferent) axons [59]. Thus morphological changes occur after transection of their nerves [27], which means that also spontaneous activity in nerves may be important for maintaining the integrity of the target neurons.

The fact that inactivity such as from deprivation of input can cause expression of neural plasticity may be regarded as the reverse of Hebb's principle in that neurons that become inactive may lose their normal established connections. This relationship may be expressed by the well-known statement "use it or lose it."

Efficacy of synapses

Change in synaptic efficacy is an important component of expression of neural plasticity. Strengthening of synaptic efficacy has similarities with long-term potentiation (LTP), and it may have similar functional signs such as increased excitability of sensory receptors, decreased threshold of synaptic transmission in central neurons or decreased inhibition. Studies of LTP in slices of hippocampus in rats or guinea pigs show that LTP is best invoked by stimulation at a high rate [103]. The effect may last from minutes to days and glutamate and the NMDA receptor have been implicated in LTP [89].

Some of the basic early studies on change in synaptic efficacy that were done in the spinal cord as a part of research on pain [121] showed similar features. These studies showed that synapses that normally could not cause their cells to fire could be activated by deprivation of input, and the investigator [121] coined the term "dormant synapses" to describe the event where synaptic connections are blocked because they have high synaptic thresholds or too low efficacy, and the opening of such synapses was described as "unmasking" of dormant synapses.

The changes described in these early studies caused cells in the dorsal horn of the spinal cord to respond to input from dermatomes from which they normally did not respond. This investigator [121] hypothesized that many synapses that exist anatomically may not normally be functional ("masked") but may become activated ("unmasked") by some abnormal event such as deprivation of input. The existence of ineffective synapses in the spinal cord of normal animals was also demonstrated by other investigators at about the same time [35]. These early results have been repeated and expanded and there is now a vast amount of literature providing evidence that expression of neural plasticity can cause re-routing of information.

Wall also showed in the same experiments as described above [121] that electrical stimulation of dorsal roots at a high rate could activate cells in the spinal cord at distant segments. Electrical stimulation can activate all fibers of a nerve at the same time, thereby activating the target neurons more coherently than is the case for natural stimulation.

The change that was demonstrated in the spinal cord neurons occurred instantaneously and it was therefore assumed to be caused by changes in synaptic efficacy rather than sprouting of axons or formation of new synapses, which have been assumed to require longer time to occur. The rapid changes that Wall observed could, however, also have been caused by changes in protein synthesis or change in protease activity. Rubel and his co-workers [108] have shown in the chick that deprivation of input from the ear caused rapid changes in protein synthesis in the target cells (cochlear nucleus), and thereby changes in their function. Other studies have shown that elimination of dendrites can occur rapidly after deafferentiation [22].

Sensitization

Hypersensitivity caused by sensitization is a common component of expression of neural plasticity that is associated with changes in the efficacy of synapses [7, 31, 132, 136]. Sensitization is involved in pain and in hyperactive disorders such as tinnitus. It can occur in the periphery and in central structures. It has been studied extensively in regard to pain (see Chapter 4).

Sensitization can occur in the periphery (peripheral sensitization) or centrally (central sensitization). Nociceptive stimulation causes a cascade of complex events to occur at the receptor and in the dorsal horn (and the trigeminal nucleus) [7] and that gives ample possibilities for changes in function through expression of neural plasticity. Increased responsiveness of receptors and cells in the CNS (peripheral and central sensitization) plays an important role in creating symptoms and signs of disease through expression of neural plasticity. Sensitization at the nociceptor level can occur because of repeated activations, which reduces the amount of depolarization that is needed to elicit an action potential in the afferent axon or by secretion of noradrenaline from sympathetic

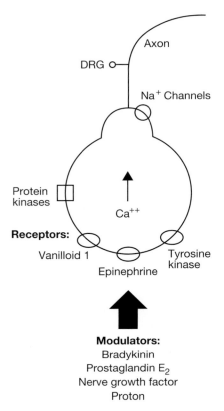

Fig. 1.2 Factors involved in peripheral sensitization. (Based on Bolay and Moskowitz, 2002 [7].)

nerve endings (Fig. 1.2). Vanilloid receptors that are located in C fibers are important for this kind of sensitization. Prostaglandins (PGE_2), serotonin, bradykinin, epinephrine (EP), adenosine and nerve growth factor (NGF) that act on receptors in the afferent axon (Fig. 1.2) can also promote sensitization at the receptor level [7]. Exposure to heat, capsaicin or protons (H^+) can cause such peripheral sensitization.

Central sensitization is evident from studies of pain [7, 136] (see Chapter 4) and studies of other hyperactive disorders such as tinnitus [14, 30, 44, 83] (see Chapter 3). Central sensitization can occur at the level of the first neuron in the dorsal horn (Fig. 1.3) (or the trigeminal nucleus), where cholecystokinin (CCK) enhances transmission of noxious stimulation while opioids and GABA have inhibitory influence [7]. Central sensitization is the cause of the wind-up phenomenon that has been studied in connection with pain [115, 133] (Chapter 4). The wind-up phenomenon is an example of changes in central processing through expression of neural plasticity [7, 39, 115]. It is believed to be

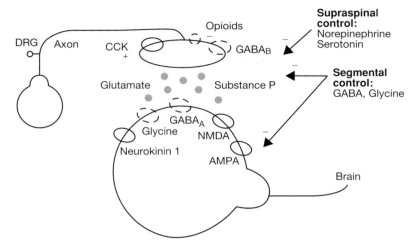

Fig. 1.3   Nociceptive stimulation of a cell in the dorsal horn. Receptors and factors involved in central (spinal cord) sensitization. (Based on Bolay and Moskowitz, 2002 [7]).

caused by repetitive firings of C fibers [115] and it changes the way neurons such as the wide dynamic range neurons (WDR) respond.

Several receptors are involved in central sensitization; especially important is the NMDA receptor [7] (Fig. 1.3) for sensitization to repeated noxious stimulations such as from heat and application of capsaicin. Vasoactive peptides such as calcitonin, gene-related peptide (CGRP), substance P (SP), and neurokinin A may also promote sensitization [7]. The NMDA receptor is involved in central sensitization of pain impulses (see Chapter 4) [133] (Fig. 1.3) [7], causing a cascade of events to occur, where calcium plays an important role. These events play an important role in creating the "wind-up" phenomenon. The release of SP and glutamate from intense sustained noxious stimulation can cause EPSPs lasting tens of seconds and removal of the magnesium blockade of the NMDA calcium channel [7].

The wind-up phenomenon is a form of altered (exaggerated) temporal integrations where the response to stimulation is abnormally affected by a preceding stimulation. Studies of temporal summation of painful (electrical) stimulation to the skin have shown signs of changed temporal integration in individuals with pain disorders [77]. This is similar to observations of changes of altered temporal summation in connection with hyperactivity in sensory systems that were assumed to be caused by expression of neural plasticity [32, 114].

Tissue injury is a frequent cause of sensitization of pain circuits. Tissue injury can initiate a chain of events involving expression of neural plasticity that cause:

1. changes in gene expression (upregulation of specific membrane channel proteins and vanilloid receptor 1),
2. phenotype switch (substance P, and calcitonin gene-related peptide, CGRP, brain derived neurotrophic factor (BDNF) by large myelinated fibers),
3. altered synaptic connections in central structures (such as the dorsal horn and trigeminal nucleus), and
4. death of interneurons due to excitotoxicity.

Availability of neural transmitters

Expression of neural plasticity in many systems depends on availability of specific neural transmitters [39, 92, 97]. The availability of glutamate, acetyl-choline and GABA has been shown to be important in sculpting the receptive field of the cells of the cerebral cortices and establishing the normal balance between excitation and inhibition [122]. Deprivation of input can cause reduced expression of GABA while increased activity can cause increased expression of GABA and thereby increased inhibition. These reactions to deprivation may be seen as self-regulating mechanisms that tend to compensate for low activity by decreasing inhibition and limit increase in activity by increasing inhibition.

The GABA receptors have been a target for pharmacological treatment of disorders using drugs of the benzodiazepine family, which are agonists to the GABA$_A$ receptors, but other agents such as ethanol and endogenous modulators can alter GABA receptors [28]. The function of the GABA$_A$ receptor is flexible and subjected to change through expression of neural plasticity.

Glutamate and the NMDA receptor plays an important role in expression of neural plasticity. Ketamine, a non-competitive antagonist of the NMDA receptor, blocks NMDA receptor mediated neural plasticity [19, 108] and administration of ketamine is known to decrease expression of neural plasticity. These neural transmitters, together with serotonin and acetylcholine, are important players in the dynamic regulation of sensory processing [25]. Other studies have shown the beta adrenergic system of the locus coeruleus, together with the GABA and NMDA receptor systems, have positive effects on the regulation of ocular dominance plasticity [49].

NMDA receptor mediated neural plasticity is affected by factors such as stress and by drugs such as antidepressants [92]. In a similar way, the noradrenergic influence from locus coeruleus has been shown to be important for modulating synaptic plasticity during critical periods of developing odor preferences (in the rat) [68]. Acetylcholine and noradrenaline are the two major neuromodulators of plastic changes in the cerebral cortex [25, 50] where the changes in function involve interplay between neural circuits in the thalamus and primary sensory cortices. Studies have demonstrated the importance of the cholinergic system of the nucleus basalis in cortical plasticity in the auditory system is well documented [51]. This cholinergic basal forebrain system that include nucleus basalis also comprises GABA, calcium-binding proteins and inhibitory neuropeptides [87] and these could also play a role in cortical plasticity. These forebrain structures are altered in Alzheimer's disease.

Change in protein synthesis and protease activity

Rubel and his co-workers have shown that insults to the nervous system such as deprivation of input can change protein synthesis in the target cell [8, 108]. These investigators showed that the changes occur rapidly [108] and that the change in protein synthesis is related to presynaptic impulse activity. However, protease activity also plays an important role in plastic changes in cells [116] and the activity of various proteases are subject to change in connection with injuries and change in input to nerve cells. Proteases of the caspase and calpain families have been implicated in neurodegenerative processes such as cell's death pathways, and it has been suggested that these proteases can also modulate synaptic plasticity [17]. Changes in protease activity can also affect how neurotrophins regulate synaptic plasticity [63]. Neurotrophines are generally assumed to be involved in synaptic plasticity and that the synthesis, secretion and action of neurotrophines are regulated by electrical activity in the nervous system [104].

Other functional changes from expressions of neural plasticity

Increased excitability of a nerve cell may occur because of a decrease in the inhibitory input to the cell. Inhibitory input may prevent cells in the cerebral cortex from firing [42, 43, 96]. Reduced inhibitory input to central neurons lower their threshold and this can have the same effect as unmasking excitatory synapses.

Changes in the threshold of firing of a nerve cell or its resting potential affects its excitability. When the threshold is lowered, input becomes more effective and it may cause some cells to become activated by input that normally would not activate the cells. Making the resting potential less negative requires a smaller EPSP to exceed the cell's threshold and thus excite the cell.

In the cells of the spinal cord, both presynaptic and postsynaptic activity can be modulated from supraspinal sources through the norepinephrine-serotonin (NE-serotonin) descending pathway (see Fig. 4.23) and from segmental levels where GABA and glycine are the important transmitter substances [7]. It is important to keep in mind that even the target cells of receptors receive input from many segmental and supraspinal sources. In fact, the most numerous connections to cells in the dorsal horn are from other cells in the spinal cord. Cells in the brainstem are also under influence from other brainstem cells and from cells at higher levels of the CNS.

There is evidence from a few published studies that temporal integration can change as a result of expression of neural plasticity [3, 30, 32, 66, 77, 114]. On the cellular level, increased temporal integration makes input more efficient and trains of impulses with lower frequency may activate cells that normally required higher frequency input.

1.4.2   Anatomical changes

Anatomical connections can be altered through expression of neural plasticity by

1.   sprouting or elimination of axons and dendrites,
2.   formation or elimination of synapses or changes of the size of synapses,
3.   apoptosis (programmed cell death).

Morphological changes can have a similar effect to change in synaptic efficacy, thus causing re-routing of information, widening of response areas and changes in neural processing. Many phenomena that are attributed to expression of neural plasticity such as the "lateral spread" may be equally well explained by sprouting of axons and dendrites as change in synaptic efficacy. It has been assumed that morphological changes take time to complete, and therefore the effect of morphological changes has been assumed to occur with some delay [121]. However, other studies show that degeneration of dendrites can occur rapidly [22].

Sprouting of dendrites and axons

Studies of pain have shown evidence of outgrowth of new connections as an expression of neural plasticity. For example, some studies indicate that Aβ fibers in the spinal cord can sprout from a location deep in the dorsal horn of the spinal cord into more superficial parts where C-fibers normally terminate (lamina II of the dorsal horn) and make synaptic contacts with neurons that normally are activated by noxious stimuli [24, 53, 54, 134]. Sprouting may explain symptoms such as allodynia that often occurs after peripheral nerve injuries but allodynia may also be explained by changes in synaptic efficacy (see Chapter 4). Several investigators have published results of animal experiments that indicate that expression of neural plasticity in the auditory system may promote outgrowth of new connections [85, 86, 129] (see Chapter 3).

Change in synaptic morphology

Synapses undergo processes of assembly and disassembly as a natural process of postnatal development and aging; and these processes are also related to activity-dependent plasticity [33]. Despite extensive research efforts relatively little is known about the dynamic processes that govern creation and elimination of synapses, and which factors control the size of synapses. It, however, has become evident that these processes are extremely important for postnatal development, and for the changes in function that occur as a result of expression of neural plasticity.

Apoptosis

Even though apoptosis is defined as programmed cell death (in contrast to causes such as injuries and asphyxia), the process of apoptosis is believed to depend on expression of neural plasticity [48]. Apoptosis is important in postnatal development where it can be affected by neural activity such as that evoked by sensory stimulation [90].

1.4.3   Effects of changes caused by expression of neural plasticity

We discussed above how expression of neural plasticity or changed input can alter processing by causing changes in synaptic efficacy, outgrowth of new connection and elimination of connections. These matters have been studied most extensively in connection with pain circuits where the sensitization of peripheral and central structures has been studied in detail. Also sensory systems can be affected in a similar way through expression of neural plasticity. Some of these processes alter the balance between inhibition and excitation, which can change neural processing and generate symptoms of diseases. Altered synaptic efficacy and change in input can also cause re-direction of neural activity.

Activation of new brain regions ("re-wiring" or re-routing)

Many connections between neurons are not functional because the activity that is delivered to a cell by an axon cannot excite the cell. In the hypothetical example in Fig. 1.4 one neuron represents the entrance of one pathway and the other neuron represents the entrance of another pathway. One of the neurons responds by an action potential whereas the other neuron does not respond to the same stimulus. This means that the information that is represented in the input will only travel in one of these two pathways. The reason that only one neuron responds can be ineffective synapses, or insufficient temporal summation, that prevent the input to generate an EPSP of sufficient amplitude to reach

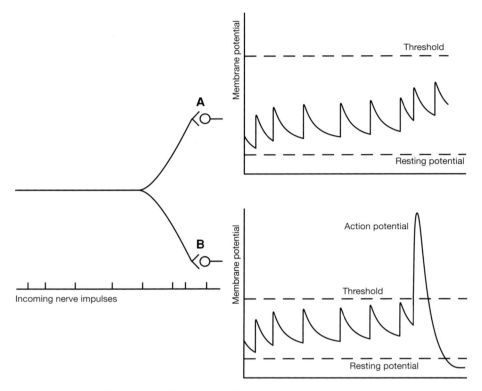

Fig. 1.4 Hypothetical illustration of how the same input to two neurons, each representing a separate pathway, causes one of the neurons (B) to open and the other (A) to remain unresponsive.

the threshold of the cell, or too high a threshold. In the example in Fig. 1.4 low frequency input is not able to cause the EPSP to exceed the threshold in neuron A, but it can cause an action potential in neuron B, making only pathway B open for low frequency input. If each of the two neurons represented the entrance to two different pathways, only one of the two pathways would carry the information that the input represented.

Increased synaptic efficacy, proliferation of synapses or decreased threshold could make it possible for the input to elicit an EPSP that could exceed the threshold of the target cell.

Making a cell that is normally not activated respond can open a path that is normally closed and it can cause information to reach populations of nerve cells that normally do not receive such information, thus re-routing information.

Figure 1.5 shows how the cell in the top illustration in Fig. 1.4 can be made to respond by changing the rate of the input impulses. At a higher rate, both cells respond and thereby allow high frequency information to travel in both

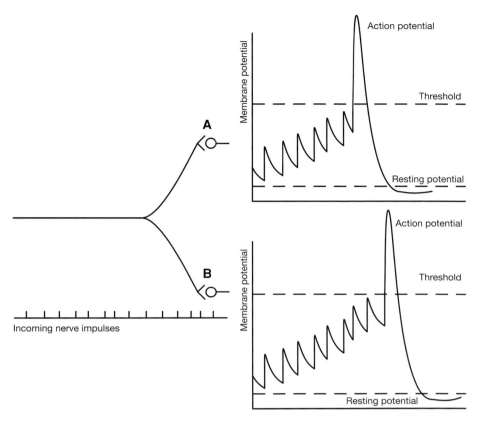

Fig. 1.5 Hypothetical re-routing by change in impulse frequency. Similar illustration as in Fig. 1.4, showing how increased frequency of the stimulation can open the A pathway that was closed to low frequency input (Fig. 1.4).

of the pathways represented by the two neurons. Change in the input from sustained firing to burst firing (Fig. 1.1) is an example of how change in input can make a normally non-responsive cell respond and open new connections, or, conversely, a change to lower discharge rate may prevent activation of cells that are normally responding (Fig. 1.4).

The examples in Figs. 1.4 and 1.5 illustrate how change of input can re-route information. Change in synaptic efficacy, change in temporal integration or change in the threshold of neurons can have the same effect. Changes in the relation between inhibition and excitation can also make neurons respond to input to which they normally do not respond.

Synapses that are not conducting (dormant) are common in all parts of the CNS thus making it possible to functional "re-wire" many parts of the CNS. Such re-organization may open new pathways and thereby activate populations of neurons that are normally not activated and change response areas of neurons.

The existence of dormant synapses means that anatomical studies only provide information about which pathways are available and physiological studies are required to determine if pathways are open for neural traffic. Anatomical studies generally give the impression of the existence of far more pathways than those that are functional but such "unused" pathways may become available to the organism through expression of neural plasticity.

The reorganization of the central nervous system that results from expression of neural plasticity may make information take alternate routes and reach structures that are normally not activated by specific sensory activation. For example, limbic structures may receive subcortical input from sensory systems such as the auditory system because of activation of the non-classical auditory pathways that use nuclei in the dorsal and medial thalamus [81] and subsequent activation of the dorsal or medial thalamus [60] (see Chapter 3, p. 68). The direct subcortical route to the amygdala nuclei may explain why central neuropathic pain and severe tinnitus often are accompanied by affective disorders such as fear and depression [80, 81, 95]. The ascending pathways from the medial and dorsal thalamus (non-classical pathways, see p. 72) project to secondary and association cortices thus bypassing the primary sensory cortices [60, 81].

The cross-modal sensory interaction between somatosensory and auditory systems that exists during childhood [81] is an indication of activation of the non-classical auditory system. These signs decrease with age and are absent in most adult individuals indicating changes in the routing of auditory information. Similar cross modal interaction can occur later in life in connection with tinnitus as indicated by re-occurrence of the abnormal cross-modal interaction between the auditory system and the somatosensory system [13, 14, 75]. A recent study indicated that the cross modal interaction observed in early childhood is maintained into adulthood in autistic individuals [84] thus supporting the hypothesis of abnormal childhood development in autism where the normal disconnection to the non-classical auditory pathway has not occurred. Blocking of normally functional synapses and elimination of connections is a normal phenomenon in postnatal development.

Re-routing of sensory information in the dorsal horn of the spinal cord has been assumed to be the cause of allodynia and hyperpathia (see Chapter 4) indicating that abnormal connections have been established between the somatosensory nervous system and pain circuitries in the spinal cord [54, 94, 95]. Phantom sensations such as typically occur after limb amputations [70] may have similar changes in the CNS as may occur in some forms of tinnitus [44].

The symptoms and signs of some vestibular disorders are caused by re-routing of information. Thus while information from the balance organ (inner ear) normally does not reach our consciousness, disorders of the auditory-vestibular nerve can cause information about movements of the head to reach consciousness and produce the sensation of dizziness and vertigo. Head motion may cause vomiting, a sign of activation of regions of the CNS that are not normally activated by the vestibular system.

Remapping the CNS

Shaping of the receptive fields of cortical neurons occur constantly in response to the state of vigilance and learning [25]. Re-mapping of cortical areas through expression of neural plasticity is a complex process in which the thalamo-cortical pathways and specific channels within these pathways are involved [25]. Remapping of sensory cortices can be initiated by sensory stimulation (adaptation to changing demands) and such remapping is facilitated by input from the nucleus basalis [50]. The nucleus basalis receives input from among other sources, the central nucleus of the amygdala (see Fig. 3.7, p. 92). The changes that occur in cortical receptive fields may be permanent such as has been demonstrated in the auditory system [51, 99] and in the somatosensory systems [46, 72] (see Chapter 3).

Changes in neural representation that occur in response to change in demand often include an increase in the response area. Extension of response areas has been demonstrated in studies in the somatosensory cortex in humans by Edward Taub and his colleagues [11, 62, 123]. The cortical representation of the body to which pain is referred also increases as a result of expression of neural plasticity [18, 24, 136]. Unmasking of inefficient (dormant) synapses can cause extension of the sensory activation areas by opening connections to adjacent neurons and thereby widen response areas. Widening of response areas is also known as "lateral spread" (see pp. 26, 363). Similar mechanisms can open connections to regions of the brain that are not normally activated. These dynamic changes may "crystallize" into long lasting or permanent changes by learning-induced plasticity [25].

Unmasking of dormant synapses may explain the results of studies of the somatosensory representation on the cerebral cortex by Merzenich and colleagues [46] who were some of the first to publish experimental studies that demonstrated widening of the cortical representation of the skin caused by altered input (deprivation) of input (amputation of a finger) [72]. Similar phenomena have been observed in the auditory cortex [99].

The extension of response areas that often occurs as a result of expression of neural plasticity can be regarded as the spatial component of neural plasticity ("where," p. 89), with changes in neural processing being the objective components ("what" component).

The dependence on vigilance (wakefulness) on neuromodulation of cerebral cortex has necessitated studies in awake animals, and the results obtained in anesthetized animals must be viewed and interpreted with that in mind.

The changes in the function of cerebral cortex that are induced by abnormal sensory input causing sensory dysfunction is accompanied by extensive changes in subcortical structures [7] that result in re-organization of sensory systems extending from the periphery to the sensory cortices. This means that the dysfunction that occurs after injuries to sensory organs, sensory nerves, spinal cord and amputations can be regarded as diseases of re-organization of large regions of the CNS [120].

1.5   Diagnosis and treatment of disorders caused by expression of neural plasticity

Plastic changes in the nervous system represent change in function and such changes cannot be detected by commonly used imaging techniques or electrophysiological tests. Chemical testing and imaging techniques are the basic diagnostic tools of modern medicine and disorders that show only functional abnormalities that cannot be documented by objective tests are often regarded with suspicion by the medical profession and consequently do not receive optimal treatment. Some diseases that may have been caused by expression of neural plasticity have been labeled "functional" in the meaning that the symptoms were generated in the patient's mind without any physiological or anatomical abnormality. This is unfortunate because there are effective treatments available for disorders that are caused by expression of neural plasticity.

Since expression of neural plasticity that causes change in the function of specific CNS structures is not accompanied by tissue damage they are potentially reversible [4, 9, 45, 46, 128]. For example, treatment using electrical stimulation (TENS) [128] to treat pain is attractive not only because of its efficiency but also because of its lack of side effects, thus different from typical pharmacological or surgical treatments. Tinnitus Retraining Therapy (TRT) [45] is another example of training in connection with sensory stimulation that can alleviate symptoms of functional changes in the CNS. The fact that synkinesis of facial muscles after injuries to the facial nerve can be successfully treated by exercise [9] is a similar example of effective treatment of a disorder of the motor system. Another disorder where the symptoms can be relieved by sensory stimulation is Ménière's disease, where the application of air puffs to the inner ear can decrease the symptoms [23]. More methods are under development for reversing the functional changes such as those causing tinnitus. Recently it was shown that electrical or magnetic stimulation of the cerebral cortex was effective in alleviating some forms of tinnitus [20, 21].

Therapy-induced expression of neural plasticity has also been shown to occur in the motor systems [55] and recent developments have shown that electrical stimulation of specific parts of the cerebral cortex can facilitate rehabilitation after strokes through training by inducing expression of neural plasticity [12, 91].

However, incomplete understanding of the mechanisms of disorders that are caused by expression of neural plasticity is a severe obstacle for being able to reverse many forms of functional changes in the performance of the nervous system. The fact that the anatomical location of the physiological abnormality that causes the symptoms and signs of the disorders that are caused by expression of neural plasticity is often different from that to which the patients refer their symptoms is an obstacle in obtaining a correct diagnosis and for instituting proper treatment of disorders caused by functional changes in the nervous system. Patients often attempt to associate their symptoms with events that they assume have precipitated the symptoms, e.g. trauma to a peripheral nerve, yet, symptoms of disorders where expression of neural plasticity is involved often seems unrelated to these events. These psychological factors are obstacles both in treatment of individual patients and in research that is aimed at developing effective treatments for disorders where the symptoms and signs are caused by expression of neural plasticity.

References

1. Ahroon, W. A. and R. P. Hamernik, Noise-Induced Hearing Loss in the Noise-Toughened Auditory System. *Hear. Res.*, 1999. **129**: pp. 101–110.

2. Altschuler, R. A., Y. Cho, J. Ylikoski, U. Pirvola, E. Magal, and J. M. Miller, Rescue and Regrowth of Sensory Nerves Following Deafferentiation by Neurotrophic Factors. *Ann. N.Y. Acad. Sci.*, 1999. **884**: pp. 305–11.

3. Arendt-Nielsen, L., J. Brennum, S. Sindrup, and P. Bak, Electrophysiological and Psychophysical Quantification of Temporal Summation in the Human Nociceptive System. *Eur. J. Appl. Physiol. Occup. Physiol.*, 1994. **68**(3): pp. 266–73.

4. Bach, S., M. F. Noreng, and N. U. Tjellden, Phantom Limb Pain in Amputees During the First 12 Months Following Limb Amputation, after Preoperative Lumbar Epidural Blockade. *Pain*, 1988. **33**: pp. 297–301.

5. Bear, M. F., L. N. Cooper, and F. F. Ebner, A Physiological Basis for a Theory of Synapse Modification. *Science*, 1987. **237**(4810): pp. 42–8.

6. Boivie, J., Central Pain, in *Textbook of Pain*, P. D. Wall and R. Melzack, Editors. 1999, Churchill Livingstone: Edinburgh. pp. 879–914.

7. Bolay, H. and M. A. Moskowitz, Mechanisms of Pain Modulation in Chronic Syndromes. *Neurology*, 2002. **59** (Suppl. 2): pp. S2–7.

8. Born, D. E. and E. W. Rubel, Afferent Influences on Brain Stem Auditory Nuclei of the Chicken: Presynaptic Action Potentials Regulate Protein Synthesis in Nucleu Magnoc 295Xellularis Neurons. *J. Neurosci.*, 1988. **8**(3): pp. 901–919.

9. Brach, J. S., J. M. Van Swearingen, J. Lenert, and P. C. Johnson, Facial Neuromuscular Retraining for Oral Synkinesis. *Plastic and Reconstructive Surgery*, 1997. **99**(7): pp. 1922–1931.

10. Brattgard, S. O., The Importance of Adequate Stimulation for the Chemical Composition of Retinal Ganglion Cells During Early Postnatal Development. *Acta Radiol. (Stockh.)*, 1952. **Suppl. 96**: pp. 1–80.

11. Braun, C., R. Schweizer, T. Elbert, N. Birbaumer, and E. Taub, Differential Activation in Somatosensory Cortex for Different Discrimination Tasks. *J. Neurosci.*, 2000. **20**(1): pp. 446–50.

12. Brown, J. A., H. L. Lutsep, S. C. Cramer, and M. Weinand, Motor Cortex Stimulation for Enhancement of Recovery after Stroke: Case Report. *Neurol. Res.*, 2003. **25**: pp. 815–818.

13. Cacace, A. T., T. J. Lovely, D. J. McFarland, S. M. Parnes, and D. F. Winter, Anomalous Cross-Modal Plasticity Following Posterior Fossa Surgery: Some Speculations on Gaze-Evoked Tinnitus. *Hear. Res.*, 1994. **81**: pp. 22–32.

14. Cacace, A. T., Expanding the Biological Basis of Tinnitus: Crossmodal Origins and the Role of Neuroplasticity. *Hear. Res.*, 2003. **175**: pp. 112–132.

15. Canlon, B., E. Borg, and A. Flock, Protection against Noise Trauma by Pre-Exposure to a Low Level Acoustic Stimulus. *Hear. Res.*, 1988. **34**: pp. 197–200.

16. Cant, N. B., Structural Development of the Mammalian Auditory Pathways, in *Development of the Auditory System*, E. W. Rubel, A. N. Popper, and R. R. Fay, Editors. 1998, Springer: New York. pp. 315–413.

17. Chan, S. L. and M. M. Mattson, Caspase and Calpain Substrates: Roles in Synaptic Plasticity and Cell Death. *J. Neurosci. Res.*, 1999. **58**(1): pp. 167–90.

18. Coderre, T. J., J. Katz, A. L. Vaccarino, and R. Melzack, Contribution of Central Neuroplasticity to Pathological Pain: Review of Clinical and Experimental Evidence. *Pain*, 1993. **52**: pp. 259–285.

19. Corbett, D., Ketamine Blocks the Plasticity Associated with Prefrontal Cortex Self-Stimulation. *Pharmacology, Biochemistry & Behavior*, 1990. **37**(4): pp. 685–8.

20. De Ridder, D., E. Verstraeten, K. van der Kelen, G. De Mulder, S. Sunaert, J. Verlooy, P. van de Heyning, and A. Møller. Transcranial Magnetic Stimulation for Tinnitus: Influence of Tinnitus Duration on Stimulation Parameter Choice and Maximal Tinnitus Suppression. *Otol Neurotol.*, 2005. Jul. 26(4): pp. 616–619.

21. De Ridder, D., G. De Mulder, V. Walsh, N. Muggleton, S. Sunaert, and A. Møller, Magnetic and Electrical Stimulation of the Auditory Cortex for Intractable Tinnitus. *J. Neurosurg*, 2004. **100**(3): pp. 560–4.

22. Deitch, J. S. and E. W. Rubel, Rapid Changes in Ultrastructure During Deafferentiation-Induced Dendritic Atrophy. *J. Comp. Neurol.*, 1989. **281**: pp. 234–258.

23. Densert, B. and K. Sass, Control of Symptoms in Patients with Ménière's Disease Using Middle Ear Pressure Applications: Two Years Follow-Up. *Acta Otolaryng. (Stockh.)*, 2001. **121**: pp. 616–621.

24. Doubell, T. P., R. J. Mannion, and C. J. Woolf, The Dorsal Horn: State-Dependent Sensory Processing, Plasticity and the Generation of Pain, in *Handbook of Pain*, P. D. Wall and R. Melzack, Editors. 1999, Churchill Livingstone: Edinburgh. pp. 165–181.

25. Edeline, J. M., The Thalamo-Cortical Auditory Receptive Fields: Regulation by the States of Vigilance, Learning and the Neuromodulatory System. *Exp. Brain Res.*, 2003. **153**(4): pp. 554–72.

26. Elbert, T., C. Pantev, C. Wienbruch, B. Rockstroh, and E. Taub, Increased Cortical Representation of the Fingers of the Left Hand in String Players. *Science*, 1995. **270**(5234): pp. 305–7.

27. Engel, A. K. and G. W. Kreutzberg, Neuronal Surface Changes in the Dorsal Vagal Motor Nucleus of the Guinea Pig in Response to Axotomy. *J. Comp. Neurol.*, 1988. **275**: pp. 181–200.

28. Fritschy, J. M. and I. Brunig, Formation and Plasticity of GABAergic Synapses: Physiological Mechanisms and Pathophysiological Implications. *Pharmacol. Ther.*, 2003. **98**(3): pp. 299–323.

29. Frost, S. B., S. Barbay, K. M. Friel, E. J. Plautz, and R. J. Nudo, Reorganization of Remote Cortical Regions after Ischemic Brain Injury: A Potential Substrate for Stroke Recovery. *J. Neurophysiol.*, 2003. **89**(6): pp. 3205–14.

30. Gerken, G. M., Temporal Summation of Pulsate Brain Stimulation in Normal and Deafened Cats. *J. Acoust. Soc. Am.*, 1979(66): pp. 728–734.

31. Gerken, G. M., S. S. Saunders, and R. E. Paul, Hypersensitivity to Electrical Stimulation of Auditory Nuclei Follows Hearing Loss in Cats. *Hear. Res.*, 1984. **13**: pp. 249–260.

32. Gerken, G. M., J. M. Solecki, and F. A. Boettcher, Temporal Integration of Electrical Stimulation of Auditory Nuclei in Normal Hearing and Hearing-Impaired Cat. *Hear. Res.*, 1991. **53**: pp. 101–112.

33. Goda, Y. and G. W. Davis, Mechanisms of Synapse Assembly and Disassembly. *Neuron*, 2003. **40**(2): pp. 243–64.

34. Goddard, G. V., Amygdaloid Stimulation and Learning in the Rat. *J. Comp. Physiol. Psychol.*, 1964. **58**: pp. 23–30.

35. Goshgarian, H. G. and L. Guth, Demonstration of Functionally Ineffective Synapses in the Guinea Pig Spinal Cord. *Exp. Neurol.*, 1977. **57**: pp. 613–21.

36. Hartmann, R., R. K. Shepherd, S. Heid, and R. Klinke, Response of the Primary Auditory Cortex to Electrical Stimulation of the Auditory Nerve in the Congenitally Deaf White Cat. *Hear Res.*, 1997. **112**: pp. 115–33.

37. Hebb, D. O., *The Organization of Behavior*. 1949, Wiley: New York.

38. Heid, S., T. K. Jahn-Siebert, R. Klinke, R. Hartmann, and G. Langner, Afferent Projection Patterns in the Auditory Brainstem in Normal and Congenitally Deaf White Cats. *Hear. Res.*, 1997. **110**: pp. 191–199.

39. Herrero, J. F., J. M. Laird, and J. A. Lopez-Garcia, Wind-up of Spinal Cord Neurones and Pain Sensation: Much Ado About Something? *Progress in Neurobiology*, 2000. **61**(2): pp. 169–203.

40. Hyson, R. L. and E. W. Rubel, Activity-Dependent Regulation of a Ribosomal RNA Epitope in the Chick Cochlear Nucleus. *Brain Res.*, 1995. **672**(1–2): pp. 196–204.

41. Illing, R. B., Activity-Dependent Plasticity in the Adult Auditory Brainstem. *Audiol. Neuro-Otol.*, 2001. **6**(6): pp. 319–345.

42. Irvine, D. R. and R. Rajan, Injury- and Use-Related Plasticity in the Primary Sensory Cortex of Adult Mammals: Possible Relationship to Perceptual Learning. *Clin. Exp. Pharmacol. Physiol.*, 1996. **23**(10–11): pp. 939–947.

43. Irvine, D. R. and R. Rajan, Injury-Induced Reorganization of Frequency Maps in Adult Auditory Cortex: The Role of Unmasking of Normally-Inhibited Inputs. *Acta Otolaryng. (Stockh.)*, 1997. **532**: pp. 39–45.

44. Jastreboff, P. J., Phantom Auditory Perception (Tinnitus): Mechanisms of Generation and Perception. *Neurosci. Res.*, 1990. **8**: pp. 221–254.

45. Jastreboff, P. J., Tinnitus as a Phantom Perception: Theories and Clinical Implications, in *Mechanisms of Tinnitus*, J. A. Vernon and A. R. Møller, Editors. 1995, Allyn & Bacon: Boston. pp. 73–93.

46. Jenkins, W. M., M. M. Merzenich, M. T. Ochs, T. Allard, and E. Guic-Robles, Functional Reorganization of Primary Somatosensory Cortex in Adult Owl Monkeys after Behaviorally Controlled Tactile Stimulation. *J. Neurophysiol.*, 1990. **63**(1): pp. 82–104.

47. Johnson, M. H., Development of Human Brain Functions. *Biol Psychiatry*, 2003. **54**(12): pp. 1312–6.

48. Johnston, M. V., Clinical Disorders of Brain Plasticity. *Brain Dev.*, 2004. **26**(2): pp. 73–80.

49. Kasamatsu, T., Adrenergic Regulation of Visuocortical Plasticity: A Role of the Locus Coeruleus System. *Prog Brain Res*, 1991. **88**: pp. 599–616.

50. Kilgard, M. P. and M. M. Merzenich, Plasticity of Temporal Information Processing in the Primary Auditory Cortex. *Nature Neurosci.*, 1998. **1**: pp. 727–731.

51. Kilgard, M. P. and M. M. Merzenich, Cortical Map Reorganization Enabled by Nucleus Basalis Activity. *Science*, 1998. **279**: pp. 1714–1718.

52. Klinke, R., R. Hartmann, S. Heid, J. Tillein, and A. Kral, Plastic Changes in the Auditory Cortex of Congenitally Deaf Cats Following Cochlear Implantation. *Audiol. Neurootol.*, 2001. **6**: pp. 203–206.

53. Koerber, H. R., K. Mirnics, A. M. Kavookjian, and A. R. Light, Ultrastructural Analysis of Ectopic Synaptic Boutons Arising from Peripherally Regenerated Primary Afferent Fibers. *J. Neurophysiol*, 1999. **81**: pp. 1636.

54. Kohama, I., K. Ishikawa, and J. D. Kocsis, Synaptic Reorganization in the Substantia Gelatinosa after Peripheral Nerve Neuroma Formation: Aberrant Innervation of Lamina II Neurons by Beta Afferents. *J. Neurosci.*, 2000. **20**: pp. 1538–1549.

55. Kopp, B., A. Kunkel, W. Muhlnickel, K. Villringer, E. Taub, and H. Flor, Plasticity in the Motor System Related to Therapy-Induced Improvement of Movement after Stroke. *NeuroReport*, 1999. **10**(4): pp. 807–10.

56. Kral, A., R. Hartmann, J. Tillein, S. Heid, and R. Klinke, Congenital Auditory Deprivation Reduces Synaptic Activity within the Auditory Cortex in Layer Specific Manner. *Cerebral Cortex*, 2000. **10**: pp. 714–726.

57. Kral, A., R. Hartmann, J. Tillein, S. Heid, and R. Klinke, Delayed Maturation and Sensitive Periods in the Auditory Cortex. *Audiol. Neurootol.*, 2001. **6**(346–362).

58. Kral, A., R. Hartmann, J. Tillein, S. Heid, and R. Klinke, Hearing after Congenital Deafness: Central Auditory Plasticity and Sensory Deprivation. *Cereb. Cortex*, 2002. **12**: pp. 797–807.

59. Kreutzberg, G. W., Neurobiology of Regeneration and Degeneration the Facial Nerve, in *The Facial Nerve*, M. May, Editor. 1986, Thieme: New York.

60. LeDoux, J. E., Brain Mechanisms of Emotion and Emotional Learning. *Curr. Opin. Neurobiol.*, 1992. **2**: pp. 191–197.

61. Lenarz, T., R. Hartrampf, R. D. Battmer, B. Bertram, and A. Lesinski, Cochlear Implant Management of Young Children. *Laryngorhinootologie*, 1996. **75**(12): pp. 719–26.

62. Lenz, F. A., J. I. Lee, I. M. Garonzik, L. H. Rowland, P. M. Dougherty, and S. E. Hua, Plasticity of Pain-Related Neuronal Activity in the Human Thalamus. *Progr. Brain Res.*, 2000. **129**: pp. 253–273.

63. Lu, B., Pro-Region of Neurotrophines: Role in Synaptic Modulation. *Neuron*, 2003. **39**(5): pp. 735–8.

64. Lu, Y., P. Monsivais, B. L. Tempel, and E. W. Rubel, 2004, 470:3–1906, Activity-Dependent Regulation of the Potassium Channel Subunits Kv1.1 and Kv3.1. *J. Comp. Neurol.*, 2004. **470**: pp. 93–106.

65. Lynch, M. A., Long-Term Potentiation and Memory. *Physiol Rev*, 2004. **84**(1): pp. 87–136.

66. Maixner, W., R. Fillingim, A. Sigurdsson, S. Kincaid, and S. Silva, Sensitivity of Patients with Painful Temporomandibular Disorders to Experimentally Evoked Pain: Evidence for Altered Temporal Summation of Pain. *Pain.*, 1998. **76**(1–2): pp. 71–81.

67. Margolis, R. L., D. M. Chuang, and R. L. M. Post, Programmed Cell Death: Implications for Neuropsychiatric Disorders. *Biol. Psychiatry.*, 1994. **35**(12): pp. 946–56.

68. McLean, J. H. and M. T. Shipley, Postnatal Development of the Noradrenergic Projection from Locus Coeruleus to the Olfactory Bulb in the Rat. *J. Comp Neurol.*, 1991. **304**(3): pp. 467–77.

69. Melzack, R. and P. D. Wall, Pain Mechanisms: A New Theory. *Science*, 1965. **150**: pp. 971–979.

70. Melzack, R., Phantom Limbs. *Sci. Am.*, 1992. **266**: pp. 120–126.

71. Mendell, L. M., Modifiability of Spinal Synapses. *Physiol Rev*, 1984. **64**: pp. 260–324.

72. Merzenich, M. M., J. H. Kaas, J. Wall, R. J. Nelson, M. Sur, and D. Felleman, Topographic Reorganization of Somatosensory Cortical Areas 3b and 1 in Adult Monkeys Following Restricted Deafferentiation. *Neuroscience*, 1983. **8**(1): pp. 3–55.

73. Miller, J. M., C. S. Watson, and W. P. Covell, Deafening Effects of Noise on the Cat. *Acta Oto Laryng. Suppl. 176*, 1963: pp. 1–91.

74. Møller, A. R. and P. J. Jannetta, On the Origin of Synkinesis in Hemifacial Spasm: Results of Intracranial Recordings. *J. Neurosurg.*, 1984. **61**: pp. 569–576.

75. Møller, A. R., M. B. Møller, and M. Yokota, Some Forms of Tinnitus May Involve the Extralemniscal Auditory Pathway. *Laryngoscope*, 1992. **102**: pp. 1165–1171.

76. Møller, A. R., Similarities between Chronic Pain and Tinnitus. *Am. J. Otol.*, 1997. **18**: pp. 577–585.

77. Møller, A. R. and T. Pinkerton, Temporal Integration of Pain from Electrical Stimulation of the Skin. *Neurol. Res*, 1997. **19**: pp. 481–488.

78. Møller, A. R., Similarities between Severe Tinnitus and Chronic Pain. *J. Amer. Acad. Audiol.*, 2000. **11**: pp. 115–124.

79. Møller, A. R., *Hearing: Its Physiology and Pathophysiology*. 2000, San Diego: Academic Press.

80. Møller, A. R., Symptoms and Signs Caused by Neural Plasticity. *Neurol. Res.*, 2001. **23**: pp. 565–572.

81. Møller, A. R. and P. Rollins, The Non-Classical Auditory System Is Active in Children but Not in Adults. *Neurosci. Lett.*, 2002. **319**: pp. 41–44.

82. Møller, A. R., *Sensory Systems: Anatomy and Physiology*. 2003, Amsterdam: Academic Press.

83. Møller, A. R., Pathophysiology of Tinnitus, in *Otolaryngologic Clinics of North America*, A. Sismanis, Editor. 2003, W. B. Saunders: Amsterdam, pp. 249–266.

84. Møller, A. R., J. K. Kern and B. Grannemann, Are the Non-Classical Auditory Pathways Involved in Autism and PDD? *Neurol. Res.*, 2005. 27.

85. Morest, D. K., M. D. Ard, and D. Yurgelun-Todd, Degeneration in the Central Auditory Pathways after Acoustic Deprivation or Over-Stimulation in the Cat. *Anat. Rec.*, 1979. **193**: pp. 750.

86. Morest, D. K. and B. A. Bohne, Noise-Induced Degeneration in the Brain and Representation of Inner and Outer Hair Cells. *Hear. Res.*, 1983. **9**: pp. 145–152.

87. Mufson, E. J., S. D. Ginsberg, M. D. Ikonomovic, and S. T. Dekosky, Human Cholinergic Basal Forebrain: Chemoanatomy and Neurologic Dysfunction. *J. Chem Neuroanat.*, 2003. **26**(4): pp. 233–42.

88. Murray, T., Eye Muscles Surgery. *Curr Opin Ophthalmol.*, 1999. **10**(5): pp. 327–32.

89. Nicoll, R. A. and R. C. Malenka, Expression Mechanisms Underlying NMDA Receptor-Dependent Long-Term Potentiation. *Ann. N.Y. Acad. Sci.*, 1999. **868**: pp. 515–25.

90. Nucci, C., S. Piccirilli, R. Nistico, L. A. Morrone, L. Cerulli, and G. Bagetta, Apoptosis in the Mechanisms of Neuronal Plasticity in the Developing Visual System. *Eur. J. Ophthalmol.*, 2003. **13**(Suppl. 3): pp. 36–43.

91. Plautz, E. J., S. Barbay, S. B. Frost, K. M. Friel, N. Dancause, E. V. Zoubina, A. M. Stowe, B. M. Quaney, and R. J. Nudo, Post-Infarct Cortical Plasticity and Behavioral Recovery Using Concurrent Cortical Stimulation and Rehabilitative Training: A Feasibility Study in Primates. *Neurol. Res.*, 2003. **25**: pp. 801–810.

92. Popoli, M., M. Gennarelli, and G. Racagni, Modulation of Synaptic Plasticity by Stress and Antidepressants. *Bipolar Disorders*, 2002. **4**(3): pp. 166–82.

93. Price, D. D., *Psychological and Neural Mechanisms of Pain*. 1988, New York: Raven.

94. Price, D. D., S. Long, and C. Huitt, Sensory Testing of Pathophysiological Mechanisms of Pain in Patients with Reflex Sympathetic Dystrophy. *Pain*, 1992. **49**: pp. 163–173.

95. Price, D. D., Psychological and Neural Mechanisms of the Affective Dimension of Pain. *Science*, 2000. **288**: pp. 1769–1772.

96. Rajan, R. and D. R. Irvine, Neuronal Responses across Cortical Field AI in Plasticity Induced by Peripheral Auditory Organ Damage. *Audiol. Neurootol.*, 1998. **3**: pp. 123–144.

97. Ren, K. and R. Dubner, Central Nervous System Plasticity and Persistent Pain. *J. Orofacial Pain*, 1999. **13**(3): pp. 164–71.

98. Rice, D. and S. J. Barone, Critical Periods of Vulnerability for the Developing Nervous System: Evidence from Humans and Animal Models. *Environ Health Perspect.*, 2000. **108 Suppl** 3: pp. 511–33.

99. Robertson, D. and D. R. Irvine, Plasticity of Frequency Organization in Auditory Cortex of Guinea Pigs with Partial Unilateral Deafness. *J. Comp. Neurol.*, 1989. **282**(3): pp. 456–471.

100. Rubel, E. and B. Fritzsch, Auditory System Development: Primary Auditory Neurons and Their Targets. *Ann. Rev. Neurosci*, 2002. **25**: pp. 51–101.

101. Rubel, E. W., A. N. Popper, and R. R. Fay, eds. *Development of the Auditory System*. 1998, Springer: New York.

102. Sanes, D. H. and E. J. Walsh, Development of Central Auditory Processing, in *Development of the Auditory System*, E. W. Rubel, A. N. Popper, and R. R. Fay, Editors. 1998, Springer: New York. pp. 271–314.

103. Sarvey, J. M., E. C. Burgard, and G. Decker, Long-Term Potentiation: Studies in the Hippocampal Slice. *J. Neurosci. Methods*, 1989. **28**(1–2): pp. 109–24.

104. Schinder, A. F. and M. Poo, The Neurotrophin Hypothesis of Synaptic Plasticity. *Trends Neurosci.*, 2000. **23**(12): pp. 639–45.

105. Sen, C. N. and A. R. Møller, Signs of Hemifacial Spasm Created by Chronic Periodic Stimulation of the Facial Nerve in the Rat. *Exp. Neurol.*, 1987. **98**: pp. 336–349.

106. Sharma, A., M. F. Dorman, and A. J. Spahr, Rapid Development of Cortical Auditory Evoked Potentials after Early Cochlear Implantation. *Neuroreport*, 2002. **13**(10): pp. 1365–8.

107. Sharma, A., M. F. Dorman, and A. J. Spahr, A Sensitive Period for the Development of the Central Auditory System in Children with Cochlear Implants: Implications for Age of Implantation. *Ear Hear.*, 2002. **23**(6): pp. 532–9.

108. Sie, K. C. Y. and E. W. Rubel, Rapid Changes in Protein Synthesis and Cell Size in the Cochlear Nucleus Following Eighth Nerve Activity Blockade and Cochlea Ablation. *J. Comp. Neurol.*, 1992. **320**: pp. 501–508.

109. Stent, G. S., A Physiological Mechanism for Hebb's Postulate of Learning. *Proc. Nat. Acad. Sci*, 1973. **70**(4): pp. 997–1001.

110. Sterr, A., M. M. Muller, T. Elbert, B. Rockstroh, C. Pantev, and E. Taub, Perceptual Correlates of Changes in Cortical Representation of Fingers in Blind Multifinger Braille Readers. *J. Neurosci.*, 1998. **18**(11): pp. 4417–23.

111. Syka, J. and J. Popelar, Noise Impairment in the Guinea Pig. I. Changes in Electrical Evoked Activity Along the Auditory Pathway. *Hear. Res.*, 1982. **8**: pp. 263–272.

112. Syka, J., N. Rybalko, and J. Popelar, Enhancement of the Auditory Cortex Evoked Responses in Awake Guinea Pigs after Noise Exposure. *Hear. Res.*, 1994. **78**: pp. 158–168.

113. Syka, J., Plastic Changes in the Central Auditory System after Hearing Loss, Restoration of Function, and During Learning. *Physiol Rev*, 2002. **82**(3): pp. 601–36.

114. Szczepaniak, W. S. and A. R. Møller, Evidence of Neuronal Plasticity within the Inferior Colliculus after Noise Exposure: A Study of Evoked Potentials in the Rat. *Electroenceph. Clin. Neurophysiol.*, 1996. **100**: pp. 158–164.

115. Thompson, S. W. N., A. E. King, and C. J. Woolf, Activity-Dependent Changes in Rat Ventral Horn Neurons in Vitro: Summation of Prolonged Afferent Evoked Post-Synaptic Depolarization Produce a d-APV Sensitive Wind-Up. *Eur. J. Neurosci.*, 1990. **2**: pp. 638–649.

116. Tomimatsu, Y., S. Idemoto, S. Moriguchi, S. Watanabe, and H. Nakanishi, Proteases Involved in Long-Term Potentiation. *Life Sci.*, 2002. **72**(4–5): pp. 355–61.

117. Turner, J. G. and J. F. Willott, Exposure to an Augmented Acoustic Environment Alters Auditory Function in Hearing-Impaired DBA/2J Mice. *Hear. Res.*, 1998. **118**: pp. 101–113.

118. Wada, J. A., *Kindling 2*. 1981, Raven Press: New York.

119. Wall, J. T., J. H. Kaas, M. Sur, R. J. Nelson, D. J. Felleman, and M. M. Merzenich, Functional Reorganization in Somatosensory Cortical Areas 3b and 1 of Adult Monkeys after Median Nerve Repair: Possible Relationships to Sensory Recovery in Humans. *J. Neurosci.*, 1986. **6**(1): pp. 218–233.

120. Wall, J. T., J. Xu, and X. Wang, Human Brain Plasticity: An Emerging View of the Multiple Substrates and Mechanisms That Cause Cortical Changes and Related Sensory Dysfunctions after Injuries of Sensory Inputs from the Body. *Brain Res. Rev.*, 2002. **39**(2–3): pp. 181–215.

121. Wall, P. D., The Presence of Ineffective Synapses and Circumstances Which Unmask Them. *Phil. Trans. Royal Soc. (Lond.)*, 1977. **278**: pp. 361–372.

122. Wang, J., S. L. McFadden, D. M. Caspary, and R. J. Salvi, Gamma-Aminobutyric Acid Circuits Shape Response Properties of Audiory Cortex Neurons. *Brain Res.*, 2002. **944**(219–31).

123. Weiss, T., W. H. Miltner, R. Huonker, R. Friedel, I. Schmidt, and E. Taub, Rapid Functional Plasticity of the Somatosensory Cortex after Finger Amputation. *Exp. Brain Res.*, 2000. **134**(2): pp. 199–203.

124. Wiesel, T. N. and D. H. Hubel, Effects of Visual Deprivation on Morphology and Physiology of Cells in the Cats Lateral Geniculate Body. *J. Neurophysiol.*, 1963. **26**: pp. 973–93.

125. Wiesel, T. N. and D. H. Hubel, Effects of Monocular Deprivation in Kittens. *Naunyn Schmiedebergs Arch Pharmacol.*, 1964. **248**: pp. 492–7.

126. Wiesel, T. N. and D. H. Hubel, Extent of Recovery from the Effects of Visual Deprivation in Kittens. *J. Neurophysiol.*, 1965. **28**: pp. 1060–1072.

127. Wiesel, T. N. and D. H. Hubel, Comparison of the Effects of Unilateral and Bilateral Eye Closure on Cortical Unit Responses in Kittens. *J. Neurophysiol.*, 1965. **28**(6): pp. 1029–40.

128. Willer, J. C., Relieving Effect of TENS on Painful Muscle Contraction Produced by an Impairment of Reciprocal Innervation: An Electrophysiological Analysis. *Pain*, 1988. **32**: pp. 271–274.

129. Willott, J. F. and S. M. Lu, Noise Induced Hearing Loss Can Alter Neural Coding and Increase Excitability in the Central Nervous System. *Science*, 1981. **16**: pp. 1331–1332.

130. Willott, J. F., T. H. Chisolm, and J. J. Lister, Modulation of Presbycusis: Current Status and Future Directions. *Audiol. Neurotol.*, 2001. **6**: pp. 231–249.

131. Wolpaw, J. R., Acquisition and Maintenance of the Simplest Motor Skill: Investigation of CNS Mechanisms. *Med. Sci. Sports Exerc.*, 1994. **26**(12): pp. 1475–9.

132. Woolf, C. J., Evidence of a Central Component of Postinjury Pain Hypersensitivity. *Nature*, 1983. **308**: pp. 686–688.

133. Woolf, C. J. and S. W. N. Thompson, The Induction and Maintenance of Central Sensitization Is Dependent on N-Methyl-D-Aspartic Acid Receptor Activation: Implications for the Treatment of Post-Injury Pain Hypersensitivity States. *Pain*, 1991. **44**: pp. 293–299.

134. Woolf, C. J., P. Shortland, and R. E. Cogershall, Peripheral Nerve Injury Triggers Central Sprouting of Myelinated Afferents. *Nature*, 1992. **355**: pp. 75–78.

135. Woolf, C. J. and R. J. Mannion, Neuropathic Pain: Aetiology, Symptoms, Mechanisms, and Managements. *The Lancet*, 1999. **353**: pp. 1959–1964.

136. Woolf, C. J. and M. W. Salter, Neural Plasticity: Increasing the Gain in Pain. *Science*, 2000. **288**: pp. 1765–1768.

137. Zwolan, T. A., C. M. Ashbaugh, A. Alarfaj, P. R. Kileny, H. A. Arts, H. K. El-Kashlan, and S. A. Telian, Pediatric Cochlear Implant Patient Performance as a Function of Age at Implantation. *Otol. Neurotol.*, 2004. **25**(2): pp. 112–20.

2

Nerves

Introduction

Symptoms and signs of disease related to nerves can be a direct result of changes in the function of the axons themselves, or the symptoms and signs can result from subsequent changes in the function of more central structures through changes in procession of information or from expression of neural plasticity. Disorders of nerves (neuropathy[1]) can therefore present many different, often complex, symptoms. Neuropathy of sensory nerves can give pain, cause paresthesia and other abnormal sensations and functions and cause expression of neural plasticity with subsequent re-organization of CNS structures. Neuropathy of motor nerves can give paresis, paralysis and abnormal muscle activity. Pathologies of motor nerves, the neuromuscular junctions (muscle endplates) or muscles themselves mostly result in reduced, or loss of, function (paresis or paralysis). Disorders of muscles and motor nerves can also cause re-organization of neural circuits in the CNS including the motor cortex through expression of neural plasticity. Interruption of mixed nerves can affect motor function indirectly when proprioceptive nerve fibers are affected because of change of proprioceptive input to the spinal cord or to cranial nerve motor circuits. (Disorders of cranial nerves are discussed in Chapter 6.)

Nerve disorders can initiate changes in the function of CNS structures through expression of neural plasticity; these changes develop gradually and may persist even after healing of the nerve injuries. The CNS changes may be permanent or reversible, with or without intervention. There are many similarities

---

[1] Neuropathy: The word neuropathy theoretically includes all disorders that affect the nervous system, but neurologists usually only use the term to describe disorders of peripheral and cranial nerves, and their roots.

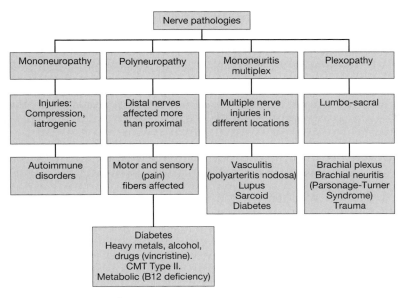

Fig. 2.1 Pathologies of nerves

between signs and symptoms of disorders affecting spinal nerves and cranial nerves, with the latter displaying slightly more variance (see Chapter 6).

2.1   Symptoms and signs of disorders of nerves

The symptoms of disorders of nerves depend on whether sensory, pain or motor fibers are involved and what kind of pathology is affecting the nerves. The pathologies of nerves have been classified according to the symptoms and signs they produce (Fig. 2.1). Some of the symptoms and signs originate directly from the pathological function of the nerve in question whereas other symptoms arise from subsequent changes in the function of CNS structures, brought about by expression of neural plasticity.

Disorders of nerves can include total interruption of neural conduction causing paresis and paralysis or loss of sensory functions, but nerves that are partially conducting (slightly injured nerves) can transform the normal impulse pattern [9, 37] or generate neural activity by themselves [9]. Disorders of motor nerves, the neuromuscular junction, muscles and alpha motoneurons normally cause paresis or paralysis without abnormal function (flaccid paresis or paralysis, see Chapter 5). Loss of function of sensory nerves can, in addition to sensory deficit, cause expression of neural plasticity that can cause complex symptoms such as paresthesia [45] and other phantom sensations such as tinnitus [6]. Even injuries to motor nerves can cause expression of neural plasticity [42]. Regeneration of motor nerves is often associated with synkinesis, perhaps caused by failure of the regenerating axons to make contact with their correct target. This occurs especially in neurotmesis. Synkinesis that occurs in connection with axonotmesis is more likely to be caused by altered central processing (in the motonucleus) that has been brought about by expression of neural plasticity [4]. Neurotmesis of motor nerves is also likely to cause expression of neural plasticity with subsequent changes in the function of CNS structures. Neurotmesis is also likely to cause expression of neural plasticity with subsequent changes in the function of CNS structures. Various forms of irritations of a nerve, especially of its root, may create symptoms and signs such as spasm [30] or pain and these symptoms are mostly caused by the expression of neural plasticity [11, 26]. Injuries to mixed nerves can cause complex motor symptoms because proprioceptive fibers are affected.

2.1.1   Causes of disorders of nerves

Injuries to nerves resulting from insults such as physical trauma (compression, stretching or wounding) can cause focal damage to a nerve. Gun shot wounds, accidents and surgery (iatrogenic incidents) are common causes of permanent damage to peripheral nerves. Nerves can be transiently or permanently injured by heat, often resulting from burns or from electrocoagulation used in surgical operations (iatrogenic injuries). Other forms of focal damage to nerves may be caused by entrapments such as from scar formation and from surgical manipulations (iatrogenic). General (global) injuries may be caused by chemical and metabolic factors such as occur in poisoning, diabetes, vitamin deficits, uremia and hepatic dysfunction, or by inflammation (neuritis) of various kinds. Such disorders that affect motor nerves are commonly studied clinically using electromyography [1]. In some nerve disorders, it is not possible to find a cause (idiopathic).

Trauma

Trauma may affect all parts of a nerve, but the central portions (the root exit or entry zones) are more sensitive to mechanical insults than the peripheral portions of nerves. The central portions of nerves are, however, protected from insults because of their location inside the spinal canal or inside the cranium. Nerve roots are at risk of injury from surgical manipulations in spinal and intracranial operations. The introduction of microneurosurgery and the use of intraoperative neurophysiologic monitoring have decreased the risk of surgical trauma to spinal nerve roots in operations on the spine as well as cranial nerves (see pp. 106, 332).

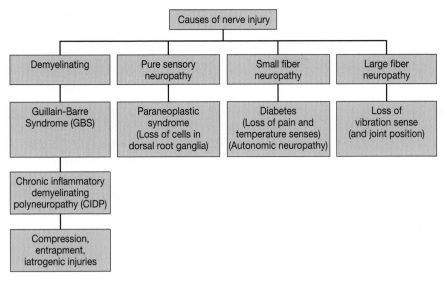

Fig. 2.2 Causes of nerve injuries

It is often difficult to discern which of the symptoms from nerve compression are caused by the changed function of the nerve in question, and which are caused by subsequent changes in the function of central structures through expression of neural plasticity or because of changes in the input to the CNS. Phantom sensations such as tingling or "pins and needles," which are common nerve compression symptoms, may be caused by altered input to the CNS or changes in the function of the CNS caused by expression of neural plasticity. The effect of increased temporal dispersion in an injured nerve is an example of how input to the CNS from sensory nerves can change central processing of sensory stimuli.

Chronic compression of nerves may cause pain but it may also occur without noticeable symptoms. For example, common symptoms of "carpal tunnel syndrome" are often assumed to be caused by compression of a nerve at the wrist, but the cause may be more complex (see pp. 56, 190). Other causes of compression or entrapment are from scar formation after trauma or because of surgical operations (such as the use of non-resorbable sutures). Some forms of common lumbar back pain is assumed to be caused by mechanical compression of the roots of spinal nerves, yet similar morphological changes can occur without noticeable symptoms [26] (see Chapter 4). However, the pathophysiology of these disorders is more complex than just conduction block in nerves [26]. The subsequent involvement of CNS structures through the expression of neural plasticity plays an important role in generating the symptoms and signs of many forms of nerve compression and injuries – it may explain the poor correlation between morphological signs of nerve entrapment and symptoms.

Inflammation

Inflammation of nerves (neuritis) is a frequent cause of symptoms and signs. Different strains of the Herpes virus are often involved in neuritis. Herpes zoster causes neuropathies of different kinds such as shingles and the Ramsey-Hunt syndrome. The varicella-zoster virus causing chicken pox has also been implicated in other diseases, where eruption of the skin occurs, especially in children. The Herpes simplex strain is known for causing disorders of the CNS, especially in children, including encephalitis; it can also cause neuropathy of single nerves. The virus is known for residing in sensory ganglia such as the trigeminal nerve ganglion in asymptomatic individuals. Some forms of neuritis are caused by unknown viral agents (idiopathic polyneuritis).

Diabetes and other causes of neuropathy

Diabetes neuropathy is a common cause of symptoms from nerves. Diabetes mainly affects small nerve fibers and therefore predominantly causes pain and deficits of the temperature sense. Deficiency of vitamins B_1, B_2 and B_{12} can also cause neuropathy. Extensive ingestion of alcohol is a common cause of neuropathy (alcohol neuropathy), but the effect is mainly caused by malnutrition and vitamin B_1 deficiency. Many other chemical agents can cause neuropathy when ingested. Some agents are transmitted from the environment. Age related factors likewise cause damage resulting in symptoms from nerves. The changes often begin in distal parts of nerves first causing symptoms from the feet and hands.

Neural plasticity may be evoked in the target nuclei of an injured nerve by abnormal firing of nerve impulses or caused by deprivation of input from sensory nerves causing changes in synaptic efficacy, formation or elimination of synapses, sprouting of dendrites and axons and even change in protein synthesis [39] (see Chapter 1). Similar changes may occur in motoneurons after injury to motor nerves [22] (see pp. 358, 1).

Demyelinating disorders

The Guillain-Barre syndrome (GBS) is a common demyelinating disorder. Symptoms of GBS often begin after a viral infection but can appear without any known infections. Patients with GBS notice ascending sensory loss and weakness that can occur over a few hours to a week or two. Severe injury that progresses to acute respiratory failure may occur. Pathophysiology of GBS is presumed to be antibody mediated since treatment with plasmaphoresis and infusions of intravenous immunoglobulin are effective. Recovery is generally good.

One of the most prominent signs of genetic inherited abnormalities of myelin occurs in the hereditary motor sensory neuropathy (HMSN-I) (also known as Charcot-Marie-Tooth disease (CMT-I). While GBS is an acquired multifocal demyelination that causes conduction block over affected segments of the nerve, HMSN-I is a hereditary disorder that causes demyelination that generally begins at the root entry (or exit) zone and later in the course of the disease primarily affects more distal segments of nerves. The pathology of GBS typically begins in the periphery and progresses proximally. This means that nerve conduction in distal parts of nerves in HMSN-I is normal and only studies which include measurement of proximal conduction such as the F wave (see pp. 62, 272), show abnormalities.

2.2   Anatomy and physiology of nerves

Spinal nerves originate or terminate in the spinal cord, while cranial nerves originate or terminate in the brainstem or cerebrum. Many spinal and cranial nerves are mixed nerves (cranial nerves are discussed in Chapter 6). Most nerves contain somatic motor fibers, sensory nerve fibers, proprioceptive fibers and pain fibers. Some nerves contain visceral and autonomic nerve fibers.

Nerves from the periphery enter the spinal cord as dorsal roots while nerves to the periphery exit the spinal cord as ventral roots. The ventral roots mostly consist of motor fibers, while the dorsal roots consist of fibers that innervate sensory receptors (including pain fibers and fibers that innervate proprioceptors). Some dorsal roots also contain fibers of the autonomic nervous system.

The central portions of nerves are different from the peripheral portions in several ways. The myelin of the central portion of nerves is generated by oligodendrocytes while the myelin of the peripheral portion is generated by Schwann cells. The peripheral and the central parts of nerves differ by the type of myelination. The transition zone between the peripheral and the central part of nerves occurs near their entry to the CNS, where the myelin changes from Schwann cell generated myelin to oligodendrocyte cell generated myelin in the central part. This transition zone is known as the Obersteiner-Redlich zone.

Sensory and motor fibers are mostly myelinated nerve fibers, while some fibers that carry pain signals and those that belong to the autonomic nervous system are unmyelinated. It is common to divide myelinated fibers into three groups according to the diameter of their axons, Aα, Aβ, Aδ. Unmyelinated fibers are C-fibers. The conduction velocity of nerve fibers is proportional to the diameter of their axons (Table 2.1).

Table 2.1 *Conduction velocity in nerve fibers of different types*

Fiber type	Function	Average axon diameter (μm)	Average conduction velocity (m/s)
Aα	Motor nerves, primary muscle-spindle afferents	15	100 (70–120)
Aβ	Mechanoreceptor afferents	8	50 (30–70)
Aδ	Temperature and pain afferents	<3	15 (12–30)
C	Pain afferents Sympathetic postganglionic fibers (Unmyelinated)	approx. 1	1 (0.5–2)

The support structure of the peripheral portion of nerves is also different from that of the central portion. Each axon of the peripheral portion of nerves is covered by endoneurium to form nerve fibers. Nerve fibers are organized in bundles (fascicles) that are covered by a sheath of perineurium (Fig. 2.3). The peripheral portion of nerves may consist of a single funiculus or can be composed of several funiculi (bundles) that are covered by perineurium. Epineurium covers nerve trunks.

Funiculi in the peripheral portion of nerves have an undulated course (Fig. 2.4) that allows the nerves to be stretched without inducing stress on the individual nerve fibers. Traction that exceeds the stretched length of a nerve will cause the typical injuries seen in traumatic nerve injuries [41].

The endoneurium that consists of collagen fibrils has finer fibrils in the central portion of a nerve than in the peripheral portion. Perineurium and epineurium are also absent in the central portion of nerves, making the central portion of nerves more vulnerable to mechanical stress. The central part of nerves therefore lacks some of the protection that peripheral portions have, and as a result, the central segments of nerves are more fragile than their peripheral counterparts. In addition, the central portion of nerves lacks a funicular support structure and proceeds in parallel without the undulations of the peripheral portion of nerves (Fig. 2.4). This means that the central portion of nerves is more fragile with regards to stretching.

The transition zone between the peripheral and central portion of nerves (the Obersteiner-Redlich zone) is important because it is the anatomical location of pathologies such as tumors (Schwannoma) (see p. 334). (This transition zone has been studied especially in cranial nerves where it has been shown to be sensitive to irritation from, for example, blood vessels; see Chapter 6, pp. 332, 334).

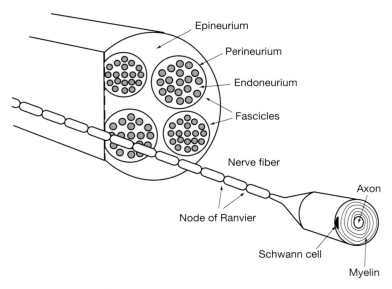

Fig. 2.3 Anatomy of a typical peripheral portion of a nerve [40].

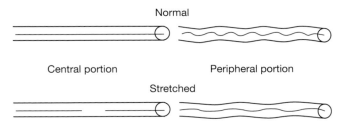

Fig. 2.4 Effect of traction and injury on the central and the peripheral portion of a nerve [41].

2.2.1   Sensory nerves

Sensory fibers from the periphery are bipolar fibers, with their cell bodies located in the dorsal root ganglia (DRG). Nerve fibers of different diameters make synaptic contact with cells in different layers of the dorsal horns. Sensory nerves from the periphery enter the dorsal horn of the spinal cord as dorsal root fibers, where they travel together with fibers that innervate pain receptors (nociceptors), proprioceptors and autonome fibers. Low threshold cutaneous receptors are innervated by Aβ fibers (6–12 μm diameter) and such fibers have conduction velocities in the range of 30–70 m/sec (Table 2.1). Aβ fibers terminate in lamina III-V (Rexed's classification [35]). Proprioceptive fibers from muscle spindles and tendon organs and receptors monitoring joint movements are large (Aα) fibers.

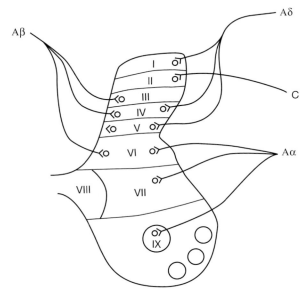

Fig. 2.5 Different types of sensory nerve fibers terminating on cells in the horn of the spinal cord [5].

Fibers carrying pain information are small diameter myelinated fibers (Aδ) and unmyelinated fibers (C fibers). The Aδ fibers enter lamina I, IV and V, and C fibers enter lamina II of the dorsal horn [5] (Fig. 2.5). Proprioceptive fibers terminate in lamina VI, of the spinal horn (Fig. 2.5).

2.2.2   Motor nerves

Motor fibers leave the spinal cord as ventral spinal roots, where some fibers innervate skeletal muscles (extrafusal muscles) while other fibers innervate muscle spindles (intrafusal muscles). The motor nerve fibers are generally larger than sensory fibers belonging mostly to the Aα group of nerve fibers. The cell bodies (alpha motoneurons) of axons that innervate skeletal muscles are located in lamina IX of the ventral horn of the spinal cord (Fig. 2.5) [5]. The cell bodies of the nerve fibers that innervate the intrafusal muscle (γ fibers) are also located in lamina IX of the ventral horn of the spinal cord.

2.2.3   Autonomic nerves

Many nerves include fibers that lead to and from the autonomic nervous system. Efferent preganglionic sympathetic innervation originates in neurons in the intermediolateral column of the lower thoracic and upper lumbar segments of the spinal cord [5]. These preganglionic fibers leave the spinal cord as ventral roots, and connect, through sympathetic cells in the sympathetic trunk, to effector organs (see Chapter 3).

The fibers of nerves of the autonomic nervous system are unmyelinated (C fibers) or myelinated fibers of small diameter (Aδ fibers) and enter the spinal cord through dorsal roots – from there, they make contact with cells in the dorsal-most parts of the dorsal horn with their cell bodies being in the dorsal root ganglion (DRG). Dorsal roots that enter the spinal cord at T_{11} and L_4 therefore contain sympathetic fibers from the body. Parasympathetic efferents that innervate the bladder and some genital organs originate in the dorsal roots of the S_3 and S_4 segments of the spinal cord (see p. 167). The afferent sympathetic innervation of viscera (visceral afferents) in the abdomen forms the greater and lesser splanchnic nerves. Afferent sympathetic nerve fibers that innervate the lower body pass uninterrupted through the sympathetic trunk, enter the spinal cord at T_{11}-L_4 levels through dorsal roots, and terminate in the dorsal-most part of the spinal cord while the vagus nerve (CN X) provides most of the parasympathetic innervation of visceral organs (see Chapter 6). Parasympathetic afferents from S_3 and S_4 segments innervate the bladder and the genital organs (see Chapter 4). Generally, afferents from visceral nociceptors follow sympathetic nerves, while autonomic afferents from other receptors follow parasympathetic nerves [5]. This would mean that the vagus nerve does not carry nociceptor afferents – which has been disputed because it has been shown that vagal stimulation can affect nociception [2, 12] (see Chapters 4 and 6).

Sympathetic innervation of the head involves the superior cervical ganglion the fibers of which follow the internal carotid artery to innervate the dura and some large intracranial arteries.

2.3   Pathologies of nerves

Various insults to nerves can produce symptoms and signs of disorders. Trauma can cause specific injuries to nerves and disorders of different kinds can cause injuries to the myelin (demyelination). Inflammation and age-related changes are other examples of insults to nerves that can cause deficits and other symptoms and signs of disorders.

2.3.1   Focal injuries

Focal injuries affect a limited portion of a (single) nerve while general injuries affect an entire nerve. Mononeuropathy describes injuries that affect a single nerve. Injuries to more than one nerve is known as polyneuropathy.

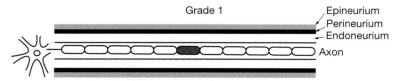

Fig. 2.6 Illustration of a nerve with a conduction block without morphological changes (neurapraxia, Sunderland grade 1) [40].

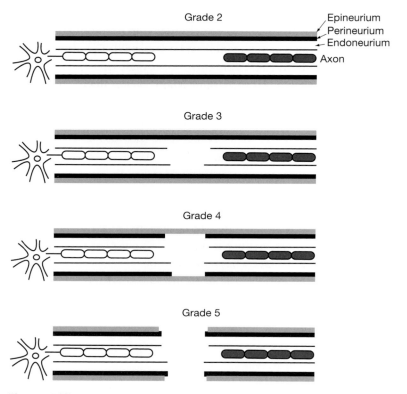

Fig. 2.7 Different types of nerve injuries (Sunderland grades 2,3, 4 and 5) [41].

Morphological changes in nerves from injuries have been classified into three main types, namely neurapraxia, axonotmesis, and neurotmesis, or in 5 groups according to Sunderland [40] (Figs. 2.6, 2.7).

The mildest form of focal lesions of a nerve is neurapraxia (Sunderland grade 1 [40]) (Fig. 2.6), which involves conduction failure without any detectable morphologic change. In neurapraxia, the morphologic structure of the nerve is preserved, but neural conduction is blocked partially or totally. Neural conduction in a nerve can recover totally from neurapraxia without any intervention.

Most nerves are mixed nerves, containing axons of different diameter. Stretching or compression of a mixed nerve affects large diameter axons more than smaller fibers. Temporary obstruction of axoplasmic flow or ischemia may cause signs of neurapraxia with large diameter fibers being affected more than small fibers. This may explain why sensation can be lost from compression of a nerve while maintaining pain sensation. Local anesthetics affect neural transmission in small (pain) fibers first, providing absence of pain while tactile sensation may be maintained.

Axonotmesis (Sunderland grade 2) involves interruption of axons of a nerve without damage to its supporting structures. Axonotmesis may be caused by crushing or pinching a nerve or after strong compression or stretching. When lesions occur distally to the location of the cell body, the parts of axons that are distal to the location of the lesion begin to degenerate immediately after the lesion (Wallerian degeneration[2]) [8]. The distal portion may conduct nerve impulses for 24–72 hours after an injury that disconnect it from the proximal portion, but the degeneration of the distal portion is usually complete within 48–72 hours after the injury, and after that the distal part of the nerve will not conduct nerve impulses. Interruption of axons proximal to the cell body causes degeneration of the proximal stump of the axons.

Neurotmesis (Sunderland grade 3, 4 and 5 [40]) (Fig. 2.7) involves interruption of not only axons, but also injury to the support structure. Grade 3 is a mixture of axon damage (axonotmesis) and damage to the support structure (loss of Schwann cell basal lamina endoneural integrity). Partial regeneration can occur without intervention and some function is regained. Grade 4 describes injuries that are more severe and involve scar formation extending the entire cross-section of the nerve but the continuity of the nerve is preserved. Regeneration is blocked by scar tissue. Grade 5 injury represents a total transection of a nerve and is often referred to as neurotmesis. It requires surgical intervention (grafting) to regain function.

Trauma to the central portion of nerves produces similar kinds of injuries to that of the peripheral portion, but the central portion of nerves is more vulnerable to injury than the peripheral portion because of the lack of support structures. The absence of the undulation of the central portion of nerves that in peripheral portions allows stretching without causing injury adds to the vulnerability of the central portion of nerves (Fig. 2.4). This makes the central portion of nerves more likely to become injured from surgical manipulations than their peripheral portions.

---

[2] Wallerian degeneration: Degenerative changes of the distal segment of a nerve fiber (axon and myelin) occurs when continuity with its cell body is interrupted.

2.3.2   *Regeneration of injured nerves*

The normal repair process of injured nerves, where axons have been interrupted, involves sprouting of axons. After interruption of an axon it begins to grow (sprout) away from its cell body and towards its normal target using the preserved support structure as a conduit. In axonotmesis, the support structure is intact, and serves as a conduit for sprouts. Many of the new axons will eventually reach their targets and form new contacts with the cells to which they were originally connected. The regeneration proceeds at a speed of approximately 1 mm per day. If the interruption of a bipolar axon occurs at a location that is proximal to the cell body, the axon will grow centrally.

The distance that a nerve can grow is limited, which can limit recovery of function from axonotmesis. Recovery of function after lesions of axons of a motor nerve that has suffered axonotmesis depends on the formation of new motor endplates when the outgrowing axon reaches the muscle that it innervated before it was interrupted. Sensory nerve fibers such as those innervating cutaneous receptors must rebuild sensory receptors.

Axons will also regenerate (sprout) after neurotmesis, but whether the sprouts will successfully reach their target depends on the condition of the support structure of the injured nerve. If some of the support structure is intact, sufficient regrowth may occur, achieving satisfactory recovery of function. If the lesion is extensive, such as in Grade 4 and 5 injury grafting, either end-to-end or with another nerve serves to provide the support structures that can act as conduits for the regenerating axons. Scar tissue that may form after injuries is an obstacle to regeneration.

In situations where interruption of the support structure of a peripheral nerve (Grade 5 lesion) has necessitated surgical grafting, the axons will not reach their correct targets and not all axons will regenerate. This means that the regenerated nerve has fewer functional nerve fibers than it had before the injury, and many of the new axons will activate their targets incorrectly. Misdirected and incomplete regeneration of sensory nerves cause abnormal sensory input (or deprivation of input) to the CNS, resulting in changed processing of sensory information and expression of neural plasticity [28].

Sprouting of motor nerves consists of multiple fine fibers, but each one of these fine fibers may not create functional motor endplates. Therefore, some of these fine filaments must be eliminated [17]. While the natural repair of damage to nerves depends on sprouting of new axons, sprouting may cause formation of neurinoma, which if excessive can cause symptoms such as pain (see Chapter 4).

Animal studies have shown signs that collateral sprouting from the undamaged part of a damaged nerve can form sensory and motor axons that rebuild endorgans for both motor (endplates) and sensory function (sensory receptors) [27]. Severed motor nerves will regenerate distally and form new neuromuscular junctions when they reach their target muscles.

2.3.3   *Symptoms and signs of focal nerve injuries*

Some symptoms from focal injury to nerves are directly related to the altered function of the injured nerves. Other (secondary) symptoms are caused by abnormalities within the CNS that are caused by reorganization or altered function of specific central structures brought about by expression of neural plasticity elicited by the altered function of the injured nerve (or nerves) in question. Impairment of conduction in sensory nerves primarily causes loss of sensory function and in motor nerves it causes paralysis of the muscles that are innervated by the nerve in question. Impaired conduction in proprioceptive fibers can affect motor functions in different ways. There are distinct differences between injuries that involve total conduction block and nerve injuries where axons are conducting nerve impulses, but abnormally. Nerve injuries often cause a mixture of these pathologies and often the degree of injury varies among the different axons in a nerve. Some axons may have total blockage of conduction while other axons conduct nerve impulses, but abnormally. Naturally, total interruption of a nerve abolishes the function of that nerve, be it a sensory or a motor nerve.

Secondarily, impaired conduction of nerves can cause many different symptoms and signs through expression of neural plasticity causing reorganization of CNS structures. It is often difficult to distinguish between the symptoms caused by physiological abnormalities in a nerve and those caused by re-organization of CNS structures, because the symptoms of both kinds of abnormalities are often referred to the injured nerves in question despite that the anatomical location of the physiological abnormality is the CNS. Changes in the function of CNS structures may persist after healing of nerve injuries.

Since activity in large fibers can modulate activity in the target neurons of smaller fibers (pain and temperature) in the dorsal horn of the spinal cord injury to a mixed somatic peripheral sensory nerve may change the processing of information that is carried in small fibers. Injury to large fibers may therefore promote pain and even cause sensation of pain without stimulation of the specific pain receptors in the skin even though large fibers do not carry information about pain (see Chapter 4).

Nerves that are slightly injured from insults such as trauma, inflammation or other external causes build a group of their own. The axons of an injured nerve may transmit nerve impulses in an abnormal way and slightly injured nerves can create many different pathological conditions. Slightly injured nerves can cause many different symptoms and signs that can be severe but difficult to treat because the cause of the symptoms is unknown. Partial conduction block in sensory nerves causes a decrease in the input to target cells. For motor nerves, a partial block can result in pareses and reduced muscle strength. Injuries to nerves often include damage to the myelin sheath, which causes decreased conduction velocity and abnormal firing pattern within nerve fibers. Since the slowing of neural conduction is likely to be different for individual fibers within a nerve, it causes an increased temporal dispersion of the nerve activity that arrives at target neurons or to target muscles for motor nerve fibers. In sensory nerves, processing of sensory information will be affected (such as in the auditory nerve, causing reduced speech discrimination, see p. 110), and if it is a motor nerve, the strength of contraction is likely to be reduced.

Mechanical compression of a sensory nerve mainly affect the large fibers that carry somatosensory information, leaving smaller fibers that carry pain and temperature information intact. Compression of a nerve causes specific changes in the morphology and function of the nerve [10], including ischemia [13, 24], narrowing of axons that impair axoplasmatic flow, and cause apoptosis and proliferation of Schwann cells [16]. The effects of ischemia are amplified by hyperventilation, which causes hypocalcaemia that lowers the threshold of nerves [25]. Nerve compression also causes proliferation of Schwann cells and increased apoptosis in addition to causing demyelination [16], which causes slowed neural conduction. The increased turnover of Schwann cells occurs with a minimum of axonal injury [16]. The effects of acute compression of a nerve are reversible, while the effects of chronic compression that causes demyelination and slowed conduction may persist after the release of the compression and only reverses slowly. Compression of motor nerves can cause muscle contractions (twitches) [23, 24]. Abnormal muscle activity is, however, more likely to be caused by changes in the function of CNS structures through expression of neural plasticity or changes in proprioceptive input.

Distal and proximal portions of a nerve are affected differently by injuries and diseases. For example, GBS affects the central parts of a nerve before affecting more distal segments of the nerve. Genetic inherited abnormalities of myelin such as HMSN-I or CMT-I cause increased conduction times in nerves.

2.3.4   Mechanosensitivity of injured nerves

Slight injury to a nerve may make a nerve more sensitive to mechanical stimulation (stretch or compression). Normal peripheral nerves are rather insensitive to moderate mechanical stimulation, but injured nerves can be very sensitive to mechanical stimulation. An example is carpal tunnel syndrome, where tapping on the skin over the median nerve produces paresthesia that is referred to the parts of the hand where the skin is innervated by the injured nerve (this phenomenon is known as the Tinel's sign[3]). Mechano-sensitivity of dorsal root ganglia and injured axons has been hypothesized to be involved in some forms of pain [18].

> Many observations have confirmed that slightly injured nerves are sensitive to mechanical stimulation. For example, surgical manipulations of the central portion of motor nerves can produce contraction of the muscles. Touching the intracranial portion of the facial nerve with surgical instruments during resection of vestibular schwannoma reveals that the facial nerve is much more sensitive to such manipulation after it has been injured than before being injured. Slight mechanical stimulation of such an injured facial nerve results in contraction of facial muscles, while similar mechanical stimulation of an uninjured nerve elicits little or no muscle contractions. This observation provides a clear indication that a nerve's sensitivity to mechanical stimulation is related to its injury.

2.4   Pathophysiology of disorders of nerves

Some of the causes of the different signs of disorders of nerves have been studied in great detail while others are less known. A wide range of changes in the function of different parts of the CNS is caused by expression of neural plasticity elicited by disorders of peripheral nerves.

2.4.1   Nerves as mechanoreceptors

It is not known in detail how axons become sensitive to mechanical deformation, but mechanoreceptors such as those of the Pacinian corpuscles are in fact modified axons that function as very sensitive mechanoreceptors [31]. This means that the axons of nerves and their roots can be transformed in such a way that they become sensitive to mechanical deformations. It is believed that changes in the permeability of specific ion channels in axons makes them more sensitive to mechanical deformations and subsequently cause changes in the membrane potentials of the altered axon. Such transformation may occur not only because of trauma, but sprouting axons from injured nerves that may form neuroma can also be very sensitive to pressure or other mechanical manipulations [18], indicating that the membranes of such premature axons are different from those of mature axons.

2.4.2   Nerves as impulse generators

Pathologies of nerves may make the affected nerve act as an impulse generator [9]. Slightly injured nerves may begin to express α adrenoreceptors

---

[3] Tinel's sign: a tingling sensation from percussion of the skin over a peripheral nerve. It is a sign of an injured nerve or a nerve under regeneration.

responding to circulating catecholamines such as epinephrine and nor-epinephrine causing the axons to discharge [3]. Sympathetic axons that project to dorsal root ganglia can sprout after injuries to the nerve in question. This is another way in which catecholamines can stimulate afferent pain fibers and cause sympathetically maintained pain [3] (see Chapter 4). After-discharges often occur in response to activity that arrives at an injured segment of a nerve [23]. Compression of a nerve may involve little physical damage to the nerve, but cause nerve impulses to be generated at the location of the compression [7, 23]. Such ectopic impulses can propagate both in the distal and central directions from the injured segment of a nerve. These aberrant impulses may interact with the normally generated nerve impulses and elicit trains of impulses when passing injured or ischemic areas of a peripheral nerve, which can act as a "trigger zone" for ectopic activity [23]. Generation of such abnormal activity is exacerbated by hyperventilation because of hypocalcemia.

2.4.3   *Ephaptic transmission*

It is been hypothesized that axons in which the myelin sheath is injured may communicate with each other directly (ephaptic transmission[4]) [14, 34, 38]. It has also been hypothesized that such ephaptic transmission is involved in creating the symptoms of several disorders of nerves and their roots. However, ephaptic transmission can only occur when the neural propagation at the site of the lesion is so slow that an action potential has a sufficient amplitude at the end of the refractory period to excite neighboring fibers [19, 34, 38]. This is a rare condition. Furthermore, the documented physiological signs of such ephaptic transmission (or cross-talk) between axons of injured nerves have been either from acutely injured nerves in humans [29] or severed nerves in animal studies [15]. The observed effect of the interaction has been small in magnitude (indicating that few fibers were involved) [29] and short lasting (few minutes) [15, 29]. Despite the lack of experimental support, ephaptic transmission has frequently been regarded as the cause of the symptoms and signs of disorders of nerves [14, 32] (see Chapter 6, p. 149).

> Signs of ephaptic transmission in injured nerves was first described by Granit and his co-workers, who showed that such direct transmission between injured (cut) nerve fibers occurs for a short period after the injury [15]. The hypothesis that neural transmission may occur directly between bare axons has been further tested experimentally by Howe and

---

[4] Ephaptic transmission: Direct transfer of impulse activity from one (denuded) axon to another (the word ephaptic is an artificial word constructed from the word synapse, partly backwards).

his co-workers [18], who used chromic sutures to create focal demyelination of the trigeminal nerve. These investigators found evidence that a single spike entering the injured zone could set up a reverberation that could generate (abnormal) high-frequency neural spike trains. Later, similar findings were made in dorsal roots of the spinal cord [34]. Brief periods of signs of ephaptic transmission in a surgically injured central portion of the facial nerve were demonstrated in studies of the abnormal muscle contraction in a patient undergoing a MVD operation for hemifacial spasm [29].

2.4.4   Reflection of neural activity

Demyelination of a segment of a nerve may cause reflection of neural activity that reaches that segment. Such abnormalities have been implicated in chronic pain [19, 33], (see Chapter 4)

2.4.5   Change in discharge pattern

Slightly injured nerves may have a longer refractory period than normal nerve fibers [21] increasing the shortest interval within which an axon can fire thus limiting the maximal frequency of firing. Such a decrease in the maximal firing rate can prevent sensory nerves to activate a target cell that requires short intervals between incoming impulses in order to become activated. For motor nerves, limitation of firing rate reduces the maximal strength of a muscle.

Normally, a nerve conducts nerve impulses that are initiated at the peripheral end of a nerve, and delivers the nerve impulses unchanged to the target of the nerve, which may be a nerve cell or a muscle. Slightly injured nerves may not be able to transmit nerve impulses without altering the discharge pattern, so the temporal pattern of the discharges that reaches a target neuron may be different from that of normal functioning nerves.

Injury to a nerve may change its discharge pattern from a steady pattern to a burst pattern. The change from a continuous firing pattern to a pattern of firing in bursts can change the central processing, even when the average number of nerve impulses remains unchanged. Firing of target neurons in which the excitatory post synaptic potential (EPSP) decays rapidly can only occur when the interval between incoming impulses is sufficiently short to allow temporal integration. This means that a target cell may not be activated by the continuous train of impulses that a nerve normally delivers but it may be activated by an injured nerve that fires in bursts. If a sensory nerve is slightly injured and fires in bursts instead of producing a continuous train of impulses, the intervals between individual nerve impulses within a bursts may be sufficiently short to generate EPSPs that exceed the threshold of firing of a target neuron that normally never fires (see Fig. 1.1). A change in the firing pattern from steady to burst activity, which often occurs in slightly injured nerves, may therefore open synapses that are normally closed (unmask dormant synapses). This is one way to open new connections in the CNS, causing re-routing of information (see Chapter 1).

2.4.6 Effect of change in conduction velocity: the importance of spatial dispersion

The effect of trauma to a nerve typically manifests as an increase in conduction time (decreased conduction velocity) which makes neural activity arrive at its target with a longer delay than normally. This may have little effect on the functions of sensory and motor systems if it affects all nerve fibers equally. However, most pathologies that cause decreased conduction velocity in axons affect different axons differently, and that can make the temporal dispersion of the neural activity that converge on a target neuron to increase. The decrease in conduction velocity (increased conduction time) that is typical for slightly injured nerves may therefore increase spatial dispersion in the input to a nerve cell on which many nerve fibers converge (Fig. 2.8). This temporal dispersion increases along a nerve, and the effect of such uneven decrease in conduction velocity will therefore be greater for long nerves than for short nerves. This may explain some of the differences in the symptoms of disorders that affect the distal portion of a nerve, compared with effects on more proximal portions.

In a normal (uninjured) nerve the temporal dispersion is a function of the variation in the conduction velocities of the group of fibers in question, and the length of the nerve. The distribution of diameters of nerve fibers differs for different nerves and thereby the dispersion differs. For example, the variation in conduction velocity is much larger for C fibers than for myelinated fibers. This means that the activity elicited at the same time in such a group of fibers will arrive at their target nuclei or muscles with a certain degree of temporal dispersion. The effect of that can determine whether the membrane potential in the target cell reaches the threshold for delivering an action potential in its axon (Fig. 2.8).

If the target neuron functions according to the "integrate and fire" model of neurons, it will only fire if the interval between nerve impulses in the fibers that converge on it is sufficiently small (see Fig. 1.1). When the variation in conduction velocity of a population of nerve fibers that converge on an individual neuron is increased, such as may occur in injured nerves, the temporal dispersion of the input to the neuron is increased and this affects the ability of the input to excite the neuron in question.

A target cell on which many axons converge integrates neural activity not only in each individual nerve fiber over time but it also integrates the input

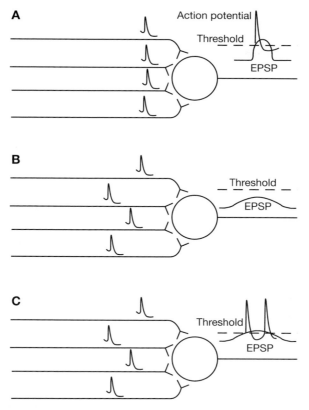

Fig. 2.8 Hypothetical illustration of the effect of spatial integration by a cell on which many axons converge.

A: Little spatial dispersion

B: Increased spatial dispersion but the high threshold of the neuron prevents it from firing.

C. Lower threshold of the neuron. The prolonged EPSP makes the neuron fire twice.

from all the axons that converge onto the cell. This means that both temporal and spatial coherence are important factors that determine whether or not a target cell will fire. If the nerve fibers that converge upon such a nerve cell are stimulated by a brief impulse, which activates all the nerve fibers at the same time, the target neuron in question will receive the nerve impulses at slightly different times and the resulting excitatory post synaptic potential (EPSP) will have a lower amplitude than it would have had if the nerve impulses arrived at exactly the same time (Fig. 2.8).

If the dispersion is small, a neuron may only fire once because the amplitude of the generated EPSP decays below that of the neuron's threshold before the end of the neuron's refractory period thus preventing the neuron from firing again (Fig. 2.8A) even when the amplitude of the EPSP exceeds the threshold of the neuron by a large amount. If the temporal or spatial dispersion is large, the activity impinged on the neuron spreads out longer over time (is diluted) and therefore may not produce an EPSP of sufficient amplitude to exceed the threshold of the target cell (Fig. 2.8B). However, if the threshold of the neuron is sufficiently low, the neuron will fire and if the duration of the prolonged EPSP exceeds the refractory period of the neuron it may fire more than once (Fig. 2.8C).

The same excitation at the distal end of a nerve may thus cause the target cell to fire once (Fig. 2.8A), twice (or multiple times) (Fig. 2.8C) or not at all (Fig. 2.8B) depending on the dispersion of the input to the neuron and the threshold of the neuron. This means that increase of temporal or the spatial dispersion of the input to a neuron, both of which may occur as a result of insults to a nerve, may in fact make the input more efficient in exciting a target neuron (Fig. 2.8). A large degree of temporal and spatial dispersion of the input to a neuron may in fact be more efficient in exciting a neuron than the same number of nerve impulses that occur with little dispersion, provided that the threshold of firing is sufficiently low.

The temporal dispersion increases with the distance between the location of excitation of a nerve and the target neuron. The effect of increased temporal dispersion through pathologies is therefore likely to be greater for long nerves than for short nerves. This may account for some of the differences in symptoms of neuropathy from distal limbs compared with the symptoms from more proximal parts of the body.

To summarize, increased temporal dispersion (decreased temporal coherence) in nerves may have widely different effects on target neurons. Disorders of sensory nerves that alter temporal or spatial dispersion of the input to a nerve cell in the CNS can therefore affect processing of information in the CNS and increased temporal dispersion can have different effects.

1. It can decrease the activation of the target neuron (Fig. 2.8).
2. It can increase the duration of firing of the target neuron, which may cause increased excitation of the following neuron.
3. Increased temporal dispersion may prevent activation of the next neuron in a chain, or it may make it possible to activate neurons that are not normally activated, which may be regarded as a form of functional re-wiring of the nervous system.
4. Increased temporal dispersion may degrade information when temporal coding is important such as in sensory systems, most pronounced in hearing (see Chapter 3).

2.4.7   *Electrophysiological signs of nerve injuries*

Measurement of nerve conduction velocity is an important tool for diagnosis of different kinds of disorders of nerves. The principles are to stimulate a nerve electrically and record the response from the same nerve at a distance from where it is being stimulated. Often clinical nerve conduction studies are performed by recording the responses from muscles (electromyography, EMG) in response to electrical stimulation of a mixed nerve [1]. Examination of EMG responses from muscles to electrical stimulation of a nerve provides quantitative information about abnormalities in the function of motor nerves including abnormal neural conduction velocity. Recording of nerve action potentials (compound action potentials, CAP) from nerves can be used for determining the neural conduction velocity in all (large) fibers in a mixed nerve and thereby provide quantitative assessment of demyelination and axonal injuries. Lower than normal amplitude of the recorded CAP and EMG response with relative preservation of conduction velocity is a sign that some axons are not conducting. Broadening of the CAP is a sign of temporal dispersion because the decrease in conduction velocity differs among axons. However, it has to be remembered that measurements of neural conduction using these methods only reflect neural conduction in large fibers and there are no feasible clinical tools available for measurement of neural conduction in $A\delta$ and C fibers. This means that the measured conduction velocity in mixed nerves in patients with small fiber neuropathies falls within normal limits because only the fastest conducting fibers are studied in nerve conduction studies.

Recording of F-response[5] is effective in measuring conduction velocity of the proximal part of motor nerves. This is important for diagnosis of disorders where conduction is normal in distal nerves but abnormal in their proximal parts such as HMSN-I.

2.4.8   *The role of neural plasticity*

Interruption of neural conduction and abnormal firing of sensory nerves may cause symptoms due to abnormal input to the CNS, or indirectly by causing changes in the function of CNS structures through expression of neural plasticity. Total blockage of neural conduction in sensory nerves causes not only sensory deficits, but the deprivation of input may also result in reorganization of central structures through expression of neural plasticity. Deprivation of input

[5] The F-response is caused by backfiring of motoneurons. It is performed in a similar way to the H-response, by stimulating mixed nerves electrically and recording from muscles that are innervated by the nerve that is stimulated [1].

may also cause phantom symptoms, such as paresthesia and pain for somatic nerves, and tinnitus for the auditory nerve (see Chapter 3).

Symptoms and signs of central involvement

The symptoms and signs of these secondary effects are different from those of primary effects, and often involve hyperactivity and reorganization of central structures. However, it can be difficult to discern which of these symptoms are directly caused by abnormal functioning of a nerve and which are caused by changes in the function of CNS structures. The change in the function of central structures may be beneficial or cause symptoms and signs of disease. The symptoms of changes in the function of central structures such as those that may occur after trauma to a nerve may persist after healing of the nerve injuries. Both the direct effects of injuries and the indirect effects may occur simultaneously but the effects of changes in the function of CNS structures can have more severe consequences than the primary effects of nerve injuries. The symptoms from either cause are almost always referred to the anatomical location of the injured nerves in question.

Intervention such as training is highly beneficial for recovery of function after grafting of severed motor or sensory nerves (grade 5 injuries), and it is normally necessary to retrain motor skills by inducing expression of neural plasticity that can reorganize central nervous structures to generate motor commands that compensate for the incorrect connections of motor nerves fibers. Training can make recovery faster and more complete such as for example after compression (entrapment) of a peripheral nerve that has caused loss of nerve fibers (such as may occur in the carpal tunnel syndrome where function can be restored by training), especially if the intervention is made early [36].

While the naturally occurring expression of neural plasticity and that induced by training are aimed at restoring normal function, it may also be misdirected causing abnormal movements (Chapters 5 and 6) or abnormal sensory perception (paresthesia) and pain (Chapter 4) may result.

The cause of expression of neural plasticity

Deprivation of sensory input such as can occur because of conduction block (or severance) of a nerve is a strong promoter of reorganization of CNS circuits [43, 44]. Change in the discharge pattern of the peripheral or central portions of nerves, or nerve roots, can also cause reorganization and change of the function of specific central structures. Alteration or absence of input can cause re-routing of information and altered processing of information from sensory organs or change motor commands through expression of neural plasticity. Changes in the function of central structures (through expression of neural plasticity may occur in order to compensate for changes in the function of nerves. The hyperactivity that often results from decreased input to the CNS may be invoked to compensate for the decreased input (by increasing the gain), but if the changes in the function of CNS structures are too large hyperactivity may be an unwanted effect (see Chapters 5 and 6), tinnitus. Injuries to motor nerves and muscles can also cause expression of neural plasticity [20].

Nerves have often been regarded as an entity separate from their own nuclei and the structures to which their nuclei communicate in the CNS. The extensive interaction between pathologies of nerves and processing of information in related CNS structures makes it more appropriate to regard nerves, their nuclei and the parts of the CNS with which the nuclei communicate, as an integrated system, where the different components interact closely with each other in normal functions as well as in the various disorders that affect these nerves.

References

1. Aminoff, M. J., *Electromyography in Clinical Practice*. 1998, Churchill Livingstone: New York.
2. Berthoud, H. R. and W. L. Neuhuber, Functional and Chemical Anatomy of the Afferent Vagal System. *Autonomic Neurosci.*, 2000. **85**(1–3): pp. 1–17.
3. Bolay, H. and M. A. Moskowitz, Mechanisms of Pain Modulation in Chronic Syndromes. *Neurology*, 2002. **59**(5 Suppl. 2): pp. S2–7.
4. Brach, J. S., J. M. Van Swearingen, J. Lenert, and P. C. Johnson, Facial Neuromuscular Retraining for Oral Synkinesis. *Plastic and Reconstructive Surgery*, 1997. **99**(7): pp. 1922–1931.
5. Brodal, P., *The Central Nervous System*. 1998, Oxford University Press: New York.
6. Cacace, A. T., T. J. Lovely, D. J. McFarland, S. M. Parnes, and D. F. Winter, Anomalous Cross-Modal Plasticity Following Posterior Fossa Surgery: Some Speculations on Gaze-Evoked Tinnitus. *Hear. Res.*, 1994. **81**: pp. 22–32.
7. Calvin, J. H., To Spike or Not to Spike? Controlling the Neuron's Rhythm, Preventing the Ectopic Beat, in *Abnormal Nerves and Muscles as Impulse Generators*, W. J. Culp and J. L. Ochoa, Editors. 1982, Oxford University Press: New York. pp. 295–321.
8. Chaudhry, V. and D. R. Cornblath, Wallerian Degeneration in Human Nerves; Serial Electrophysiological Studies. *Muscle & Nerve*, 1992. **15**(6): pp. 687–693.
9. Culp, W. J., J. Ochoa, and H. E. Torebjoerk, Ectopic Impulse Generation in Myelinated Sensory Nerve Fibers in Man, in *Abnormal Nerves and Muscles as Impulse Generators*, W. J. Culp and J. Ochoa, Editors. 1982, Oxford University Press: New York. pp. 490–512.
10. Dahlin, L. B., Aspects on Pathophysiology of Nerve Entrapments and Nerve Compression Injuries. *Neurosurgery Clinics of North America*, 1991. **2**(1): pp. 21–9.

11. Fromm, G. H., Pathophysiology of Trigeminal Neuralgia, in *Trigeminal Neuralgia*, G. H. Fromm and B. J. Sessle, Editors. 1991, Butterworth-Heinemann: Boston. pp. 105–130.

12. Fu, Q. G., M. J. Chandler, D. L. McNeill, and R. D. Foreman, Vagal Afferent Fibers Excite Upper Cervical Neurons and Inhibit Activity of Lumbar Spinal Cord Neurons in the Rat. *Pain*, 1992. **51**: pp. 91–100.

13. Fullerton, P. M., The Effect of Ischemia on Nerve Conduction in the Carpal Tunnel Syndrome. *J. Neurol. Neurosurg. Psych.*, 1963. **26**: pp. 385.

14. Gardner, W., Crosstalk – the Paradoxical Transmission of a Nerve Impulse. *Arch. Neurol.*, 1966(14): pp. 149–156.

15. Granit, R., L. Leksell, and C. R. Skoglund, Fibre Interaction in Injured or Compressed Region of Nerve. *Brain*, 1944(67): pp. 125–140.

16. Gupta, R. and O. Steward, Chronic Nerve Compression Induces Concurrent Apoptosis and Proliferation of Schwann Cells. *J. Comp. Neurol.*, 2003. **461**(2): pp. 174–86.

17. Happel, L. and D. Kline, Intraoperative Neurophysiology of the Peripheral Nervous System, in *Neurophysiology in Neurosurgery*, V. Deletis and J. L. Shils, Editors. 2002, Academic Press: Amsterdam. pp. 169–195.

18. Howe, J. E., J. D. Loeser, and J. H. Calvin, Mechanosensitivity of Dorsal Root Ganglia and Chronically Injured Axons: A Physiologic Basis for Radical Pain of Nerve Root Compression. *Pain*, 1977. **3**: pp. 25–41.

19. Howe, J. F., W. H. Calvin, and J. D. Loeser, Impulses Reflected from Dorsal Root Ganglia and from Focal Nerve Injuries. *Brain Res.*, 1976: pp. 116–144.

20. Jacobs, K. M. and J. P. Donoghue, Reshaping the Cortical Motor Map by Unmasking Latent Intracortical Connections. *Science*, 1991. **251**: pp. 944–947.

21. Kimura, J., A Method for Estimating the Refractory Period of Motor Fibers in the Human Peripheral Nerve. *J. Neurol. Sci.*, 1976. **28**: pp. 485–90.

22. Kreutzberg, G. W., Neurobiology of Regeneration and Degeneration of the Facial Nerve, in *The Facial Nerve*, M. May, Editor. 1986, Thieme: New York.

23. Kugelberg, E., "Injury Activity" and "Trigger Zones" in Human Nerves. *Brain*, 1946(69): pp. 310–324.

24. Kugelberg, E., Activation of Human Nerves by Ischemia. *Arch. Neurol. Psychiat.*, 1948. **60**: pp. 140–152.

25. Kugelberg, E., Activation of Human Nerves by Hyperventilation and Hypocalcemia. *Arch. Neurol. Psychiat.*, 1948. **60**: pp. 153–164.

26. Long, D. M., Chronic Back Pain, in *Handbook of Pain*, P. D. Wall and R. Melzack, Editors. 1999, Churchill Livingstone: Edinburgh. pp. 539–538.

27. Lundborg, G., Q. Zhao, M. Kanje, N. Danielsen, and J. M. Kerns, Can Sensory and Motor Collateral Sprouting Be Induced from Intact Peripheral Nerve by End-to-Side Anastomosis? *J. Hand Surg. – [Br.]*, 1994. **19**(3): pp. 277–82.

28. Lundborg, G., Brain Plasticity and Hand Surgery: An Overview. *J. Hand Surg. – Brit. Vol.*, 2000. **25**(3): pp. 242–52.

29. Møller, A. R., Hemifacial Spasm: Ephaptic Transmission or Hyperexcitability of the Facial Motor Nucleus? *Exp. Neurol.*, 1987. **98**: pp. 110–119.

30. Møller, A. R., Cranial Nerve Dysfunction Syndromes: Pathophysiology of Microvascular Compression, in *Neurosurgical Topics Book 13, 'Surgery of Cranial Nerves of the Posterior Fossa,' Chapter 2*, D. L. Barrow, Editor. 1993, American Association of Neurological Surgeons: Park Ridge. IL. pp. 105–129.

31. Møller, A. R., *Sensory Systems: Anatomy and Physiology*. 2003, Academic Press: Amsterdam.

32. Nielsen, V., Pathophysiological Aspects of Hemifacial Spasm. Part I. Evidence of Ectopic Excitation and Ephaptic Transmission. *Neurology*, 1984(34): pp. 418–426.

33. Ochoa, J. L., The Newly Recognized Painful ABC Syndrome: Thermographic Aspects. *Thermology*, 1986. **2**: pp. 65–107.

34. Rasminsky, M., Ephaptic Transmission between Single Nerve Fibers in the Spinal Nerve Roots of Dystrophic Mice. *J. Physiol. (Lond.)*, 1980. **305**: pp. 151–169.

35. Rexed, B. A., Cytoarchitectonic Atlas of the Spinal Cord. *J. Comp. Neurol.*, 1954. **100**: pp. 297–379.

36. Rosen, B., G. Lundborg, S. O. Abrahamsson, L. Hagberg, and I. Rosen, Sensory Function after Median Nerve Decompression in Carpal Tunnel Syndrome. Preoperative Vs Postoperative Findings. *J. Hand Surg. – [Br.]*, 1997. **22**(5): pp. 602–6.

37. Scadding, J. W., Peripheral Neuropathies, in *Textbook of Pain*, P. D. Wall and R. Melzack, Editors. 1999, Churchill Livingstone: Edinburgh. pp. 815–834.

38. Seltzer, Z. and M. Devor, Ephaptic Transmission in Chronically Damaged Peripheral Nerves. *Neurology*, 1979. **29**: pp. 1061–1064.

39. Sie, K. C. Y. and E. W. Rubel, Rapid Changes in Protein Synthesis and Cell Size in the Cochlear Nucleus Following Eighth Nerve Activity Blockade and Cochlea Ablation. *J. Comp. Neurol.*, 1992. **320**: pp. 501–508.

40. Sunderland, S., A Classification of Peripheral Nerve Injuries Producing Loss of Function. *Brain*, 1951. **74**: pp. 491–516.

41. Sunderland, S., Cranial Nerve Injury. Structural and Pathophysiological Considerations and a Classification of Nerve Injury, in *The Cranial Nerves*, M. Samii and P. J. Jannetta, Editors. 1981, Springer-Verlag: Heidelberg, Germany. pp. 16–26.

42. Tetzlaff, W., M. B. Graeber, and G. W. Kreutzberg, Reaction on Motoneurons and Their Microenvironment to Axotomy. *Exp Brain Res*, 1986. **3**(Suppl,13): pp. 3–8.

43. Wall, J. T., J. H. Kaas, M. Sur, R. J. Nelson, D. J. Felleman, and M. M. Merzenich, Functional Reorganization in Somatosensory Cortical Areas 3b and 1 of Adult Monkeys after Median Nerve Repair: Possible Relationships to Sensory Recovery in Humans. *J. Neurosci.*, 1986. **6**(1): pp. 218–233.

44. Wall, P. D., The Presence of Ineffective Synapses and Circumstances Which Unmask Them. *Phil. Trans. Royal Soc. (Lond.)*, 1977. **278**: pp. 361–372.

45. Weiss, T., W. H. Miltner, R. Huonker, R. Friedel, I. Schmidt, and E. Taub, Rapid Functional Plasticity of the Somatosensory Cortex after Finger Amputation. *Exp. Brain Res.*, 2000. **134**(2): pp. 199–203.

3

Sensory systems

Introduction

The five sensory systems, hearing, vision, tactile (somatosensory), smell and taste, provide conscious perceptions of physical stimuli from the environment. In addition to these five senses, temperature receptors in the skin and the mouth mediate the sensations of warmth and cool. These senses, together with motor systems, serve the purpose of communications between an organism and the environment. In fact, all input that the central nervous system (CNS) receives from the environment comes through sensory systems. Several disorders are directly associated with sensory systems. Some disorders are caused by various kinds of insults such as trauma and inflammation. Age-related changes are perhaps the most important cause of disorders of sensory systems. The symptoms of many of these disorders are caused by functional changes in the CNS induced by expression of neural plasticity.

The vestibular system that monitors head movements and proprioceptive systems that monitor motor activity may also be regarded as sensory systems, but many authors include these systems in their description of motor systems. The balance system and proprioception, together with vision and somesthesia, contribute to our perception of our body position. (The vestibular system, and disorders associated with it, is covered separately in Chapter 6.) Proprioceptive somatosensory systems, the receptors of which are found in muscles, tendons and joints, monitor the motor systems and other bodily functions. The role of the vestibular system in control of posture and walking is discussed in Chapter 5 where other forms of proprioception are also discussed.

Pain receptors (nociceptors) detect events that pose a danger to the organism in various ways. Pain is not usually regarded as a sense, but because of its similarities with the somatosensory system, many authors cover pain together with the somatosensory system. The high prevalence of various forms of pain and its enormous impact on the life of many individuals, make it important to understand the function of the pain systems for all who are active in the field of healthcare. Therefore, in this book, a separate chapter is devoted to the pathophysiology underlying the perception of pain (Chapter 4).

The internal working of the body is controlled and monitored by the autonomic nervous system – discussion of which is outside the topic of this book – except when it concerns sensory systems, pain, and motor systems. Thirst, hunger and mental fatigue are definite sensations but are usually not regarded as parts of our senses.

This chapter begins with a description of the anatomy and normal function of sensory systems, followed by discussions of the symptoms and signs of disorders of sensory systems, their cause and treatment. The emphasis is on disorders in which neural plasticity is involved. The third section of this chapter concerns the pathophysiology of disorders of sensory systems with emphasis on the role of neural plasticity in causing the symptoms and signs. For a more detailed description of the anatomy and physiology of sensory systems, see Møller, 2003 [156].)

3.1   General organization and function of sensory systems

Sensory systems consist of

1. sensory receptors,
2. the media that conduct the physical stimuli to the receptors,
3. sensory nerves,
4. structures of the CNS that respond to sensory stimuli.

In hearing, vision and olfaction, the receptor cells are located in special sensory organs together with the media that conduct the physical stimulus to the receptors. We will discuss three of the five principal sensory systems (somesthesia, hearing, and vision) first and then only briefly discuss gustation and olfaction because few disorders are associated with these two senses.

3.1.1   Sensory organs

Sensory organs consist of the receptors and the media that conduct sensory stimuli to the receptors. The eye, in addition, contains some of the neural structures that process visual stimuli. The structures that conduct auditory stimuli to the sensory cells are more complex than those of other sensory organs.

3.1.2   Media that conduct the stimuli to the receptors

The media that conduct stimuli to the receptors are important causes of disorders. In hearing, the structures that conduct sound to the sensory receptors are complex, consisting of the middle ear that acts as an impedance matching device that improves the sound transmission to the cochlea [154], and the cochlea, which separates sound according to their frequency (filtering) and amplifies weak sounds by as much as 50 dB. Stronger sounds are amplified less than weaker sounds, which provide amplitude compression that allows sounds within a large range of intensities to be coded in the discharge pattern of auditory nerve fibers. The dynamic range of neural coding is far less than that of the sounds that can be processed by the auditory system.

The middle ear improves sound conduction to the fluid-filled cochlea by approximately 30 dB, and this provides a large difference between the forces that act on the two windows of the cochlea (round and oval windows). This difference causes the cochlear fluid to move, and thus provides the basis for activating the sensory cells of the cochlea. The acoustic middle ear reflex provides some amplitude compression [154]. Many of the disorders of the auditory system are related to the middle ear and the cochlea [154], with disorders of the middle ear being the only ones that can be successfully treated via surgical or pharmacological means.

The structures that conduct light to the visual receptors provide the ability to focus an image on the retina (at least in young individuals) and some intensity compression through the action of the pupil. Tactile information is conducted through the skin that functions as a relatively simple mechanical system, but some receptors, i.e. the Pacinian corpuscles, have a more complex mechanical structure that filters the stimuli with regard to their frequency. (For more details see [156].)

3.1.3   Receptors

Sensory receptors convert physical stimuli into a neural code. The receptors can be divided into two groups based on their morphology. One group consists of transformed axons, the membranes of which are specialized to sense specific mechanical stimuli. These transformed axons continue as regular axons of the respective sensory nerves. Mechanoreceptors in the skin belong to this type of receptor. The other type of sensory receptor cells is more complex, and consists of a complete cell to which the afferent axon connects via synapses or synapse-like structures. Such receptor cells are found in the ear and the eye. (Taste and olfactory receptors also belong to this type of receptors.) Protuberance on the receptor cell such as the stereocilia of the hair cells in the cochlea or the outer segments of visual receptor cells are sensitive to a specific physical stimulus. Visual receptors have an elaborate structure, with discs that contain a light sensitive substance. These receptor cells connect to a complex neural network of the retina, the last stage of which is ganglion cells that give rise to the axons of the optic nerve.

The two types of auditory receptor cells (inner and outer hair cells) have completely different functions; only the inner hair cells convert sound into a neural code, whereas the outer hair cells have a mechanical function (see p. 99). Both types of hair cells receive inhibitory input from the CNS but in different ways. The efferent fibers from the CNS terminate on the cell bodies of outer hair cells through a synapse, while most efferent fibers that target the inner hair cells terminate on the afferent dendrites that become the axons of the afferent nerve [211]. (For more detail about sensory receptors, see Møller, 2003 [156].)

3.1.4   *Sensory nerves*

Sensory nerve fibers travel in cranial nerves (see Chapter 6) and in peripheral nerves (see Chapter 2). The sensory nerves enter the CNS and make synaptic contact with target cells in the gray matter of the spinal cord or sensory nuclei of the brainstem and in the thalamus for vision. The axons that innervate receptors in the skin, muscles, joints and tendons are bipolar cells that enter the spinal cord as dorsal roots, with their cell bodies located in the dorsal root ganglia. These axons travel in the dorsal column of the spinal cord to reach cells in the dorsal column nuclei. Prior to this point these axons give rise to collateral axons that terminate on cells in the dorsal horn of the segment where the axons enter, as well as in other segments of the spinal cord. Sensory nerves of the face are also bipolar fibers, and most belong to the sensory trigeminal nerve (portio major of cranial nerve (CN V), the axons of which enter the pons and terminate on cells in the sensory part of the trigeminal nucleus. Some nerve fibers that innervate receptors of the face travel in the glossopharyngeal and vagus nerves and terminate in the trigeminal nucleus.

CN II and CN VIII are purely sensory nerves innervating visual and auditory-vestibular sensory organs, respectively. The axons of the optic nerve terminate in cells in the visual portion of the thalamus (the lateral geniculate nucleus, LGN). Auditory nerve fibers form collaterals that terminate in all three divisions of the cochlear nucleus. The cell bodies of the auditory nerve fibers are located in the spiral ganglion. The axons that innervate the vestibular organ have their cell bodies in Scarpa's ganglion, and the axons terminate on cells in the vestibular nucleus (see Chapter 6).

Sensory nerves, except the optic nerve, terminate in nuclei that are located on the same side of the body (ipsilateral) as the sensory organs. The axons that innervate the sensory cells in the eye terminate in a network of neurons within the retina that give rise to the optic nerve, the axons of which make synaptic contact with cells in the LGN. In humans, approximately half of the axons terminate on cells in the ipsilateral LGN, and the other half make synaptic contact with cells in the LGN on the opposite side or the contralateral side. The nerve fibers of taste receptors travel in portions of cranial nerves VII, IX and X, and terminate on cells in the nucleus of the solitary tract. The nerve fibers of the olfactory nerve terminate in the olfactory bulb, the morphology of which is similar to that of the retina [156].

3.1.5   Neural pathways

Sensory neural pathways consist of ascending and descending pathways. Much more is known about the ascending pathways than the descending pathways. Ascending sensory pathways connect sensory organs with specific regions of the cerebral neocortex through a series of nuclei that are arranged in a hierarchical way. The number of such nuclei is different for different sensory systems. Descending pathways connect cells of the cerebral cortex with various nuclei of the ascending pathways, and in some systems, even connecting to the respective sensory receptors. Some descending pathways originate from subcortical nuclei.

Ascending sensory pathways

The auditory, somatosensory and visual systems have two distinctly different ascending pathways (Fig. 3.1) making it possible for sensory information to ascend in at least two parallel pathways. We will use the terms classical and non-classical pathways to distinguish between these two different pathways [156], but other names have been used. The classical pathways are much better known than the non-classical pathways. In some sensory systems, the branching of the pathways into such distinctly different routes begins at a rather peripheral level (cochlear nucleus, see p. 80).

> These two parallel pathways have been referred to by different names by different investigators. In the auditory system, the classical and the non-classical pathways have been known as the "lemniscal" and the "extralemniscal" systems, respectively [60, 148]. Some authors have named the two auditory pathways, the "specific" and the "non-specific" pathways. Other investigators distinguish between two parts of the non-classical auditory pathways, namely the "diffuse" system [217] and the "polysensory" system [188]. In the somatosensory system, the term paralemniscal system has been used. Neurons in non-classical auditory systems and paralemniscal somatosensory system have poor spatial

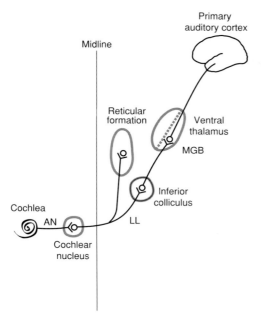

Fig. 3.1A Simplified schematic drawings of the classical ascending auditory pathways.

resolution [2] but can encode temporal patterns of stimulation into a rate code. The paralemniscal pathways use the posterior medial division of the thalamus, while the lemniscal (classical system) uses the ventral posterior medial (VPM) nucleus of the thalamus and project to the primary somatosensory cortex in complimentary patterns [109] indicating two parallel thalamocortical pathways with different processing properties [129].

The thalamus is the common pathway for sensory information to the cerebral cortex. The two ascending pathways use different regions of the thalamus and their cortical projections are different. The ventral nuclei of the thalamus are the common thalamic relays for classical sensory pathways. The neurons of these nuclei project to the respective primary sensory cortices. The non-classical pathways use the dorsomedial nuclei in the thalamus the neurons of which project to secondary cortices and association cortices and thereby bypass the primary cortices [156] (see Figs. 3.1, 3.2, 3.3). In fact, dorsal thalamic sensory nuclei project to most sensory cortical areas except primary cortex. Processing of sensory information that occurs in these two pathways is different. There is evidence that some symptoms and signs of disease are related to an abnormal activation of non-classical ascending sensory pathways (see pp. 91, 83, 56).

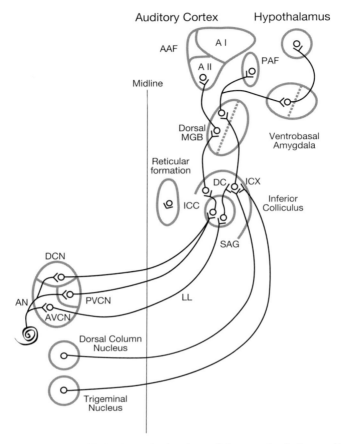

Fig. 3.1B Simplified schematic drawings of the non-classical ascending auditory pathways. (Adapted from Møller 2003[156].)

The primary cerebral cortices are the second common pathways of the classical ascending sensory pathways after the thalamic nuclei (Fig. 3.1A). From there, information is distributed to higher cortical regions and other parts of the brain. Nuclei in the dorsal and medial thalamus are the final common pathways for the non-classical sensory pathways. From this point the information branches out to higher cortical regions such as the secondary and association cortices, and to other parts of the brain (Fig. 3.1B). The subcortical connections of the non-classical pathways reach structures such as those of the limbic system that are only reached by the classical pathways through high cortical pathways, including secondary and association cortices.

Both the classical and the non-classical pathways have collaterals that project to other systems. Of particular importance are the collaterals of the lemniscal tracts in the auditory and somatosensory systems that project to neurons in the

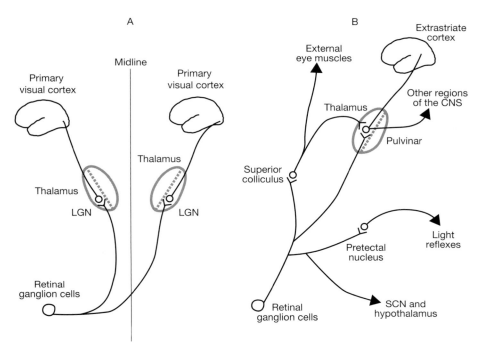

Fig. 3.2 Simplified schematic drawing of the classical (reticulogeniculocortical) and non-classical (SC and pulvinar) (B) visual pathways. (Adapted from Møller 2003[156].)

reticular formation. These collaterals are more abundant in the non-classical systems than the classical systems (Fig. 3.1, Fig. 3.3).

In the visual system, the classical and the non-classical pathways are the retinogeniculocortical and the non-geniculate pathways respectively [23]. The non-geniculate pathway has at least two parts, the superior colliculus (SC) and the pulvinar pathways (Fig. 3.2).

The classical pathway of the somatosensory system is the dorsal column pathway, and in this book we regard the anteriorlateral system, that consists of several separate pathways mediating pain and temperature and some deep touch (Fig. 3.3), to be the non-classical pathway to the somatosensory system. We will discuss the anteriorlateral system in detail in the chapter on pain (Chapter 4).

The non-classical sensory pathways are phylogenetically older than those of the classical pathways. There may be similarities with the two parallel sensory pathways and the two motor tracts, where the medial system is regarded to be phylogenetically older than the lateral system (corticospinal and rubrospinal systems) (see Chapter 5).

The parallel nature of thalamo-cortical connections have been studied extensively and it has been found that these parallel pathways in the auditory,

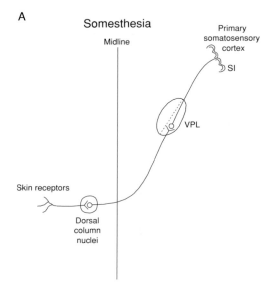

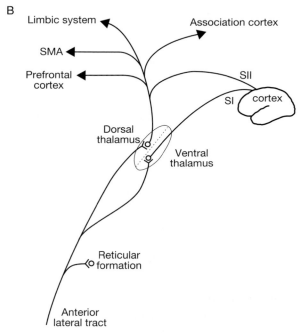

Fig. 3.3 Simplified and schematic drawing of the classical (A) and non-classical (pain) somatosensory pathways (B). (Adapted from Møller 2003[156].)

somatosensory and visual pathways perform different kinds of processing of sensory information [44, 45]. The cells of the classical pathways that originate in the ventral part of the thalamus respond more distinctly to the physical properties of sensory stimuli, than neurons of the non-classical pathways that use the dorsal thalamus.

Some neurons in the subcortical nuclei of non-classical auditory pathways receive input from other sensory systems (Fig. 3.1B) [3, 74, 202], while such cross-modal interaction is absent in subcortical nuclei of the classical pathways [156]. Neurons in the classical ascending pathways (up to and including the primary sensory cortex) only respond to stimulation of one specific sensory modality, while some neurons in the non-classical pathways respond to more than one modality of sensory stimulation. Interaction between different sensory modalities occurs in some cells of the subcortical nuclei of the non-classical pathways [3, 222]. This difference between the classical and the non-classical pathways is important for understanding some pathology of sensory systems where the non-classical pathways may be involved. Integration of sensory input of different modalities occurs generally in the association cortices.

> It has recently been shown that some neurons in an area of the auditory cortex that is located close to the primary auditory cortex (A1), respond to stimulation of other sensory systems [59]. These studies, performed in monkeys, showed that neurons in the caudomedial auditory cortex, that is located adjacent to the ipsilateral A1 cortex, respond to somatosensory stimulation. These neurons receive direct projections from neurons in the ipsilateral A1 cortex and from several thalamic nuclei such as dorsal thalamus (medial geniculate body (MGB), and magnocellular part of the MGB), as well as other thalamic regions such as the medial pulvinar [77]. The finding that neurons in caudomedial auditory cortex respond to somatosensory stimulation [59] may be a sign of activation of the non-classical auditory system, which involves the dorsal MGB (see Fig. 3.1), and it is not in conflict with the hypothesis that neurons of the classical ascending auditory systems, up to and including the primary auditory cortex, respond only to one sensory modality (sound).

Classical ascending pathways

The organization of the classical ascending sensory pathways for hearing, somesthesia and vision, has many similarities [156] (Figs. 3.1, 3.2, 3.3). These pathways all consist of a chain of well-defined nuclei that are connected by fiber tracts. The number of nuclei is different in the ascending pathways of sensory systems. All axons in the ascending tracts make synaptic contacts with neurons in specific nuclei in the ventral part of the thalamus. The neurons in these thalamic nuclei project to neurons in primary sensory cerebral cortices of the respective senses. For hearing and somesthesia, the first nucleus, which receives its input from the sensory organ through the respective sensory nerves, is located on the same side as the sensory organ and most connections from this nucleus cross the midline to make connection with other nuclei. In vision, a neural network in the retina performs the first stage of information processing of visual inputs that is similar to that of the first nuclei of the auditory and somatosensory pathways. The optic nerve in humans projects to the thalamic visual nuclei (LGN) bilaterally.

The complexity of the classical ascending sensory pathways differs; those of the auditory and the visual systems being the most complex. The fibers of the ascending sensory pathways have many collaterals. Each axon in these ascending pathways makes synaptic connections with many nerve cells in the sensory nuclei, and each cell receives many inputs, facts that usually are not apparent from the traditionally simplified drawings of ascending pathways. There are many connections between the two sides of the auditory pathways, but similar connections are absent in vision and the somatosensory systems.

The collateral connections are important for the normal function of the sensory systems as well as for pathologies, but their extensions are not normally documented in neuroanatomical textbooks. Whether connections are functional or not depends on the strength of the synapses with which they connect to their target cells. The synaptic strength differs, and it can vary from time to time and it may change because of the expression of neural plasticity (see Chapter 1). Expression of neural plasticity may also cause changes in protein synthesis in nerve cells [203] and that can affect nerve cells' excitability.

Somatosensory system All fibers that carry somatosensory information from the skin of the body, and which enter the spinal cord as dorsal roots, are interrupted by synaptic transmission in the dorsal column nuclei [23, 168] (Fig. 3.3) (the gracilis and cuneatus nuclei) that are located in the medulla oblongata. The axons of these cells form the medial lemniscus, cross to the opposite side, and terminate on cells in the ventral thalamus (ventral posterior lateral nuclei, VPL). The axons that innervate somatosensory receptors give off many collaterals, which make synaptic contact with cells in the gray matter of the spinal cord (mostly the dorsal horns) where considerable processing occurs (most input to cells in the spinal cord comes from other cells in the same or other segments of the spinal cord).

Somatosensory information from the face and the inside of the mouth [95] enters the brainstem through the trigeminal nerve. These fibers make synaptic contact with cells in the sensory division of the trigeminal nucleus [95]. The trigeminal sensory nucleus (Fig. 3.4) [95, 197] has a rostral and a caudal part.

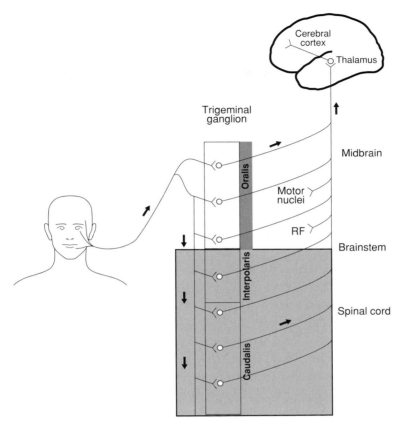

Fig. 3.4 Schematic drawings of the pathways through the trigeminal sensory nucleus. The upper part is the sensory part and the lower (shaded) part is mainly involved in processing noxious stimuli (pain processing). RF: Reticular formation. (Adapted from Sessle, 1986 [196].)

The rostral part of the trigeminal sensory nucleus has similarities with the dorsal column nuclei, thus belonging to the classical sensory pathways communicating innocuous somatosensory information. The caudal part of the trigeminal sensory nucleus has similarities with the parts of the dorsal horn of the spinal cord that are involved in processing noxious (pain) stimuli (see Chapter 4, p. 149).

The axons from the neurons of the trigeminal nucleus ascend in the medial lemniscus, together with those from the dorsal column nuclei. The fibers of the medial lemniscus enter the thalamic nuclei that are involved in somesthesia (the ventrobasal nuclei, VB); the VPM for the face region, and the VPL for the body. The fibers of the medial lemniscus have many collaterals that terminate on neurons of the brainstem reticular formation.

Proprioceptive input from the lower body, and some input from low threshold skin receptors, are not interrupted in the dorsal column nuclei but rather in the nucleus Z [73, 117], which is located slightly more rostral and medial than the gracilis nucleus [117]. The axons of the cells of the nucleus Z cross to the opposite side and join the medial lemniscus [15, 23].

Auditory system Auditory information enters the brainstem through the auditory nerve (part of CN VIII). Axons bifurcate twice and each one of the axons of the resulting three branches make synaptic contact with neurons in separate divisions of the cochlear nucleus (anterior ventral, AVCN, and posterior ventral, PVCN, nuclei, and dorsal division) [154]. The axons of the neurons of the three divisions of the cochlear nucleus form the lateral lemniscus that crosses the midline to reach the midbrain relay of auditory information (the inferior colliculus, IC) (Fig. 3.1). The axons of the lateral lemniscus project to neurons in the central nucleus of the inferior colliculus (ICC), where almost all fibers are interrupted by synaptic contact. (Other parts of the IC are involved in the non-classical auditory pathways, see p. 81.) Some of the axons of the cells in the cochlear nucleus are interrupted by synaptic connections in cells in the nuclei of the superior olivary complex (SOC), and some collateral fibers of these axons make synaptic contact with cells in the nuclei of the SOC. Some of the cells in the nuclei of the SOC receive input from both ears and these cells are important for directional hearing. The axons of the cells in the SOC join the medial lemniscus and terminate on cells in the ICC. Some collateral fibers of the lateral lemniscus make synaptic contact with cells in the nuclei of the lateral lemniscus, the cells of which project to the ipsilateral and contralateral IC [156].

The axons of the ICC ascend as the brachium of the IC and reach the thalamus where all fibers are interrupted making synaptic contact with cells of the MGB, the cells of which project to the AI cortex. There are many connections between the ascending pathways of the two sides at all levels including the cochlear nucleus but except that of the thalamus [154, 156].

Visual system Information from visual receptors is interrupted by synaptic conduction in the neural network within the retina before it enters the optic nerve and the optic tract, the axons of which are interrupted by synaptic transmission in the (ventral) visual thalamic nucleus (LGN). The axons of the cells in the LGN terminate on cells in the primary (striate) visual cortex (V1) [23] (Fig. 3.2). In humans and in animals with forward pointing eyes, the part of the optic nerve that carries information from the medial (nasal) part of the retina (the temporal visual field) crosses the midline at the optic chiasm and reaches the contralateral LGN (Fig. 3.2). The portion of the optic nerve that innervates the lateral retina continues uncrossed through the optic chiasm and its axons make synaptic contact with cells in the ipsilateral LGN.

Non-classical ascending pathways

Each one of the three sensory systems, hearing, vision and somesthesia has distinct non-classical pathways. The axons of these non-classical pathways are interrupted by synaptic transmission in the medial and dorsal divisions of the thalamus (Figs. 3.1, 3.2, 3.3). The non-classical ascending somatosensory pathway (the anterior lateral system) that mediates sensations of pain, cold and heat and some deep touch, is discussed in a separate chapter of this book (Chapter 4, p. 149).

Neurons in the external nucleus and dorsal cortex of the IC belong to the non-classical auditory system [3]. These neurons receive auditory input from the lateral lemniscus and from neurons in the ICC. Many of these neurons also receive input from somatosensory and visual systems, as indicated by the fact that they respond to somatosensory or visual input in addition to responding to auditory input [3, 13, 114]. Anatomical studies have shown that neurons in the cochlear nucleus receive connections from the somatosensory system (trigeminal nucleus [202], and via the dorsal column nuclei [91]).

While the neurons of the nuclei of the ventral portion of the thalamus mainly project to primary sensory regions of the cerebral cortex, the neurons of the medial and lateral portions of the thalamic sensory nuclei mainly project to secondary and association cortices [188], and thus bypass the primary sensory cortices. In the auditory system, these same regions of the association cortices also receive auditory information through the classical auditory pathways via the primary auditory cortex. That means that there exists an anatomical basis for interaction between the auditory information that travels in the two ascending pathways. Information that travels in the classical pathways may arrive earlier at the association cortices than the information that travels in the classical pathways and that may cause unwanted effects.

It is known that the non-classical pathways, at least of the auditory system, provide subcortical connections to many structures in the brain that are otherwise only reached by sensory information through long cortico-cortical routes. The neurons in the medial and dorsal thalamus project directly (subcortical) to limbic structures [119, 156]. This is of specific interest because this route provides subcortical connections to the amygdala (the "low route" [120]) which are normally only reached through cortico-cortical connections (the "high route" [120]).

There are indications that the subcortical connections from dorsal and medial thalamic sensory nuclei may be involved in causing symptoms and signs of diseases. Most neurophysiologic studies of the sensory systems have concerned the classical sensory systems; only a few studies have concerned the functional involvement of the non-classical pathways [3, 58, 60, 222], and only a few studies have been done in humans [148, 155]. Incomplete knowledge about the anatomy of the non-classical pathways has hampered understanding of both their normal and pathological function.

> The fact that (at least) two parallel tracts of ascending sensory pathways project to the sensory cortices has been known for a long time [58, 60]. The names and the definition of these tracts given by different investigators has varied. The two main sensory tracts that originate in the dorsal and the ventral portion of the thalamus have been referred to as the lemniscal and the extralemniscal pathways [3], and more recently as the classical and non-classical pathways [156]. The non-classical system has also been known as the diffuse system [216]. It has also been shown that the classical pathway (that originates in the ventral part of the thalamus) has two functional parts, one consisting of fibers that terminate in cells in layer IV of the primary sensory cortices (layer IV is the main receiving layer of the cerebral cortex for the classical pathways, while the fibers of other ascending pathways avoid layer IV and instead terminate in more superficial layers [45].

In the rat somatosensory system, two ascending tracts, from the ventral thalamus, the lemniscal and paralemniscal pathways have been identified. These two tracts terminate in different parts of the cerebral cortex. The fibers of the lemniscal tract respond distinctly (temporally and spatially) to somatosensory stimuli and terminate in layer IV of the cortical columns whereas the paralemniscal fibers that respond less distinctly to somatosensory stimuli terminate outside cortical columns (in septa between the columns), above and beneath layer IV [45]. The paralemniscal fibers, originating in the posterior complex of the PO part of the thalamus in rodents (corresponding to the ventral posterior nucleus in other animals) have a modulating effect on activity in the cortex and promote neural plasticity (learning) [45].

The paralemniscal channel of the pathway from the ventral thalamus also provides facilitatory input to the cortex. The two different channels that constitute the ventral thalamic-cortical connection are separated anatomically in rodents while these two channels in other animals are anatomically integrated and appear as the thalamo-cortical pathway that originates in the VPL and VPM.

Recent studies have indicated that the non-classical auditory system may be activated through expression of neural plasticity, and that activation of the non-classical system may result in symptoms and signs of disease such as tinnitus, hyperacusis and phonophobia [148] (see pp. 134, 96). (The involvement of neural plasticity in many forms of pain is well known, see Chapter 4.)

While neurons in subcortical nuclei of the classical sensory pathways only respond to stimulation with one sensory modality, neurons in the non-classical pathways respond to more than one sensory modality [3, 222] (see p. 133). That fact has been used in studies of the activation of non-classical pathways. Cross modal interaction between the auditory and the somatosensory system occurs as a constant phenomenon in young children [155] but rarely in adults [148, 155] indicating that suppression of certain connections occurs during normal childhood development. Other studies have shown evidence that these connections may re-appear in individuals with severe tinnitus [25, 148] and that is taken as a sign that re-routing of information has occurred.

Re-routing of sensory information may also be involved in producing some of the signs in some forms of autism [159]. The presence of signs of cross-modal interaction means that different sensory modalities interact abnormally. Such interaction is caused by a change in the function of the central nervous system that is caused by expression of neural plasticity [25, 100].

Re-routing of information in sensory systems including an abnormal involvement of the dorsal and medial thalamus provides a sensory pathway that bypasses the primary cortical areas and that has been demonstrated to occur in vision and hearing but it may also occur in other sensory systems. The dorsal and medial thalamic sensory nuclei provide subcortical connections to parts of the CNS such as limbic structures that are not usually reached through a subcortical route. This subcortical pathway has been implicated in such signs as phonophobia in severe tinnitus and it may also be involved in the development of depression that often accompanies severe pain and tinnitus [148, 153, 155]. Studies using functional imaging to measure changes in blood flow have shown that some tinnitus patients have an abnormally strong activation of the amygdala [128]. These subcortical connections would allow unprocessed information to reach the amygdala bypassing the primary and secondary sensory cortices and association cortices, which is the normal route to the amygdala ("high route"). The high route offers ample possibilities of modulation of the information before it reaches the amygdala while the subcortical route from the dorsal and medial thalamus provides raw sensory input to the amygdala.

The non-classical pathways of the visual system have two parts, namely the superior colliculus (SC) pathway and the pulvinar pathway [23]. The parvicellular and the magnocellular channels are parts of the lemniscal system that are anatomically integrated with the pulvinar system and referred to as the paralemniscal pathways by some investigators [45] while other investigators have used different names for these two separate pathways, such as the classical and the non-classical systems [156].

The SC pathway projects to the SC and mainly involves visual reflexes (Fig. 3.2). The pulvinar pathway involves the pulvinar of the thalamus and the lateral posterior nucleus of the thalamus. Connections from the thalamic nuclei bypass the primary visual cortex and their axons make synaptic contact with neurons in the MT/V5 association region of the visual cortex. This means that visual information that travels in the non-classical visual pathways arrives at the MT/V5 cortex earlier than information that travels in the classical pathways which reaches the MT/V5 cortical region via the V1 and secondary cortices (V2-V4). Information that travels through the classical visual pathways may therefore interact in the MT/V5 cortex with an earlier version of the information that reaches that area through the non-classical (pulvinar) pathways.

Descending pathways

The descending pathways have often been described as separate systems but it may be more appropriate to regard the descending sensory pathways as being reciprocal pathways to the ascending pathways. Both classical and non-classical ascending sensory pathways have reciprocal descending pathways. The descending pathways from the sensory cortices to the thalamic sensory nuclei are especially abundant [240], but also descending pathways that reach other more caudal sensory nuclei are extensive [239]. Some descending pathways reach as caudal as the first nucleus (spinal cord and cochlear nucleus [80, 209]), and even the sensory cells in the cochlea have been shown to receive abundant efferent innervation [231] (for details see [156]). Little is known about the function of descending sensory systems, and their role in pathologies remains unknown.

3.1.6   Olfaction and gustation

The pathways for olfaction and gustation are different from those of hearing, vision and the somatosensory sense (for information about these systems see [156]). Gustation has two parallel pathways that may be regarded as the classical and non-classical pathways (the specific and the non-specific pathways [23, 200]).

It is questionable if there are any sensory neo-cortical projections from olfaction, and few disorders are known to be related to olfaction. One aspect of olfaction, namely the heavy projection to the amygdala and other limbic structures, makes odors provide strong emotional reactions in addition to eliciting conscious perceptions. The vomeronasal (pheromone) pathway may be of clinical interest [156] because the vomeronasal organ projects via the olfactory bulb directly to the nuclei of the amygdala without having any known projection to cortical sensory regions [78, 138]. This means that pheromones may have an unconscious influence on vital functions such as sexual behavior (see [156]).

Little is known about the role of taste and olfactory pathways in disorders of the nervous system, and these sensory systems will not be considered further in this book.

3.1.7   *Organization of sensory cerebral cortices*

Sensory cortices consist of primary, secondary and higher order cortices that connect to association cortices and other parts of the CNS. The sensory cortices receive input from the ascending sensory pathways, process this information, and then send it to other regions of the cerebral cortex and to other parts of the brain. Extensive processing occurs within the sensory cortices. For example, the majority of the synapses on cells in sensory cortices are connections from other cells in the cortex. Association cortices coordinate input from different sensory systems and mediate sensory information to motor centers and other parts of the CNS. The primary sensory cortices also send information to more peripheral parts of the sensory nervous system through extensive descending pathways that are parallel to the ascending sensory pathways (see above). Cells in primary cortices respond to only one modality of sensory stimuli, while cells in higher order cortices (including secondary (auditory) cortices [59]) may respond to more than one modality.

Somatotopic organization

Cells in the sensory cortices are organized according to the spatial organization of sensory receptor surfaces; in the ear the basilar membrane of the cochlea is projected onto the surface of the auditory cortex. Neurons that are located in specific places on the auditory cortex respond best to tones of a certain frequency, therefore the auditory cortex is anatomically organized according to the frequency of sounds to which the neurons respond best (tonotopic organization). Similarly, a representation (homunculus) of the body can be laid out on the surface of the somatosensory cortex, and likewise, the receptor surface of the retina is projected onto the visual cortex. The V1 cortex is organized according to the visual field. (For details see [156].)

> The earliest quantitative information about the somatotopical organization of the somatosensory system was published by Penfield [173]. Penfield was a neurosurgeon, who had trained with the eminent physiologist Sherrington in Oxford, England, and became interested (and knowledgeable) about neurophysiology. Penfield became the first to make extensive

use of the opportunities that are available in the neurosurgical operating room for studies of the functioning nervous system in humans.
Specifically, he used the knowledge and understanding of the function
of the nervous system he had acquired from Sherrington to study the
somatosensory cortex in patients on whom he operated. Penfield's functional mapping of the somatosensory cortex has not been significantly
improved upon, or repeated to an extent that has replaced the maps he
published in the 1930s. Penfield's maps still currently appear in modern
textbooks. Additions have been made subsequently, and it is now recognized that there are many subdivisions of the somatosensory cortex that
have separate maps (see [156])

It is an interesting question to what extent the spatial mapping of the cerebral
cortices and nuclei of sensory systems is based on the anatomical relation to
the receptor surfaces and to what extent it is influenced by stimulation. It has
been known for a long time that the frequency mapping of the auditory cortex
can be molded by stimulation (in animals with hearing) [105, 186], but it has
been difficult to study to what extent such mapping existed in the absence of
any stimulation at all. The advent of cochlear implants has not only made the
question of practical importance with regards to the auditory system, but also it
has made it possible to study the origin of tonotopic organization of the auditory
cortex [46].

The tonotopic organization that may exist in deaf animals that have intact
auditory nerves but no functional hair cells must be based on the anatomical
relationship between the innervation of the receptor surface (the basilar membrane of the cochlea) and structures of the ascending auditory pathways. Only
a few studies have addressed the question about how much tonotopic organization exists without input, thus being based on the anatomical projection of
the receptor surface. Published studies, however, show that deaf animals with
deprived stimulation of the auditory nerve have a rudimentary cochleotopic
organization in brainstem nuclei [84] and in the auditory cortex [81]. There is
thus no question that sensory stimulation is important for organization of the
nervous system [107, 111]. How fast such organization occurs after sound exposure is not known but experience from individuals who have received cochlear
implants seems to show that it occurs rapidly. A similar question can be applied
to the mapping of the somatosensory system and the retina on respective cortical areas.

Sound input is thus necessary for proper development of the auditory nervous system [35, 112, 113, 190], but cortical maps in the adult organism are not
static either, and they can be modified by various means such as through expression of neural plasticity or by changes in the relationship between inhibition

and excitation. The response of individual cells depends on the convergence of input and the balance between inhibitory and excitatory input. Increased convergence widens a cell's response area, lateral inhibition makes cells' response areas narrower. Furthermore, other complex interactions between the input to different cortical cells affect their response to sensory stimuli and the appearance of cortical maps.

In the auditory system, expression of neural plasticity may be caused by sounds, or the absence of sounds (deprivation of input). Cortical maps of other sensory systems can also be altered through the expression of neural plasticity [105, 186].

Other forms of cortical organization

In addition to spatial organization, cells of sensory cortices are organized anatomically according to the properties of sensory stimuli. Cortical maps that reflect functional properties of stimuli are known as functional maps, or computational maps. An example of computational maps is the mapping of auditory space [156]. Computational maps are equally dynamic and modifiable by expression of neural plasticity as well.

3.1.8   Parallel processing

Parallel processing means that the same sensory information is processed in different populations of neurons in sensory systems, or that information can follow several routes as it travels in ascending sensory pathways. The anatomical basis for such parallel processing is repeated bifurcation of fibers in the ascending sensory pathways. For example, each auditory nerve fiber innervates neurons in three different parts of the cochlear nucleus (Fig. 3.5), which is the first relay nucleus for auditory information. A similar anatomical basis for parallel processing occurs at more central locations of ascending sensory pathways; examples are the lateral lemniscus and the medial lemniscus that send collaterals to several structures of the brainstem, such as the reticular formation, before reaching the thalamus [154] (see Figs. 3.1 and 3.3). Axons that carry somatosensory input to the spinal cord and the trigeminal nucleus, give off many collateral axons that make synaptic contact with cells in many different locations in the spinal cord and brainstem. The separation of pathways in classical and non-classical pathways is also an example of parallel processing, where the same information is processed in different populations of nerve cells. Parallel processing is abundant in the sensory cortices.

While bifurcation of nerve fibers is the anatomical basis for parallel processing, not all fibers that bifurcate form functional connections because some

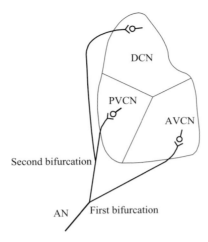

Fig. 3.5 Branching of auditory nerve (AN) fibers before they enter the cochlear nucleus. (Adapted from Møller 2003[156].)

connections terminate in dormant synapses[1]. When dormant synapses become activated (unmasked), for example, through expression of neural plasticity it may alter processing or open new routes for information. This means that not all routes that can be verified anatomically are functional. Parallel routes may therefore offer redundancy that can be activated after injury, or because of change in demand by expression of neural plasticity. Activation of such dormant connections may also cause symptoms of diseases (see pp. 83, 149).

3.1.9   Stream segregation

Stream segregation is different from parallel processing in that it implies that different kinds of information is processed in different populations of neurons. While parallel processing is evident at peripheral levels of the ascending sensory pathways, stream segregation has been associated with higher levels of the nervous system. For example, the processing of information that occurs in association cortices is divided into streams, where different kinds of information are processed in different parts of the association cortices. This separation according to the kind of sensory information received was first described in the visual system [144, 227], where it was observed that spatial information was processed in a dorsal stream while object information was processed in

---

[1] The term "dormant synapses" was coined by Patrick Wall 1977 [230] to describe synapses that were anatomically present but which could not activate the neurons on which they terminate. Such "dormant" synapses can be "unmasked" through the expression of neural plasticity or through changes of the input, from for example, low rate to high rate, or from continuous firing to burst firing.

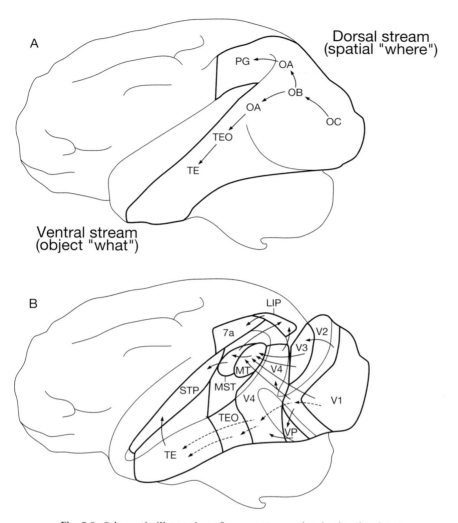

Fig. 3.6 Schematic illustration of stream segregation in the visual system.

A: Schematic diagram of the monkey brain. OC, OB, OA, TEO, TE and PG: different areas of the visual cortex[16].

B: More detailed drawing. V1–4: Visual cortex; MT: Middle temporal area; MST: Medial superior temporal area; STP: Superior temporal area; TEO: Posterior inferior temporal area. (Adapted from Gross *et al.* 1993[75].)

a ventral (or temporal) stream (Fig. 3.6). This separation in processing of spatial and object information became known as the "where" and "what" types of information.

Similar forms of stream segregation as occur in the visual system have been found to occur in the auditory system [184]. As studies of stream segregation have progressed, it has been clear that segregation of several different qualities of sensory stimuli occurs, and that stream segregation is not simply limited to separation of spatial and object information (for details see [156]).

3.1.10   Connections to other parts of the CNS

Sensory systems connect to many different parts of the CNS that are not anatomically regarded as being sensory regions. Sensory pathways connect to autonomic centers of the brain, and to the motor system. We have already mentioned that the limbic system (the emotional brain) receives sensory input. Likewise the reticular system of the brainstem receives sensory input that is important for control of wakefulness.

Motor system

The motor system is the output organ (effector organ) for sensory communication. For humans, speech is the main output medium, but the mimic muscles play an important role in communications. Limb and body movements are subjected to conscious commands that often depend on sensory input, or use sensory input as feedback. Sensory input to spinal motor systems is mainly proprioceptive, and parts of reflexes, but also nociceptors, supply input to motor systems such as through the withdrawal reflex. (Reflexes are discussed in Chapter 5.) Sensory stimulation can elicit general motor activity such as the startle reflex (see p. 282). Eye muscles are activated by sound, as are neck muscles in righting reflexes. The proprioceptive system's input to the motor system is especially important, but tactile and visual feedback is also important for control of movements. Also other sensory systems supply important input to the motor system for feedback and coordination.

> The streams of visual information in the association cortices that are involved in the feedback of hand movement (reaching) are different from those streams that concern perception [71, 143]. Injury to one of the two streams of visual information (dorsal or ventral) while leaving the other intact, causes deficits either of visual feedback (when the dorsal stream was injured) with intact perception of visual images; or injury to the other stream (ventral stream) causes deficits in visual perception, leaving visual feedback for hand movements intact. (These studies [71] were done in patients with strokes that were limited to the anatomical regions that processed one of the two main visual streams.)

Reticular formation

The axons of the fiber tracts of ascending sensory pathways that pass through the brainstem, send collaterals to the reticular formation. The reticular formation controls the excitability of cortical neurons, and sensory activation of the reticular formation is necessary to elicit responses from cortical cells to sensory stimulation. This means that perception of sensory stimuli requires activation of sensory receptors by a physical stimulus, *and* activation of the sensory cortices from the reticular formation. Non-classical pathways provide more extensive input to the reticular formation than the classical pathways. Arousal of the cerebral cortex can also occur through the amygdala via the nucleus basalis (Fig. 3.7), which means that emotional activation and attention can increase the excitability of sensory cortices.

Limbic system

Sensory systems have ample anatomical connections to nuclei of the limbic system, mainly the amygdala nuclei (Fig. 3.7). The lateral nucleus of the amygdala is the main receiving nucleus for input from the auditory, somatosensory and visual systems (Fig. 3.7). The lateral nucleus projects to the basolateral nucleus, which connects to the central nucleus of the amygdala. The central nucleus is the main output nucleus of the amygdala, and its neurons connect to endocrine, behavioral and autonomic centers of the brain. The central nucleus also projects to the nucleus basalis, which plays an important role in controlling arousal of the cerebral cortex. Input to cortical cells from the nucleus basalis facilitates plastic changes in cerebral sensory cortices [104, 105].

There are two main routes that sensory information can take to the amygdala: One is through a long chain of neurons, from primary somatosensory cortices, through secondary and association cortices to the lateral nucleus of the amygdala. This route is known as the "high route" [120]. The other route, known as the "low route", is a subcortical route that originates in the medial and dorsal thalamus, where neurons project directly to the lateral nucleus of the amygdala [120] (Fig. 3.7). (In the auditory and visual systems, the dorsal and medial thalamic nuclei are parts of the non-classical ascending sensory pathways [see pp. 81, 72].) The dorsomedial thalamus has strong influence on the nucleus basalis and thereby on the ability of sensory cortices to reorganize through the expression of neural plasticity. This pathway also provides arousal to the neocortex (see Fig. 3.7).

> While the anatomy of the connections from sensory systems to the amygdala is relatively well known, the functional connections are much less well understood. Some studies have shown evidence that the non-classical auditory pathways may not be activated by sensory information in adult humans [148, 155], and consequently, the subcortical route to the amygdala may not be functional under normal conditions in adults. There is evidence that the non-classical auditory pathways are active in children

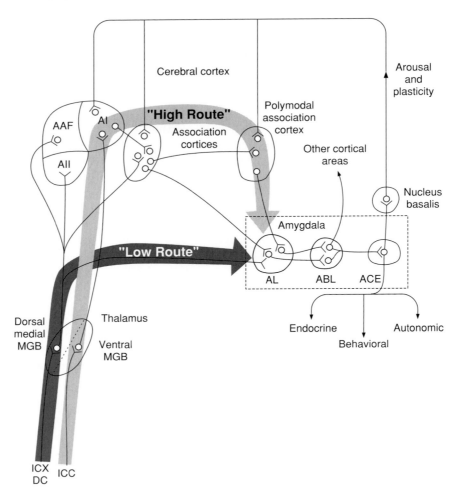

Fig. 3.7 Schematic drawing illustrating the "high route" and the "low route" from sensory systems to the lateral nucleus of the amygdala. The drawing shows connections from the auditory system to the lateral nucleus of the amygdala. ABL: Basolateral nucleus of the amygdala; ACE: Central nucleus of the amygdala; AL: Lateral nucleus of the amygdala. Connections between the different nuclei of the amygdala and connections from these nuclei to different parts of the CNS are also shown. (From Møller 2003[156], based on LeDoux [120].)

[155]. The finding that some individuals with severe tinnitus have signs of activation of the non-classical auditory pathways [25, 28, 148] indicates that a subcortical route to the amygdala can become functional under pathological conditions opening the possibility of subcortical sensory activation of the amygdala. Functional imaging studies have also

provided evidence of increased activation of limbic structures in some individuals with tinnitus [128], which may occur through the "low route". (There is also evidence that the non-classical auditory system may be abnormally active in some developmental disorders (autism) [159].)

Autonomic nervous system

The autonomic nervous system can be activated by sensory input in several ways. Autonomic activation of the autonomic system is most pronounced for the chemical senses, where taste can control secretion in the mouth and the digestive organs. Sensory systems connect to autonomic systems through the limbic system by which sensory input can change the function of the vascular system (blood pressure and heart rate) and cause sweating. Certain sounds can in some individuals cause autonomic reactions such as salivation and contraction of muscles in the skin. Bright light can elicit sneezing. Some of these reactions may occur without any conscious awareness, while others elicit distinct perceptions and can be aborted by conscious efforts.

Many of the connections from sensory systems to non-sensory systems are reciprocal. Thus, the autonomic nervous system projects to sensory system affecting (or modulating) their function. For example, sympathetic nerve fibers that terminate near mechanoreceptors in the skin can secrete norepinephrine, which changes (increases) the sensitivity of sensory receptors. Sympathetic nerve fibers also terminate close to other receptor cells such as the hair cells in the ear [43] and in the vestibular organs [53], but the function of these connections is unknown. The autonomic nervous system can also affect the function of sensory receptors by its effect on the blood flow to sensory organs.

Adrenergic nerve fibers terminate in sensory ganglia [86, 115], where they can alter processing of sensory information. Anatomically these adrenergic fibers are different from those that are innervating blood vessels. The functional significance of the adrenergic innervation of the sensory ganglia is unknown but it is reasonable to assume that this innervation plays a role in altering (increasing) the sensitivity of sensory receptors during stress. There is also autonomic innervation of cells that processes innocuous and noxious (pain) sensory information in the dorsal horn of the spinal cord, and the sympathetic nervous system is known to influence neural processing of pain signals (see Chapter 4, p. 149).

3.1.11 *Organization of sensory systems is dynamic*

Descriptions of the structure of the sensory pathways such as those shown in Figs. 3.1–3.7 are based on anatomical studies. Anatomically verified connections may not be functional, however, under normal conditions because they terminate in synapses that are ineffective at a given time. The efficacy of synapses can increase or decrease through the expression of neural plasticity. Unmasking of normally dormant synapses can alter processing of sensory information and open connections within sensory systems and thereby re-route information to neurons that normally do not receive such information. In a similar way, masking of functional synapses can interrupt connections that are normally functional and eliminate processing of sensory information in neurons that normally perform such processing (see Chapters 4 and 5). Connections from sensory systems to other systems in the CNS are also subjected to changes through the expression of neural plasticity. Neural plasticity can be initiated by changing demands of sensory systems, or as compensatory measures after injuries. (We discussed neural plasticity in more detail in Chapter 1.)

The information that flows in some parts of sensory pathways can be consciously modulated; whereas other ascending information is subject to unconscious control. We have already mentioned that there are connections to the limbic system from different nuclei of sensory pathways ("low route") and from the cerebral cortex (association cortices, the "high route"). The classical pathways provide the most central connections and the non-classical pathways provide subcortical connections to the amygdala but these (anatomically verified) connections may not always be functional. The flow of information in the "high route" to the amygdala can be modulated consciously, whereas information that reaches the amygdala through subcortical connections is probably not subjected to similar conscious modulation. Activation of the amygdala through the "high route" that may mediate fear can thereby be controlled consciously (see p. 91) while the flow of information in the "low route" is largely beyond such conscious control.

3.2   Disorders of sensory systems

Sensory disorders can affect the conductive apparatus of sensory organs, the sensory receptors, the sensory nerve and the central nervous system. Disorders that affect each one of these four main steps of sensory processing have specific symptoms and signs. Some disorders that affect sensory systems are complex, and the symptoms may be referred to anatomically different locations than those where the physiological abnormal neural activity is generated. This not only makes diagnosis difficult, but it also complicates studies of the pathophysiology of sensory systems.

Disorders of sensory systems can cause decreased sensitivity (increased threshold), change in processing of sensory stimuli, and sensations that occur without physical stimulation of sensory receptors (such as paresthesia,[2] tinnitus, and other phantom sensations. Some disorders cause changes in the processing of sensory stimuli in the nervous system resulting in symptoms such as hyper-esthesia, hyperacusis, dysesthesia[3] and allodynia.[4] Phantom sensations such as tinnitus, paresthesia and central neuropathic pain, are caused by neural activity that is generated in the central nervous system and thus not at the anatomical location to which the sensation is referred. These symptoms are typically caused by reorganization of the CNS and redirection of information through expression of neural plasticity. In fact, neural plasticity is involved in generating the symptoms of many disorders of sensory systems.

The symptoms and signs of disorders of sensory systems can be caused by changes in function that have no detectable morphological correlates. For example, there are strong indications that many forms of tinnitus and other phantom sensations are caused by plastic changes of the nervous system. Neural plasticity may even be involved in the loss of sensitivity of sensory systems including those that occur with aging.

Expression of neural plasticity may cause reorganization of the nervous system that can change neural processing of sensory stimuli, or re-routing of information. Such functional changes may cause the generation of sensations without any physical stimuli reaching sensory receptors. Phantom limb sensations are examples of sensations that are generated in the CNS but referred to a peripheral anatomical location (that no longer exists). Another example is tinnitus in individuals with a severed auditory nerve, where the sensation of sound is referred to the ear but obviously not generated in the ear.

Age-related changes in sensory function affect sensory receptor cells, sensory nerves and CNS structures. In general, the sensitivity and the acuity of sensory functions decreases with age. Age-related changes are perhaps the most common causes of sensory deficits [236].

In this section, we will first discuss disorders that are related to the structures that conduct sensory stimuli to the receptors and thereafter discuss disorders that are specifically related to sensory receptors. That is followed by deeper discussions of changes in the function of the central nervous system that cause hyperactive symptoms and phantom sensations, and changes in processing of

---

[2] Paresthesia: Abnormal (somatic) sensations that occur without physical stimulation. The term is mostly used in connection with the somatosensory system to describe sensations such as tingling, tickling or pricking.

[3] Dysesthesia: An unpleasant sensation from stimulations that are normally innocuous.

[4] Allodynia: Painful perception of normally innocuous sensory stimulation such as that of the skin (see Chapter 4).

sensory information. We will discuss further how some of these changes in the function of the central nervous system may be caused by expression of neural plasticity that is induced by changes in the input from receptors. Last, we will discuss disorders that are caused by specific injuries to the sensory nervous system. Disorders that are specifically related to sensory nerves are discussed in Chapter 2 for peripheral nerves, and in Chapter 6 for cranial nerves.

3.2.1   *Disorders of the conductive apparatus*

Disorders of the conductive apparatus of sensory systems can affect the transmission of the physical stimuli to the sensory receptor. Disorders of the visual system are mainly related to the conductive part of the eye, either cataracts that affect the corneas or macular degeneration that affect the retina. Macular degeneration, consisting of blood vessels obstructing the passage of light in the retina, can impair visual perception. Such changes are commonly age-related and little is known about their effect on central mechanism (expression of neural plasticity).

> Macular degeneration is a common age-related progressive disorder that causes visual deficits in the form of blurred vision. It affects the macula of the eye either by causing bleeding (wet macular degeneration) or by causing a breakdown of cones in the retina. It is associated with small bright (yellow) spots (drusen) in the retina. It is assumed to be caused by oxidative stress, but unlike similar age-related degeneration of auditory sensory cells, macular degeneration is not known to cause phantom phenomena (phosphenes).

Disorders of the middle ear (and obstruction of the ear canal) impair sound transmission to the cochlea and cause elevated hearing thresholds [154]. Conduction of sound through the middle ear is impaired when the air pressure in the middle ear is different from the ambient pressure because of changes in the mechanical properties of the middle ear. The air pressure in the middle ear cavity decreases if the middle ear cavity is not ventilated properly because of resorption of oxygen by the mucosa that lines the middle ear cavity. This occurs when the Eustachian tube does not open and equalize the pressure. Inability of the Eustachian tube to open often accompanies the common cold because of swelling of the mucosa in the pharynx. More severe middle ear disorders such as middle ear infection cause fluid accumulation in the middle ear cavity resulting in greater conductive hearing loss. Inflammatory processes of the middle ear may cause the middle ear cavity to become filled with fluid (otitis media with effusion [12]), which will cause transmission of sound to the cochlea to become impaired if the fluid covers the backside of the tympanic membrane [154]. Such disorders are common in childhood and if not remedied may cause deprivation of input to the ear that can hamper normal development of the auditory nervous system [111].

Perforation of the tympanic membrane is another cause of conductive hearing loss. A hole in the tympanic membrane lets sound into the middle ear cavity making the difference between the sound pressure on the two sides of the tympanic membrane to become less than it is normally, and consequently the vibration of the tympanic membrane is reduced and less sound is conducted to the cochlea. A small hole affects low frequencies more than high frequencies because it acts as a low-pass filter that lets low frequencies pass into the middle ear cavity [154]. Disease processes such as otosclerosis involve growth of bone around the stapes footplate, which impairs its normal motion [21].

The cochlea, including the outer hair cells, can be regarded as a part of the conductive apparatus of the ear. However, the action of the outer hair cells is non-linear [154] (see p. 99), in contrast to other conductive media such as the middle ear, which acts as a linear system. Impairment of the function of outer hair cells decreases the dynamic range over which the ear can function [154]. This is because the active function of outer hair cells normally causes a compression of the intensity range of sounds that activate inner hair cells, and thereby increases the ear's dynamic range (see p. 99). Because of their nonlinear action, loss of function of outer hair cells impairs the frequency selectivity of the cochlea, which can impair discrimination of complex sounds such as speech sounds. Therefore, injuries to outer hair cells cause changes in the processing of sounds that occur in the cochlea in addition to causing an elevation of the hearing threshold. These changes in the function of the cochlea explain some forms of hyperacusis that often accompany hearing loss of cochlear origin. (Other causes of hyperacusis are changes in the function of the auditory nervous system, see p. 83).

3.2.2   *Disorders that primarily affect sensory receptors*

Disorders of sensory receptors primarily cause reduced sensitivity of the affected sensory organ. Most sensory receptors are affected by overload, first by reducing their sensitivity temporarily. Permanent damage occurs from exposure above a certain intensity of the physical stimuli that reach the receptors. In the ear outer hair cells are most vulnerable to overexposure but outer hair cells do not act as sensory cells with respect to converting sound into a neural code. As mentioned above, outer hair cells may rather be regarded as a part of the sound conducting apparatus. That means that noise induced hearing loss (NIHL) may be regarded as being caused by a complex impairment of sound conduction in the cochlea. Sensory receptors in the eye can be damaged permanently from looking without protection at the sun. Temporary reduction in sensitivity occurs from normal light exposure, which is not regarded as a trauma but rather an adaptation[5] to light.

Age-related decreases in sensitivity of sensory receptors occur in all sensory systems [236], perhaps most pronounced in the auditory system where it is known as presbycusis (see p. 103) [214]. Again, it is the outer hair cells that are most vulnerable, and inner hair cells are rarely affected [82]. Age-related loss of sensitivity also occurs in the somatosensory system, but probably has its greatest effect in connection with proprioception because reduction of proprioception contributes to the impairment of movement (see Chapter 5). Age-related changes in the function of sensory receptors are often followed by compensatory plastic changes, which may give symptoms that are more troublesome than the deficits in sensitivity. Reduction in the sensitivity of olfaction and taste with age has implications for nutrition because it may cause lack of appetite.

Impairment of sensory sensitivity (elevated threshold) has earlier been closely related to deficits in the conduction of the stimulus to the sensory receptors, and injuries or other deficits of these receptors. However, more recently it has become evident that the sensitivity of a given sensory system is affected by complex factors that are not restricted to the receptors. Examples include the finding that an enriched environment of sensory stimulation can affect the progression of age-related sensory deficits, both in the somatosensory system [87] and the auditory system (augmented acoustic environment [237]). Obviously, sensory sensitivity depends on more complex factors than impaired function of sensory cells, or obstruction of conduction of the sensory stimuli to the receptors. In the following, we will discuss hearing in some detail because that is the sense that has been studied most extensively. The ear is also a more complex organ than that of the other senses. We will discuss the role of neural plasticity and the source of the large individual variation in the effect of pathologies, including age-related changes in the function of sensory systems.

Hearing

Auditory receptors can be injured by sound exposure; chemical agents including pharmaceutical drugs; and age-related processes – outer hair cells being more vulnerable than inner hair cells. In fact, most of the common causes of sensorineural hearing impairment are deficits in the function of outer hair cells.

---

[5] The term adaptation is used differently in perceptual literature and physiology literature. In vision, dark adaptation means the gradual increase in sensitivity that occurs in darkness, while light adaptation means a decrease in sensitivity because of exposure to light. In other sensory systems, adaptation means a decrease in sensitivity caused by exposure to stimulation. In physiology, the term adaptation is often used to describe the decrease in firing of nerve fibers or nerve cells that occurs after applying a stimulus.

Temporary or permanent hearing loss can occur after exposure to loud sounds (NIHL) [24, 40]. The degree of the hearing loss depends on the intensity of the sound that reaches the ear and its duration. The effect on sensory receptors in the cochlea (hair cells) from noise exposure is damage to outer hair cells as evidenced from morphological studies. Outer hair cells in the basal (high frequency) part of the cochlea are normally damaged to a greater extent than hair cells in more apical (lower frequency) parts of the cochlea [154, 212]. Detectable injury to inner hair cells, which perform the neural transduction of the vibration of the basilar membrane, is rare. The fact that outer hair cells are more prone to damage than inner hair cells indicates that these hair cells are different from inner hair cells despite their morphological similarities. A higher metabolic rate may be one reason for the greater vulnerability than that of inner hair cells. While these morphological changes were earlier regarded as the (sole) cause of NIHL, it has become evident that the cause of NIHL is more complex than just damage to hair cells that can be detected by morphological techniques (see pp. 99, 118).

It has recently been shown that hair cells may regenerate after injury, and that there is a potential for alleviating hearing loss from injuries to hair cells [101].

While impairment of the function of receptors in the eye, skin, tongue and the nose mainly causes decreased sensitivity to the stimuli of the particular sense, impairment of auditory receptors is more complex. This is because the two types of hair cells, the outer and inner hair cells, have completely different functions.

> The outer hair cells act as active mechanical elements that are parts of the mechanical system of the cochlea. The outer hair cells are thus involved in the transmission of sound to the inner hair cells, which are the sensory cells that convert sounds into a neural code in the auditory nerve. The outer hair cells act as "motors" that provide energy to the motion of the basilar membrane of the cochlea. Since the outer hair cells serve a mechanical function in the cochlea rather than transduction of sound into a neural code, impairment of the function of outer hair cells affects the conduction of the stimulus to the inner hair cells that transduces the motion of the basilar membrane into a neural code. Impairment of outer hair cells may therefore be regarded as a (complex) form of conductive hearing impairment.
>
> The outer hair cells normally provide amplification of approximately 50 dB and destruction of outer hair cells can consequently cause a hearing loss of up to 50 dB [154]. However, outer hair cells are nonlinear elements of sound conduction and the gain they provide is different at different sound intensities. Unlike disorders of the middle ear, which affect all sound intensities equally, injury to outer hair cells mainly affects sounds of low intensity because the gain they normally provide is greatest at low sound intensities. Through their non-linear function,

the outer hair cells provide amplitude compression, and injuries to the outer hair cells therefore affect the ability of the cochlea to compress the amplitude of sounds that reach the ear.[6] Reduced amplitude compression affects processing sounds, especially complex sounds such as speech sounds. Amplitude compression is important for processing of sounds such as speech over a large sound intensity range.

Impairment of the function of outer hair cells not only reduces the sensitivity of the ear, but it also affects the way the cochlear frequency analyzer works. Since the outer hair cells sharpen the frequency selectivity of the basilar membrane for low sound intensities, impaired function of the outer hair cells affects the ability of the cochlea to separate sounds according to their frequencies.

Cochlear hearing loss normally affects hearing at high frequencies more than low frequencies. Activity in nerve cells that respond to high frequencies generally exerts more inhibitory influence on other nerve cells than cells that are tuned to low frequencies. This means that reduced activation of hair cells that are tuned to high frequencies reduce the inhibition in the auditory system, and that has been regarded as one of the reasons why high frequency hearing loss is often associated with tinnitus that may be caused by the lack of inhibitory input to the auditory nervous system.

Experiments in animals have shown that localized injury to sensory cells along the basilar membrane causes re-mapping of the basilar membrane [186]. Similar results were obtained in humans with different degrees of hearing loss [194].

Noise induced hearing loss

The adverse effect of exposure of the ear to sounds of high intensity (noise[7]) can be a temporary increase in the hearing threshold (temporary threshold shift, TTS). If the exposure is above a certain level and of certain duration, the hearing loss does not recover completely. The component of hearing that does not recover (is present a long time after the end of the exposure) is known as permanent threshold shift (PTS).

The acquired elevation of the hearing threshold (TTS and PTS) from noise exposure depends on both the level and duration of the exposure, and to some

---

[6] Amplitude compression in the cochlea means that the range of sound amplitudes that activates the inner hair cells is smaller than the range of sound amplitudes that reaches the ear. This is important because the discharge pattern in auditory nerve fibers is not able to code the entire range of sounds that the auditory system can process.

[7] Noise actually means "undesired or unwanted" sounds. The word is also normally used for sounds that can cause hearing loss such as industrial noise. Music and other "desired and wanted" sounds can cause hearing loss equally well if sufficiently loud, but such sounds are normally not called noise.

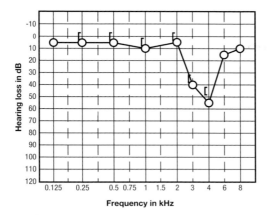

Fig. 3.8 Typical audiogram of an individual who has suffered NIHL. (Data from Lidén, 1985[127].)

extent the physical characteristics of the sound. The sound level taken together with the duration of the exposure is known as the immission level [24].[8] High frequency and impulsive sounds are more effective in producing NIHL than low frequency sounds and continuous sounds.

NIHL usually affects hearing more in the frequency range around 4 kHz than at any other frequency (Fig. 3.8). The reason for this is the amplifying effect of the ear canal together with the effect of non-linearity of the cochlea that makes location of the maximal vibration of the basilar membrane of the cochlea shift towards the base of the cochlea when the sound intensity is increased (for details, see [154]). The resonance of the ear canal increases the sound level at the tympanic membrane by 7–10 dB in the frequency range between 3 and 5 kHz. The effect of the head on the sound that reaches the ear, together with that of the resonance of the ear canal, increases the intensity of the sound at the tympanic membrane by approximately 15 dB in the frequency range from 2.5 to 4 kHz, relative to the sound that is measured at the place of the observer (see [154]).

> The resonance frequency of the ear canal varies between individuals because its length varies. A study of NIHL in individuals with ear canals of different length (and thus different resonance frequency) showed a high correlation between the resonance frequency of the ear canal and the frequency where the individuals had the greatest hearing loss [176]. The study by Pierson et al. [176] showed a mean resonance frequency of 2814 Hz in a group of individuals with NIHL. The average frequency of

---

[8] Immission level is the (average) noise level (in dB) plus 10 times the logarithm of the duration of the exposure (in months).

the greatest hearing loss occurred at 4481 Hz in these individuals. If it is assumed that the maximal sound energy that was delivered to the ear in the individuals in this study occurred at the resonance frequency of the ear canal (2814 Hz), the frequency of maximal hearing loss (at 4481 Hz) was 1.59 times the frequency of the maximal sound energy that reaches the tympanic membrane. This is in good agreement with the observation that exposure to pure tones or narrow band noise of high intensity, causes the greatest hearing loss at a frequency that is approximately one half-octave above the frequency of the sound that caused the hearing loss (assuming maximal sound energy that reaches the tympanic membrane was located at the frequency of resonance of the ear canal).

These observations were taken to support the hypothesis that the 4 kHz dip in the audiogram in individuals with NIHL is caused by peculiarities in the sound conduction apparatus and not by specific weakness of hair cells that are located at the 4 kHz location of the basilar membrane.

The difference between the frequency of maximal sound energy and the maximal hearing loss is a result of the non-linear function of the basilar membrane, which makes the frequency tuning of the basilar membrane become dependent on the sound intensity. The maximal amplitude of vibration of the basilar membrane caused by a tone of a certain frequency shifts towards the base of the cochlea when the intensity of the tone is increased from near threshold to levels where injury to hair cells may occur (for details, see [154] and p. 99). Damage to outer hair cells of the cochlea from sound exposure occurs at the location along the basilar membrane where high intensity sounds produce the greatest vibration amplitude, but the measurement of the hearing threshold is done at a low sound intensity. The threshold shift from noise exposure therefore occurs at a more basal location on the basilar membrane thus at a higher frequency than that of the maximal energy of the noise that caused the damage. This explains why the frequency of the largest hearing loss from noise exposure occurs at approximately 1/2 octave higher frequency than the frequency of the highest energy of the sound that caused the damage.

When averaged over a large population of individuals, NIHL is a function of the intensity of the sound that reaches the ear, the duration of the exposure and the character (continuous, impulsive, narrow spectrum or wide spectrum) of the noise to which the ear is exposed. However, the hearing loss that individual persons acquire varies widely, even under similar exposure conditions [24, 79] (Fig. 3.9).

Ototoxic drugs

It is well known that pharmacological agents, such as aspirin (acetylsalicylate), and aminoglycoside antibiotics can cause hearing loss (and tinnitus)

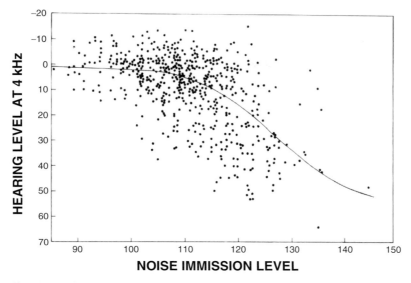

Fig. 3.9 Hearing loss at 4,000 Hz as a function of immission level. (Data from Burns and Robertson, 1970[24].)

in some individuals if given at sufficient dosages (for a review, see Forge and Schacht, 2000 [56]. Other drugs, such as loop diuretics (furosemide, ethacrynic acid), quinine, indomethacin, and cytostatica such as cisplatin can also cause tinnitus and hearing loss [195, 206].

Age-related hearing loss (presbycusis)

Age-related hearing loss (presbycusis[9]) affects high frequencies more than low frequencies, and it increases gradually with age (Fig. 3.10). The degree of age-related hearing loss in individuals who have not been exposed to known excessive noise varies considerably (Fig. 3.11). This means that endogenous and perhaps unknown exogenous causes may affect the hearing loss that occurs with age.

The pathophysiology of age-related changes of hearing (presbycusis) is not well understood. Morphological studies have shown loss of outer hair cells [82, 96], and therefore some of the hearing loss can be explained by impaired function of the cochlear amplifier that is based on the normal function of outer hair cells. Age-related changes of cochlear hair cells mostly affect the outer hair cells in the basal part of the cochlea, causing high frequency hearing loss. Oxidative stress is likely to play a role in developing presbycusis in a similar way as NIHL is affected by the content of melanin in the stria vascularis [9], and this may

[9] Presbycusis (or presbyacusis) means hearing deficits due to aging.

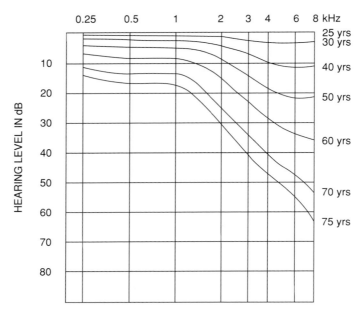

Fig. 3.10 Average hearing threshold for different age groups of men. Combined results from eight studies based on a total of 7617 ears. (Adapted from Spoor 1967[214].)

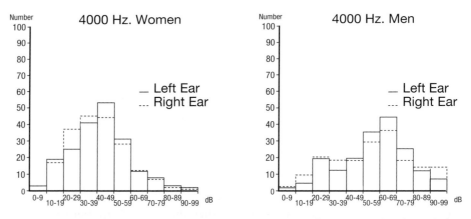

Fig. 3.11A Variation in hearing threshold at 4,000 Hz in a cross-sectional population study of non-selected individuals aged 70 years. (Data from Møller 1981 [160].)

confirm the role of melanin as a free radical scavenger. However, these morphological changes in the cochlea cannot explain all aspects of presbycusis. In some individuals, the loss in the ability to understand speech is greater than what is expected from their pure tone threshold shift, which mainly reflects impairment of the function of outer hair cells. Age-related hearing impairment is therefore

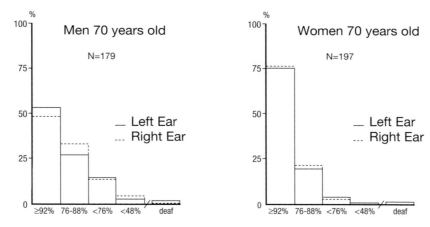

Fig. 3.11B Individual variation in speech discrimination in the same population as in Fig. 3.11A[160].

not restricted to the loss of sensitivity of the ear caused by loss of outer hair cells, but changes in the function of the nervous system may also contribute.

The difference in the age-related hearing loss between male and female has often been attributed to the fact that men are often more exposed to loud noise than women but hormonal differences may also contribute to the observed difference between presbycusis in men and women.

It is not surprising that age-related hearing loss may be linked to genetic factors [61], but this alone cannot explain the enormous difference in the hearing loss that individuals acquire with age. While animal studies confirm that genetic factors are an important factor in age-related hearing loss such studies also reveal that even inbred animals (such as certain strains of laboratory mice) that are assumed to have no genetic variation acquire different degrees of age-related hearing loss when reared under identical conditions in the laboratory [238]. Many other factors are undoubtedly involved. Different expression of the same gene in different mice (epigenetics) is one such factor that has the potential to create differences in genetically identical mice (see Chapter 1).

Another factor that can affect the development of age-related hearing loss is prior exposure to sound. Recent animal studies showed [238] that animals that are reared in an environment with sound ("augmented acoustic environment") have less age-related hearing loss than animals that are reared in a silent environment [226, 237]. The reason for that is unknown, but it does indicate that the process of age-related hearing loss is complex.

Ménière's disease

Ménière's disease [62, 172, 233, 241] is a progressive disorder that affects both the auditory and the vestibular systems. It is defined as a triad of symptoms

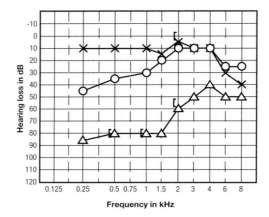

Fig. 3.12 Typical audiograms from a person with Ménière's disease. Triangles: hearing loss during an attack, open circles: hearing loss between attacks. Crosses show hearing loss in the unaffected (left) ear. (Data from Møller MB 1994[162].)

consisting of episodic vertigo, fluctuating hearing loss and tinnitus. The vestibular aspects of the disease are discussed in Chapter 6 and the auditory aspects are discussed in this chapter.

The hearing loss during attacks of Ménière's disease is greatest for low frequencies (Fig. 3.12), and tinnitus occurs at the same time. In the beginning of the disease, hearing returns to normal or near normal thresholds between attacks, and tinnitus is absent, but the hearing loss after attacks increases over time, and the frequency range of the hearing loss widens to include higher frequencies (Fig. 3.12).

The signs of Ménière's disease are supposed to be caused by an imbalance of the fluid system in the inner ear, which is shared by the auditory and the vestibular system. More specifically, it has been suggested that increased volume in the endolymphatic space causes the disease [191], but the exact pathophysiology of the disorder has eluded researchers and clinicians, and it is unknown how these abnormalities in pressure (or rather in volume) are created, and their effect on the sensory cells is not completely understood.

Many different treatments are in use to alleviate the symptoms of Ménière's disease including section of the vestibular nerve [69, 204], decompression of the endolymphatic sac [179, 199], destruction of vestibular sensory cells using ototoxic antibiotics (local application of gentamycin [205]), diuretics, diet restrictions, etc. More recent treatments use application of air puffs to the middle ear cavity [42] thereby exposing the inner ear fluid system to varying pressure. The success of that treatment indicates that the symptoms may be caused by expression of neural plasticity, thus involvement of the CNS.

Some forms of treatment aim at correcting the assumed imbalance of fluid systems in the inner ear. The relative inefficiency of such treatments indicates that the symptoms may have other causes. The relative high success rate of treatment with placebos supports the hypothesis that the anatomical location of the physiological abnormalities may be the central nervous system. There are also indications that the sympathetic nervous system may be involved in generating the symptoms and signs of Ménière's disease [172, 233].

Somatosensory system

Somatosensory senses include light touch, vibration and temperature (heat and cold are regarded as noxious stimuli and discussed in Chapter 4, p. 149). Disorders of the somatosensory system are less profound than disorders of hearing, and deficits of touch, vibration or temperature can progress further without the individual noticing any deficits as compared to those related to hearing. Much less is known about deficits of the somatosensory system than of the auditory system. Reduced sensibility in the hand and fingers affects dexterity because of the importance of somatosensory feedback for proper use of the hand and fingers. Age-related changes include changes in the function of receptors and changes in the somatosensory nervous system [70]. The somatosensory system also includes proprioception, which is involved in motor control (discussed in Chapter 5, p. 256).

The somatosensory system provides important modulation of other functions such as pain. Loss of somatosensory input can therefore cause pain (see p. 124). Loss of sensibility in the trigeminal system (CN V) can cause injuries to the cornea and biting of the lips. Loss of somatosensory function in the mouth and throat (CN IX) can cause swallowing problems and result in choking.

Lack of, or reduction of, somatosensory input can cause many different symptoms from the CNS through expression of neural plasticity such as tingling and dysesthesia.

Somatosensory input from different parts of the body is integrated to form a general picture of our body. For example, probing of a location of the body by one's finger not only provides information through tactile stimulation of receptors in the finger, but the concomitant stimulation of receptors in the skin at the location being probed contribute to the sensation. That is normally not obvious but it can become apparent when a part of the body is rendered without tactile sensation by local anesthesia. For example, probing one's face that has been numbed by a nerve block by a dentist with one's finger, provides a different impression of the size of parts of the face than it does without the effect of the local anesthesia (or comparison with the unaffected side of the face).

Other sensory organs

Disorders of visual receptors and the visual nervous system are few. Disorders of the olfactory and gustatory systems have attracted little attention. Age-related changes occur particularly in olfaction.

3.3   Disorders of the sensory nervous system

Disorders of the central sensory nervous system can be caused by trauma, strokes, tumors and inflammation. Side effects to drug therapies often include symptoms from sensory systems including dysesthesia, hyperacusis and balance disturbances. The symptoms and signs of disorders of central sensory nervous structures include deficits and altered processing of sensory information.

Some of the disorders of sensory nervous systems are caused by trauma and other insults, but many disorders are caused by expression of neural plasticity. We have already indicated how deficits of sensory receptors can affect the function of CNS structures through the expression of neural plasticity. Also trauma and other insults to the nervous system are normally accompanied by expression of neural plasticity, some of which may be compensatory for deficits, while other plastic changes may cause symptoms and signs of disease such as phantom sensations (including pain, see Chapter 4).

Many of the disorders of the somatosensory nervous system are caused by spinal cord injuries (SCI). Such injuries are morphological by nature and dominated by the symptoms from the motor system (see Chapter 5). While injury to sensory systems can affect motor systems, the sensory components of SCI are mainly neuropathic pain (Chapter 4), but also other phantom sensations occur often in SCI. Other disorders of the central somatosensory nervous system may cause phantom sensations, which are closely related to expression of neural plasticity.

Strokes can cause various forms of sensory deficits. Age-related changes in the nervous system may be regarded as an insult to nerves and the CNS but can also be regarded as a normal process similar to the postnatal development of the nervous system. Age-related changes in sensory nervous systems have complex symptoms and some few objective signs.

Morphological changes in the CNS such as from injuries and other insults to nervous structures, including sensory nerves, cause abnormal processing of sensory input. Morphological changes are almost always accompanied by functional re-organization of CNS structures through expression of neural plasticity and these changes may produce more prominent symptoms than the primary injuries.

3.3.1   Disorders of sensory nerves

Some disorders of cranial sensory nerves have prominent symptoms from the respective sensory systems. (Disorders of cranial nerves are discussed in detail in Chapter 6.) Disorders of the auditory nerve can be caused by tumors (such as vestibular schwannoma) and close contact with one or more blood vessels in the subarachnoidal space [161]. Inflammatory and other processes affect the auditory nerve in a similar way as it affects other nerves resulting in various forms of neuropathies. Auditory nerve aplasia occurs as a congenital malformation [37, 136].

> Disorders of the auditory nerve and central nervous system are known as retrocochlear disorders. More recently, the term auditory neuropathy has come into use to describe disorders of the auditory nerve [10, 215], thus adapting the terminology commonly used by neurologists for disorders of nerves.

Iatrogenic[10] causes of hearing loss from surgical manipulations when operating in the cerebello-pontine angle were common before the introduction of microneurosurgery and intraoperative neurophysiologic monitoring [150] (Fig. 3.13).

Pathologies of the auditory nerve generally cause more complex forms of hearing loss than pathologies that affect the conductive apparatus or the cochlea, and the impairment of speech discrimination from auditory nerve disorder is greater than that caused by the same degree of threshold shift from pathologies of the cochlea (or the conductive apparatus).

A particular type of hearing loss, known as sudden hearing loss, may be caused by pathology of the auditory nerve. Sudden hearing loss is a form of sensorineural hearing loss that occurs with rapid onset and without any noticed cause. It is rarely total, and it has been defined (empirically) as hearing loss of 30 dB or more at least three contiguous frequencies [234]. Hearing loss that occurs progressively over a relatively short time probably has a similar etiology [225]. The incidence of sudden hearing loss in the USA is 1.5/100 000. Other investigators have estimated that 4,000 cases of such hearing loss occur annually in the USA [135].

The cause of sudden hearing loss is unknown. Infectious diseases (bacterial or viral), circulatory, immunologic, toxic and traumatic injures have been suggested as causes. Auto-immune disease, Ménière's disease, trauma, vestibular schwannoma, multiple sclerosis, perilymphatic fistula, and vascular disorders have also been suggested as causes of sudden hearing loss [54], as has microvascular

---

[10] Iatrogenic: Unfavorable response to treatment such as injuries through surgical operations.

A

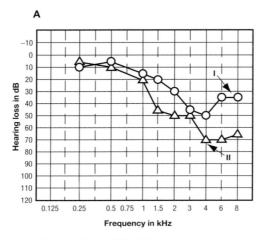

I: Pre-op   Discr.=80%   AS
II: 7 days post-op   Discr.=30%   AS

B

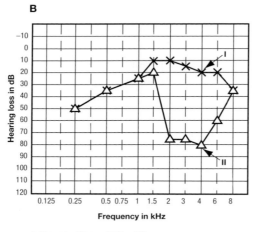

I: Pre-op   Discr.=96%   AS
II: 5 days post-op   Discr.=0%   AS

Fig. 3.13 Illustration of the effect on the tone threshold and speech discrimination from iatrogenic injury to the auditory nerve. A: Large changes in speech discrimination with relatively small changes in the pure tone audiogram. I: Preoperative audiogram, II: Audiogram obtained 7 days after an operation in the cerebello-pontine angle where the eighth cranial nerve was manipulated. The speech discrimination decreased from 80% to 30% after the operation. B: Similar data as in A, obtained before (I) and 5 days after (II) and after an operation in the cerebello-pontine angle where the eighth cranial nerve was manipulated. The speech discrimination decreased from 96% before the operation to 0% after the operation.

compression of the root of the auditory nerve [180, 229]. Two thirds of individuals with sudden hearing loss recover within days, and most recover within 2 weeks without treatment. The prognosis is worse for the most severe cases and those with downward-sloping audiograms and vertigo in addition to the hearing loss [135].

Many treatments that often include steroids, acyclovir and hyperbaric oxygen therapy have been tried without any noticeable effect on the natural history of the disease [116]. A recent study [94] using antioxidant (Vitamin E; d–tocopherol acetate, 400 mg twice daily) in addition to other treatments showed some benefit (79% recovered compared with 45% in the group who did not get Vitamin E). The fact that antioxidants seem to improve recovery from sudden hearing loss indicates that oxidative processes may be involved.

Age-related changes in sensory nerves can cause different kinds of symptoms and signs, either alone or by the concomitant change in central structures through expression of neural plasticity. For example, the variation of diameters of auditory nerve fibers increases with age [213], and this can be expected to impair the temporal coherence of nerve impulses that arrive at the cochlear nucleus. Since the time pattern of the neural code of speech sounds is important for speech intelligibility, these changes in the auditory nerve may contribute to the decrease in the ability to understand speech, especially in a noisy environment or when more than one person is talking at the same time.

Disorders of somatosensory nerves may cause different forms of paresthesia, either transient, such as may occur from compression of the sciatic nerve when sitting on a hard surface, or more persistent, as may occur from nerve entrapment, such as in carpal tunnel syndrome (see Chapter 4, p. 189). Again, it must be pointed out that the symptoms of such injuries and insults to nerves are often accompanied (and even dominated) by symptoms that are caused by changes in the function of CNS structures through expression of neural plasticity.

3.3.2   Trauma and other insults to CNS structures

Traumatic head injuries can cause vestibular symptoms and symptoms from different sensory systems such as oversensitivity to light and hyperacusis, depending on which CNS regions are affected. Head injuries often result in pain (see Chapter 4).

Neonatal jaundice that is associated with high levels of unconjugated bilirubin causes sensorineural hearing loss specifically because of lesions of auditory brainstem nuclei (the cochlear nucleus). Studies in humans indicate that lesions in the basal ganglia may also occur [134].

> Hyperbilirubinemia occurs because of immaturity of a hepatic enzyme, uridine diphosphate glucuronosyl transferase, which converts unconjugated bilirubin to conjugated bilirubin [11]. The neurotoxic effect may be

caused by altered expression of calcium binding proteins [210]. Studies of the mechanisms of neural damage from hyperbilirubinemia have been done mainly in the Gunn rat [210], which is a mutant Wistar rat that has a genetic deficiency in the glucuronyl transferase enzyme.

The symptoms of lesions of central structures of the sensory nervous system such as the cerebral cortex are less distinct than those that are caused by lesions to peripheral structures. For example, the deficits from tumors or strokes that affect the auditory cortex are subtle and speech discrimination is not affected unless in tests using low-redundancy speech [14, 110]. Other forms of lesions such as strokes and space-occupying lesions may also affect the auditory area in the temporal lobe, and cause tinnitus. Reports of meningiomas causing deafness are usually related to cerebello-pontine tumors with direct involvement of the vestibulo-cochlear nerve [174]. Brainstem tumors that affect nuclei in the ascending sensory pathways usually affect other systems to a degree that makes symptoms from sensory systems minor.

3.3.3   *Phantom sensations*

Phantom sensations are defined as sensations that are not elicited by physical stimuli reaching sensory receptors. Phantom sensations [92] occur in all senses. There are two kinds of phantom sensations, one type involves meaningless sensory perception and the other, also known as hallucinations, involves meaningful sensory perceptions such as music or speech [22]. Meaningless sensory sensations that occur without any physical input to the sensory organs [92] are most common in the auditory system (tinnitus [158]) and the somatosensory system (tingling etc.). Visual phantom eye sensations are rare and can consist of different forms of light sensations (phosphens and scotoma).

The phantom limb syndrome, and tinnitus in individuals with a severed auditory nerve, are clear examples of sensations that are not evoked by physical stimulation of sensory organs but rather by changes in the function of CNS structures, often caused by expression of neural plasticity. Deprivation of sensory input (such as occurs in limb amputations or severance of nerves such as the auditory nerve) is a strong promoter of neural plasticity. Likewise, other causes of deprivation of input to CNS structures can cause expression of neural plasticity. For example, hearing loss may cause subjective tinnitus.

Several forms of paresthesia also belong to this category of pathologies. Central neuropathic pain is another example of sensations that are not caused by any known physical stimulation of peripheral structures, and it can therefore be regarded as a phantom sensation (pain is discussed in detail in Chapter 4). Vertigo and dizziness are other examples of sensations that are evoked by stimulation of receptors that normally do not mediate conscious sensations (see Chapter 6). Scotoma is a phantom visual sensation that typically occurs in conjunction with lesions in central parts of the visual nervous system.

Phantom sensations are often accompanied by changes in the perception of physical sensory stimuli that activate sensory receptors in a normal way, indicating changes in the way that ordinary sensory stimuli are processed. These changes in function of the sensory nervous system vary between sensory systems and between different individuals, but they generally involve exaggerated responses to sensory stimuli (such as hyperacusis and hypersensitivity) or cross-modal interaction such as allodynia (pain from normally innocuous stimulation) (see Chapter 4).

Sensory hallucinations (meaningful sensations such as music, speech and pictures) often occur in connection with psychiatric disorders such as schizophrenia as well as lesions of various kinds to the brain [22]. Auditory hallucinations are rare but may occur in conjunction with psychiatric disorders [22], and can be treated successfully by psychoactive drugs [85]. Auditory hallucinations may also occur in conjunction with lesions of the temporal lobe [22].

Tinnitus

The prevalence and the consequences of tinnitus may qualify it as a separate disease of the auditory system. There are three types of tinnitus [158], objective tinnitus, subjective tinnitus and auditory hallucinations. Objective tinnitus is caused by sounds that are generated in the body and sensed by the receptors in the cochlea. Objective tinnitus can often be heard by an observer while subjective tinnitus can only be heard by the person in question. Subjective tinnitus consists of meaningless sounds. Together with neuropathic pain, subjective tinnitus is one of the most frequent and most debilitating forms of phantom sensations.

Objective tinnitus

Objective tinnitus [192] is often caused by blood flow in arteries that are close to the cochlea. Blood flow generates sound when it is turbulent such as may occur when blood flows through narrow passages. The sound that is generated by the blood flow may be transmitted to the cochlea via bone conduction. Tinnitus that is caused by blood flow is pulsatile in nature and is synchronous with the heartbeat, which makes it easy to identify. Such tinnitus may be a sign of an underlying disorder that requires medical attention. Temporomandibular joint (TMJ) disorders, spontaneous contractions of the middle ear muscles, or palatal myoclonus are examples of phenomena that may generate other kinds of sounds that can be perceived by the person in question and appear as clicking sounds

[6, 192]. The intensity of objective tinnitus is usually low and when the patient gets to know what causes the tinnitus it can often be ignored by the patient.

Subjective tinnitus

Subjective tinnitus is a common disorder that can have many forms and many causes. The intensity and the nature of the sounds that individuals with tinnitus perceive varies widely, from being barely noticeable in a quiet environment to being so loud that it disturbs work and sleep [154, 158]. In some individuals, the tinnitus is not affected much by external factors, whereas in other individuals the intensity and character of the tinnitus depends on factors such as for example stress and diet. Some forms of severe tinnitus are accompanied by changes in the processing of sounds (hypersensitivity, hyperacusis or distortion of sounds and impaired speech discrimination) [149, 157]. In some individuals, tinnitus is associated with affective disorders such as phonophobia and depression (see pp. 83, 125) [151, 156].

Various forms of injuries to the cochlea have been associated with tinnitus. For example, Ménière's disease, exposure to loud noise, or administration of ototoxic drugs that cause morphological changes in the sensory epithelium in the cochlea are disorders that are associated with hearing loss in addition to tinnitus. Tinnitus often occurs together with high frequency hearing loss. While individuals with tinnitus with few exceptions have hearing loss, individuals with hearing loss rarely have tinnitus. The hearing loss that occurs together with tinnitus may not be caused by the same morphological changes in the cochlea as those causing the tinnitus, and the anatomical location of the anomalies that cause the tinnitus may not be the same as that of the hearing loss.

Subjective tinnitus may occur after exposure to loud sounds, especially impulsive or high frequency sounds. Often this kind of tinnitus abates gradually after the end of the exposure, over minutes, hours or days depending on the intensity and the duration of the exposure but in some cases the tinnitus may last for a lifetime. There is a considerable individual variation in getting tinnitus from sound exposure.

Pharmacological agents such as aspirin (acetylsalicylate), and aminoglycoside antibiotics can cause tinnitus in some individuals if given in sufficiently large dosages [52, 56, 243]. Other drugs such as loop diuretics (furosemide, ethacrynic acid), quinine, indomethacin, cisplatin, and other cytostatica used in cancer treatment can also cause tinnitus in addition to hearing loss [195, 206]. Carbamazepine, tetracycline, antipsychotic drugs, lithium, tricyclic antidepressants, monoamine oxidase inhibitors, antihistamines, beta-adrenergic receptor blockers, local anesthetics, and steroids (to name only a few) can also induce tinnitus, but rarely hearing loss. Caffeine and alcohol can also cause tinnitus. Tinnitus caused by pharmacological agents usually disappears after cessation of administration of the agent that caused the tinnitus but, in some cases, the tinnitus becomes permanent. This is in particular the case for tinnitus caused by cytostatica and aminoglycoside antibiotics [206].

Some specific disorders are associated with tinnitus (and abnormal processing of sound). For example, individuals with Williams-Beuren (WBS) syndrome, (infantile hypocalcemia), have a high incidence of hyperacusis [20, 106]. Tinnitus is usually the first symptom of vestibular schwannoma (acoustic tumors) but individuals with tinnitus rarely have vestibular schwannoma.

> Subjective tinnitus is a symptom that cannot be evaluated through the use of tests, and only the patient's own description can be used to characterize the strength and character of the tinnitus from which an individual suffers. Tests such as loudness matching and masking tend to produce very low estimates of loudness of tinnitus, even when the tinnitus causes severe annoyance to the patient [72, 228].
>
> In one study [228] 75% of the patients with tinnitus on one side (one ear) matched the loudness of their tinnitus to a (physical) sound that was presented to the other ear at only 10-dB sensation level (SL)[11] or less. Approximately half of the patients matched their tinnitus to a sound that was only 5-dB SL. These values are low compared to the degree of annoyance from the tinnitus that was reported by the patients. Such estimates can therefore not be used to obtain estimates of the severity of tinnitus [57, 185].

The search for physiological verifiable abnormalities in the auditory nervous system in individuals with subjective tinnitus has been disappointing. Short latency auditory evoked potentials do not show the degree of abnormalities that could be expected when studied in individuals with severe tinnitus [147]. Middle latency responses (MLR) obtained in individuals with severe tinnitus (defined as "problem tinnitus" [66] had abnormally large amplitude in as many as 56% of the individuals who were tested. Similar abnormalities, but smaller, were found in elderly individuals [66] and in animals after noise exposure [219, 221].

Classification of the severity of subjective tinnitus must therefore be based solely on the patients' own estimates of the severity of the tinnitus. One classification [185] defines three degrees of severity, "slight," "moderate," or "severe," where "slight" describes intermittent tinnitus that only bothers the patient in a quiet environment; "moderate" describes tinnitus that is constant and more intense, disturbs sleep and bothering the patient when trying to concentrate. The classification "severe" is reserved for tinnitus that is a constant annoyance,

---

[11] Sensation level (SL): Sound level (in dB) above an individual person's threshold of hearing.

interferes greatly with the ability to concentrate and inhibits sleep. Individuals with tinnitus that is classified as "severe" are often incapacitated, and some patients with that degree of tinnitus resign from work as disabled persons. This form of tinnitus may cause a patient to commit suicide. The affective response to severe tinnitus differs among individuals and the condition is more severe if the tinnitus is regarded to be inescapable.

Tinnitus has many similarities to pain, and in particular, central neuropathic pain [151, 155]. There may also be similarities with pain regarding the way individuals are coping with tinnitus. Studies have found that pain that is regarded inescapable has a worse emotional impact that pain that is escapable and that these two forms of pain are represented by different hypothalamic-midbrain circuits [102, 130] (see p. 174). That tinnitus has a worse impact on a person than exposure to noise may have a similar reason, namely tinnitus being regarded as inescapable. We will show later that there are other similarities between severe tinnitus and central neuropathic pain (see p. 203).

Paresthesia of the somatosensory system

The term paresthesia is commonly used to describe abnormal sensations from the somatosensory system. The symptoms may be tingling, feeling of "pins and needles," burning, etc., often occurring in the limbs, particularly in the lower limbs in the presence of diseases that affect peripheral nerves such as diabetes. Paresthesia also occurs frequently in elderly individuals without any other known diseases (except perhaps subclinical forms of polyneuropathy). Pathologies of the CNS can also cause paresthesia, and paresthesia often occurs together with pain and itch.

Dysesthesia, hyperesthesia, neuropathic pain and pruritus[12] are examples of altered processing of information that are often symptoms of disorders of the somatosensory nervous system.

Phantom limb syndrome

The phantom limb syndrome is a form of dysesthesia that consists of sensations including tingling and pain, that are referred to specific anatomical locations on an amputated limb [8, 55, 140]. The neural activity that causes the phantom limb sensations is obviously not evoked by physical stimulation at the locations from which the sensations are felt, but instead the neural activity that causes these sensations is generated in the central nervous system. This abnormal activity can be a result of reorganization of the nervous system caused by expression of neural plasticity elicited by the absence of normal sensory input

---

[12] Pruritus: Itching.

from the periphery. The existence of the phantom limb syndrome is a clear sign that neural circuits in the CNS can produce sensations that are referred to specific anatomical locations on the body without any physical stimulus being applied to that location.

3.4   Pathophysiology of disorders of sensory systems

Research in recent years has brought insight into the pathophysiology of disorders of sensory receptors, especially those of the ear. The increased understanding of how expression of neural plasticity can alter the function of the nervous system has had an impact on understanding of disorders of sensory systems, again most pronounced for the auditory system. It has also become apparent that the division of sensory systems in the conductive apparatus, sensory receptor, nerves and the central sensory nervous system is not beneficial regarding understanding of pathophysiology of disorders of the sensory system. Instead it should be taken into account that all these components act as an integrated system with regard to the pathophysiology of disorders of sensory systems. This means that, for example, disorders of the conductive apparatus and sensory receptors are not only affecting the function of these components, but also the function of the nervous system. In fact, disorders of the nervous system may alter the function of sensory receptors by efferent connections as well. We will, however, in the following section first discuss the pathophysiology of the specific components of sensory systems, then later, discuss the integrated effect at the end of the section.

3.4.1   Disorders of sensory cells

The pathophysiology of sensory cells of the cochlea has been studied to a greater extent than that of any other sensory cells. Cochlear hair cells are more complex than most other sensory cells, and are subjected to insults from overexposure, and from administration of drugs such as certain antibiotics and diuretics (ototoxic drugs). Cochlear hair cells are also subjected to age-related deterioration, causing significant hearing deficits – the most common of the known age-related sensory deficits. In general, outer hair cells are more susceptible to injury than inner hair cells. Recalling that outer hair cells do not participate in coding of sounds in the auditory nerve but rather play a mechanical role (see p. 99), thus, pathologies of outer hair cells affect the mechanical function of the cochlea rather than directly affecting neural transduction in the cochlea. This means that these types of insults mainly impair the "cochlear amplifier," causing reduced sensitivity, reduced frequency selectivity and impairment of amplitude compression. The reason that outer hair cells are much more susceptible to insults such as from ototoxic antibiotics, aging and noise exposure than the inner hair cells, has been explained by the differences in metabolism between outer hair cells and inner hair cells [56, 88]. It is also characteristic that the cells that are located in the basal (high frequency) part of the cochlea are the most sensitive to injuries. The mechanisms of hair cell damage is best known for injuries caused by ototoxic drugs such as aminoglycoside antibiotics.

Ototoxic antibiotics

Oxidative stress is assumed to play an important role in the ototoxic effect of substance such as aminoglycoside antibiotics and studies have shown that aminoglycoside antibiotics stimulate free radical formation [198, 242]. Other studies in animals have shown that administration of free radical scavengers can reduce the hearing loss that ototoxic antibiotic causes [39, 56, 177, 243], supporting the hypothesis that oxygen free radicals are involved in the process of causing hearing loss by ototoxic antibiotics. In vitro experiments have shown evidence that reactive oxygen species cause the damage from administration of aminoglycoside antibiotics [88]. The effect of ototoxic antibiotics is different in different strains of mice, and related to the presence of Ahl1Ahl2 genes [242].

> The molecular mechanisms for the ototoxic action of ototoxic antibiotics are beginning to be better understood [243]. It is believed that they involve a block of calcium channels [175, 242] and it has been proposed that the ototoxic action depends on the ability of aminoglycosides to form chelates with iron [181]. The redox-active aminoglycoside-iron complex activates oxygen and reduces it to a superoxide radical [243]. The electron donor in this process is assumed to be a polyunsaturated fatty acid. These discoveries have opened up the possibility to reduce the ototoxic effect by iron chelation therapy [38, 207].

It has been suggested that melanin plays a role in acquiring hair cell loss from ototoxic antibiotics, showing that the degree of skin pigmentation plays a role in acquiring hair cell loss from ototoxic antibiotics, and thus suggesting an effect of melanin on the status of antioxidants in the cochlea [242]. (Ototoxic aminoglycosides are also affecting the vestibular system, and the same substances that are ototoxic are often nephrotoxic.)

Noise induced hearing loss

The pathophysiology of hearing loss from overstimulation (NIHL), is complex [187] and poorly understood. It seems to consist of at least two components: one is morphological change to hair cells in the cochlea, and the other component is (morphological or functional) change in the nervous system. Studies in animals show that the degree of NIHL is to some extent correlated with the degree of morphological damage to the sensory cells [47], but the cause of the damage to hair cells from noise exposure is poorly understood. Metabolic factors such as metabolic overload are likely to contribute to the structural damage to hair cells from exposure to loud sounds. Evidence has been presented that indicates that the pigmentation (melanin of the stria vascularis) plays a role in NIHL [9], which would point to the involvement of oxidative processes in noise induced damage to hair cells.

Evidence that damage to hair cells causes changes in central nervous system structures has emerged from studies that have shown morphological changes occur in the cochlear nucleus in connection with NIHL [164, 165]. Other studies have shown evidence that functional changes occur in parts of the CNS in connection with NIHL [64, 65, 154, 235].

The different measures of the degree of noise-induced damage that have been used in animal experiments, namely counts of damaged hair cells [82], and measurements of the elevation of the threshold of hearing [125], are correlated but do not give identical results [126].

The threshold elevation (hearing loss) caused by similar noise exposure in humans varies widely [24] (Fig. 3.9). This difference in susceptibility to noise exposure is another sign of the complexity of NIHL. Genetic factors undoubtedly affect the amount of NIHL that an individual person may acquire after exposure to noise but other factors are also affecting NIHL. Studies in animals have shown that the variability in NIHL is less in the same strain of animals [245] than in humans but still considerable (Fig. 3.14A). This is probably because laboratory animals have less genetic variation. The fact that exposure conditions are better controlled in laboratory studies than in the field for humans (workplace) also contribute to the smaller individual variations in NIHL in laboratory tests. When the genetic variation is further decreased such as in heavily inbred animals the variability in NIHL decreases further (Fig. 3.14B), but even such genetically identical animals suffer different degrees of NIHL when exposed to the same sounds under controlled laboratory conditions.

Although these studies show clearly that the genetic makeup is important there seem to be other reasons for the variability in NIHL. One such factor may be imprinting, which can silence or activate a specific gene (see Chapter 1). This would mean that NIHL is not only affected by the genetic makeup of an animal (or human) but also affected by epigenetics. The implication of these findings is that the effect of noise exposure on hearing (NIHL) can only be predicted to a certain degree even in genetically identical animals under ideal (laboratory) conditions. Perhaps there are also purely stochastic components involved in the cause of biological events such as NIHL.

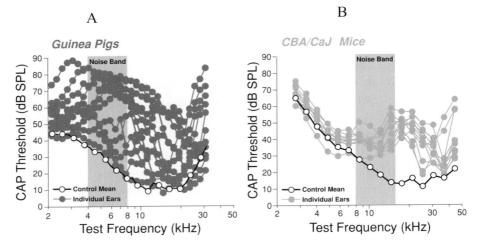

Fig. 3.14 NIHL in animals of various degrees of genetic variations. A: Data obtained in male guinea pigs (400–500 g); the exposure was a 2–4 kHz octave band of noise at 109 dB SPL for 4 hrs with a 1-week survival. The mean peak PTS was 35.1 dB at 7.6 kHz (SD of 21.33 dB)[131]. B: Inbred mice, males (23–29 g) exposed to octave band noise (8–16 kHz) at 100 dB for 2 hrs with a 1-week survival. The mean peak PTS was 38 dB at 17.5 kHz (SD of 4.06 dB) [245]. (Data, courtesy, Charles Liberman.)

Further evidence of genetic effect on the cause of NIHL comes from a study of the effect of lifetime noise exposure in two strains of rats, the Sprague Dawley strain, and the Wistar, Okamoto strain. The Sprague Dawley rats had normal development of blood pressure with age (normotensive) while the Wistar rats were spontaneously hypertensive rats [17]. Rats that were genetically disposed for hypertension (spontaneous hypertensive rats) acquired a greater degree of NIHL than normotensive rats [19] under the same circumstances. After 3 months of exposure to 105 dB SPL noise,[13] young (3 months) normotensive rats had acquired a mean hearing loss at 6 and 12 kHz of 38.5 dB, while spontaneous hypertensive rats had an average hearing loss of 56 dB under the same conditions. The normotensive rats had less loss of hair cells than spontaneously hypertensive rats [19]. Normotensive young rats exposed to noise for 1 month had no detectable morphological changes in their cochleae, while spontaneous hypertensive rats had considerable losses of hair cells under the same conditions. This is a further indication of the complexity of NIHL. The fact that renal hypertension (induced by ligating a renal artery) did not make (normotensive) rats more susceptible to NIHL [18] indicates that the greater NIHL in spontaneous hypertensive rats is

---

[13] The noise consisted of a 1640 Hz wide band of noise, sweeping from a center frequency of 3 kHz to 30 kHz every 2 seconds, and with a duty-cycle of 1 second on and 1 second off, at 100 dB Leq for 10 hours daily.

caused by genetic differences between these two strains of rats rather than the hypertension as such. In these studies, spontaneous hypertensive rats that were not exposed to noise, also had slightly larger hearing loss with age than normotensive rats.

That the mechanism of NIHL is complex is evidenced by studies in animals that have shown that the amount of acquired NIHL depends on previous exposure to sounds. The acquired NIHL from a certain noise exposure can be reduced by exposing the ear to sounds before exposure to the noise that causes NIHL. The intensity of the sounds used for such pre-exposure is lower than that which causes NIHL. This "toughening" of the ear with regard to acquiring NIHL was first demonstrated in studies in cats by Miller [142], and later many studies have confirmed the existence of this peculiar effect [30, 244]. The mechanisms of such toughening are poorly understood, but it may involve the CNS. The increased resistance to NIHL may be a result of expression of neural plasticity involving descending auditory pathways that terminate on outer hair cells.

Age-related hearing loss

Age-related changes of sensitivity occur in most sensory systems, perhaps most prominently in the auditory system. Are age-related changes normal, or pathological? Some will claim that there are normal age-related changes and if such changes occur earlier in life than "normal," then the changes are regarded as being pathological. There may be a gray area where these changes in function can be affected in one direction or the other.

Studies of the pathophysiology of age-related hearing loss have mainly focused on the cochlea, where loss of hair cells have been assumed to be the cause of age-related hearing loss [96]. The typical changes in the cochlea consist of loss of outer hair cells, most prominent in the basal parts of the cochlea. These morphological changes have been associated with age-related hearing threshold elevations. However, the causes of these changes in the hair cells are not known in detail but it is assumed that oxidative stress is involved. Some of the sensory deficits may be caused by changes in the auditory nerve [213] (p. 111), and some of the age-related changes may be caused by morphological changes in the CNS (see p. 119). Animal experiments have shown that age-related hearing loss is affected by sound exposure [226], and that indicates a more complex cause of age-related hearing loss. Genetic factors are also involved in age-related hearing loss [61].

3.4.2   Disorders related to sensory nerves and the CNS

The pathophysiology of most disorders of central sensory nervous structures is poorly understood. The symptoms of inflammation (of sensory nerves), strokes or tumors are not only related to the morphological changes but also to a great extent related to functional changes that occur from expression of neural plasticity. Many forms of changes in the function of the central sensory nervous systems are induced by disorders of peripheral structures through expression of neural plasticity. Such changes can be beneficial in that they alter function to compensate for deficits, but they can also cause symptoms and signs of disease.

Recent studies have broadened the search for causes of age-related sensory deficits to include the nervous system. Several studies have shown indications that some of the age-related deficits may originate in the CNS. It is known that the auditory nerve undergoes age-related changes that may explain some of the decrease in speech discrimination that typically occurs with age (see p. 111) but also other changes occur in the nervous system with age. For example, animal experiments have shown age-related changes in the somatosensory cortex [70]. Whether age-related changes in the function of the nervous system are caused by the changes in the receptors (through expression of neural plasticity caused by decreased input), or whether the changes in the CNS are parallel age-related changes, is not well understood. Change in GABAergic inhibition may explain some change in auditory function, and perhaps also changes that occur in other sensory systems with advancing age.

Some of the first studies that showed that the GABA systems change systematically with age were those of Caspary (1990) [31]. Caspary and coworkers found evidence of age-related decrease in the production of GABA in the IC in experiments in rats [31–33]. Other investigators have shown that age-related changes occur in the GABA systems such as the vestibular system [67]. Recent studies have indicated that reduced release of GABA can result in increased sensitivity of GABA$_A$ receptors and a proliferation of GABA receptor sites.

On the basis of studies of GABA$_A$ receptors in the IC in rats, it has been hypothesized that the age-related changes in the composition of the GABA$_A$ receptor units is a result of a compensatory change in response to lowered presynaptic GABA release [33]. It has been found that the sensitivity of GABA$_A$ receptors increases with age, and GABA$_A$ receptor sites proliferate. The increased sensitivity to benzodiazepines with age may be a form of compensatory change of the sensitivity of GABA$_A$ receptors that occurs as expression of neural plasticity in response to decreased production of GABA. Indications of abnormally strong GABAergic tone during aging may not contradict the findings of reduced production of GABA with age [31].

Other evidence that GABA is involved in compensation for reduced sensory input comes from animal experiments on vestibular injuries [29, 67]. A study using hemilabyrinthectomy showed that the GABAergic tone in old (24 month) rats, which had significant behavioral deficits after hemilabyrinthectomy, was elevated [67], and the density of benzodiazepine receptors in the lateral vestibular nuclei was higher than normal. Higher mRNA levels for glutamic acid decarboxylase (GAD) were found in the cerebral cortex and the medial vestibular nucleus. In young (3 month) rats, which had compensated for their vestibular loss, the benzodiazepine receptor density was normal in the vestibular nuclei.

Other studies have indicated that the increased GABAergic tone that some investigators have reported to occur with age, promotes neurodegeneration [170]. This would be the opposite of what occurs with other transmitter substance systems such as dopamine, and cholinergic systems, which decrease with age.

A somewhat different hypothesis about the role of GABA in age-related changes states that declining mitochondrial ATP synthesis promotes GABA synthesis [133]. This process may cause several changes that are associated with age-related symptoms such as constantly hyperpolarized cells, cell death, and blockage of axonal transport.

The involvement of GABA as promoter of age-related changes has been supported by studies that show that administration of flumazenil, a benzodiazepine antagonist, can extend the lifespan of animals (rats), and decrease age-related deterioration of memory [132], indicating that a benzodiazepine antagonist can both increase lifetime, and protect against loss of cognitive abilities.

Studies have shown evidence of loss, or reduction, of inhibition, in the cerebral cortex [123] with aging, and some investigators believe that much of the age-related change of cortical function is a result of degradation of intracortical inhibition. This is supported by findings that application of the $GABA_A$ antagonist bicuculine had less effect on the properties of cells in the monkey V1 cortex of older animals, than in younger animals [123], and administration of GABA and the $GABA_A$ agonist muscimol resulted in improved visual function. In this study, many of the treated cells behaved similarly to cells in young animals [123]. The results of these studies suggest that it would make physiological sense to administrate benzodiazepines to elderly individuals to increase the sensitivity of $GABA_A$ receptors, and that such treatment may even enhance memory and cognitive functions.

3.4.3   The role of neural plasticity

We have already mentioned that impairment of the function of sensory receptors can cause changes of the function of CNS structures through expression of neural plasticity. Decreased, or otherwise altered, input to the CNS causing expression of neural plasticity may result in hypersensitivity, hyperactivity, and other changes in processing of sensory information in the CNS. Disorders of sensory nerves may alter the information that reaches the nervous system; this may also cause expression of neural plasticity resulting in symptoms and signs of disease such as abnormal processing of sensory information, phantom sensations (tinnitus and paresthesia) and re-direction of sensory information in the CNS. Some receptors provide inhibitory input to central sensory structures, and reduction in the sensitivity of such receptors can likewise cause hyperactivity in central nervous system structures. It was discussed above that overstimulation can cause injury to sensory receptor cells, such as the cochlear hair cells, resulting in elevation of the threshold of hearing. However, overstimulation can also promote expression of neural plasticity and it is possible that overstimulation, with or without injuring sensory cells, can cause changes in neural processing through expression of neural plasticity.

Reduced sensory input can affect normal childhood development of sensory systems. For example, hearing loss due to middle ear pathologies (middle ear infection) that often occur in childhood, decreases sound input to the cochlea, and this can impair language development because of decreased CNS activation. Sound input is necessary for normal childhood development of the auditory nervous system (through activation of neural plasticity) [113]. It has been documented in animal studies that absence of input to the auditory system, such as occurs in congenital deafness, can cause anatomical and functional abnormalities in the primary auditory cortex, indicating abnormal postnatal development [107]. Lack of adequate stimulation probably also interferes with other aspects of childhood development of the nervous system.

Like other forms of morphological changes to peripheral structures, age-related changes may also cause expression of neural plasticity that can act as compensation for deficits but, in addition, produce symptoms and signs of disease. For example, the beneficial effect of an "augmented acoustic environment" on the development of age-related hearing loss [226, 237] may be mediated through plastic changes in the CNS. The mechanisms of the beneficial effect of sound exposure on age-related hearing loss may be similar to that of sound exposure that can reduce NIHL ("toughening of the ear"). The extensive efferent innervation of outer hair cells [211, 231, 232] (see pp. 71, 84) may be involved in these mechanisms because this innervation makes it possible to control the function of outer hair cells by descending neural activity. This means that input from the CNS, or results of changes in the function of CNS structures, can affect events that occur at the receptor level, and possibly affect the development of injuries and deficits of sensory cells such as the outer hair cells in the cochlea.

Hyperactive disorders and phantom sensations

It has often been assumed that hyperactive disorders such as tinnitus, paresthesia, vertigo and other vestibular disorders, were caused by morphological abnormalities of either the sensory organs or their nerves. However, it is now believed that the anatomical location of the physiological abnormalities that cause such symptoms and signs is the CNS, and that these functional abnormalities are caused by expression of neural plasticity [92] [158]. Abnormalities that cause hyperactive symptoms and signs may consist of synaptic efficacy, elimination or creation of synapses, or sprouting or elimination of axons (see Chapter 2), leading to altered balance between inhibition and excitation and re-routing of sensory information to parts of the nervous system that are normally not activated by such stimulation. For example, the observed interaction between auditory and somatosensory modalities has been interpreted as a sign of re-routing of auditory information to the non-classical auditory system [158] [156] that has been demonstrated in individuals with tinnitus [148]. The non-classical ascending auditory pathway projects to the dorsal thalamus that provides a subcortical route to the amygdala [120, 158] (p. 81), and that may explain emotional symptoms such as phonophobia and depression that often accompany severe tinnitus [158] (see Chapter 2).

The anatomical location of the physiological abnormalities of sensory deficits that are caused by changes in the CNS may be difficult to identify because the symptoms are sensory in nature and therefore referred to the respective sensory organ.

Disorders of the auditory sensory nervous system where neural plasticity is involved often have more complex signs than those of other sensory systems. Neural plasticity in the auditory system has been described more extensively than in other sensory systems. In the following, we will discuss symptoms and signs that are related to expression of neural plasticity in the different sensory systems. We will first discuss hyperactive disorders such as tinnitus, the phantom limb syndrome and paresthesia; and after that we will discuss age-related changes in the CNS, and the role of the balance between inhibition and excitation. We have already discussed the role of changes in the GABA system (p. 122).

Subjective tinnitus

The pathophysiology of subjective tinnitus is poorly understood, and since there are so many forms of tinnitus, a single mechanism cannot explain the pathophysiology for all its various forms and some of these different pathologies affect different parts of the auditory system. Difficulties differentiating between tinnitus with different pathophysiology have hampered efforts to find effective treatment for tinnitus. The early concepts assuming the pathophysiology of subjective tinnitus as being caused by pathologies of the ear, had to be revised when it became evident that some forms of subjective tinnitus occurred in deaf individuals, and in individuals with a severed auditory nerve [25] [158]. These observations provided the strongest evidence for the concept that tinnitus can be caused by physiological abnormalities in the CNS. However, since tinnitus is perceived as a sound, it is intuitively referred to the ear, and the attention directed to the ear as the site of the abnormality that causes the tinnitus has prevailed, despite the fact that many studies have shown that the central nervous system is the location of the physiological abnormality of many forms of tinnitus [158]. Despite progress in understanding the pathophysiology of subjective tinnitus it is still difficult to determine the exact location in the CNS of the physiological abnormality that causes many forms of tinnitus, and it is likely to be different in different forms of tinnitus.

> Animal experiments have shown that overexposure to sound, similar to that which is known to cause tinnitus in humans, causes signs of hyperactivity in the cochlear nucleus [99] and altered temporal integration in the IC [224]. Other animal studies have shown that injury to the peripheral auditory system can cause central auditory structures (IC and cochlear nucleus) to become hyperactive [63, 64]. The observed changes in function are most likely induced by expression of neural plasticity, either as a result of the overstimulation, or, more likely, as a result of deprivation that was caused by the NIHL from the sound stimulation that was used in these experiments. Some studies indicate that the prefrontal cortex is involved [92] as the site of the abnormalities that cause tinnitus.
>
> The hypothesis that expression of neural plasticity plays an important role in many forms of tinnitus, and that tinnitus may be caused by a compensatory mechanism for loss of sensitivity that has overreached and caused "self oscillation," is thus supported by many studies. The fact that tinnitus can be affected by psychological means (such as the tinnitus retraining program [93]) supports that hypothesis.

As we have discussed in other parts of this book there are similarities between tinnitus and neuropathic pain [151] (see p. 214). The effect of reduced high frequency input to the auditory system in individuals with cochlear type of high frequency hearing loss (such as that which occurs from noise exposure) may be similar to pain that is caused by reduced sensory input to neurons in the dorsal horn of the spinal cord. (Sensory input normally has an inhibitory influence on neurons that mediate pain signals, see Chapter 4, p. 221.) It is not known why only a few individuals with high frequency hearing loss experience severe tinnitus. Like other pathologies, some yet unknown factors seem to be necessary for the development of tinnitus in patients with high frequency hearing loss. (In fact, few disorders are caused by any one single factor.)

> That some forms of tinnitus is caused by deprivation of high frequency input from the cochlea is supported by the finding that cochlear implants that are set to generate high frequency stimulation of the cochlea (4,800 pps) are beneficial to some tinnitus patients [189].

Age-related changes that affect the auditory nerve or other insults to the nerve can cause impairment of temporal coherence and it has been suggested that tinnitus may be related to abnormal temporal correlations between the neural activity in individual auditory nerve fibers [49, 146]. Abnormal temporal correlations may result from abnormal communication between auditory nerve fibers (ephaptic transmission, see p. 58) [146] or similar direct communication between hair cells. When no sound is present, the time pattern of the spontaneous neural activity in the axons of the auditory nerve is normally uncorrelated. Sounds elicit neural activity that is phase-locked to the waveform of a sound, and the neural discharges in individual axons consequently become correlated. Such correlation may be important for detection of the presence of sounds [50, 146]. Abnormal correlation of activity in auditory nerve fibers that is not a result of the presence of sound, may therefore be perceived in the same way as sounds, thus tinnitus [49, 146].

A few studies have shown indications that re-organization of the auditory cortex is involved in some forms of tinnitus [169]. Other studies have shown that re-organization of the cerebral cortex may occur because of deprivation of input [186, 194] in a similar way as has been shown for other sensory cortices [183]. That means that expression of neural plasticity by deprivation of input may cause reorganization of the auditory cerebral cortex.

Studies dated in the 1950s and 1960s have shown that stellate ganglion block was effective in treating the tinnitus in some patients with Ménière's disease [1, 172, 233] indicating that the sympathetic nervous system is involved in generating the tinnitus in such patients. Beneficial effects (56% relief) were obtained in these patients, while patients with other causes of tinnitus had less benefit (27% relief) from that procedure [172, 233]. This again emphasizes the importance of regarding tinnitus as a heterogeneous group of disorders rather than a single entity. It is not known exactly how the sympathetic nervous system is involved in generating the tinnitus. Sympathetic activation affects the blood flow to the cochlea [118], which may affect the function of the cochlea. Sympathetic fibers are located close to the hair cells of the cochlea [43], and noradrenalin secreted from these adrenergic fibers may sensitize cochlear hair cells in a similar manner as that of adrenergic fibers that are located close to mechanoreceptors of the skin (see p. 93). Reduction of secretion of noradrenalin through sympathectomy and subsequent reduction of the sensitization of hair cells, could then explain the beneficial effect of sympathectomy on tinnitus.

Some patients with otosclerosis have tinnitus, and it has been reported that 40% of such individuals obtain relief from successful stapedectomy [68]. This would indicate that the cause of the tinnitus was located in the conductive apparatus of the ear. If the tinnitus was caused by sound deprivation due to the (conductive) hearing loss, the reduction of the tinnitus may be explained by the increased sound stimulation after stapedectomy, thus reducing the deprivation effect that caused expression of neural plasticity before the stapedectomy.

Treatment of subjective tinnitus   The effectiveness of specific treatments of disorders such as tinnitus can provide information about the pathophysiology of the disorder in question. With regard to tinnitus valuable information has been gained by such treatments as electrical stimulation of the ear and the nervous system, and from such procedures as sympathectomy.

Many forms of treatment have been tried for tinnitus, but the diversity of the pathophysiology and causes of tinnitus makes it unlikely that a single treatment will have a beneficial effect on all forms of tinnitus. The focus on treatment has moved from the ear and the periphery of the nervous system, to more central parts of the nervous system. This means that the treatments of tinnitus have been directed towards correcting the functional changes in the nervous system either by reversing the plastic changes that caused the pathologic signs and symptoms or by correcting the balance between inhibition and excitation by appropriate medications.

Some individuals experience relief of their tinnitus from administration of benzodiazepines (GABA$_A$ agonists) such as Alprazolam or Clonazepam [206], a clear sign that the anatomical location of the physiological abnormality is the CNS. Baclofen, a GABA$_B$ agonist has also been tried but with poor effect, nor has gabapentine been shown to be effective although theoretically these two drugs should also enhance GABAergic inhibition. In animal experiments, the (-)-isomer of baclofen is more effective in reducing signs of hyperactivity in the IC (induced by sound stimulation) than benzodiazepines [223]. Lidocaine given intravenously [139] can relieve tinnitus in some individuals [121], but the effect of the oral forms of the drug (tocainide) [121] on tinnitus have been disappointing, and are associated with serious side effects when given in therapeutic dosages. A similar drug, Mexilitine, has been tried [137] but the beneficial effect has been difficult to prove. In general, pharmacological treatment of tinnitus has been disappointing, and when drugs that have had beneficial effects in some patients have been tested in double blind studies, the beneficial effect has not been much better than placebos. Again, one reason for the poor results in population studies may be that patients with tinnitus are a heterogeneous group with regard to pathophysiology, and subsequently different kinds of treatment would be effective to the different groups of tinnitus patients.

Some patients get relief from their tinnitus after moving a blood vessel off the auditory nerve (microvascular decompression, MVD, operations) [108, 152, 161]. Clinical studies show that MVD of the auditory portion of the CN VIII is effective in alleviating tinnitus in a selected population of tinnitus patients [161]. This has been taken to indicate that tinnitus in these patients was caused by the compression of the auditory nerve by a blood vessel (see Chapter 6, p. 149).

Electrical stimulation by electrodes placed on the cochlea [7, 34], or behind the ear [193] has been used with some success. Electrical stimulation of the skin behind the ear probably has its effect by stimulation of the trigeminal system. In fact, it has been shown that stimulation of the somatosensory system (fingers) [97, 182] can affect (decrease) tinnitus [51].

More recently, transcranial magnetic stimulation of the auditory cerebral cortex has been successful in eliminating tinnitus in some individuals [41, 178]. Chronically implanted electrodes for electrical stimulation of the cortex can also alleviate tinnitus in selected groups of patients [41]. Such treatment is based on the observation that the auditory cortex is reorganized in patients with some forms of tinnitus [169]. Treatment of tinnitus by stimulation of the cerebral cortex is another example of such shift in focus of treatment from the periphery to central structures.

The beneficial effect of cortical stimulation is based on the assumption that the auditory cortex has re-organized in patients with tinnitus (as a result of expression of neural plasticity) [169], and that this reorganization causes the tinnitus. Electrical stimulation is assumed to reverse these changes. Similar reorganization occurs in other sensory systems after lesions of sensory organs. The visual cortex shows reorganization after lesions were made in the retina [98], and the somatosensory cortex reorganizes after selective deafferentiation [141]. A study has shown that tinnitus in patients who can switch their tinnitus on and off voluntarily activate only the cortex on one side, while sound stimulation activates the auditory cortex bilaterally [128], indicating that the auditory cerebral cortex is responding in an abnormal way to tinnitus as compared with activation from sound stimulation of the ear, further supporting the hypothesis that the cerebral cortex is involved in some forms of tinnitus.

The beneficial effect that some patients with tinnitus get from stimulation of the auditory cortex (see p. 84) might be caused by activation of thalamic cells through the descending cortico-thalamic tracts, rather than from activation (or deactivation) of cells in the primary auditory cortex. Other evidence points to the thalamus as being involved in tinnitus (perhaps through non-classical pathways) (for details, see [156]).

Whether electrodes placed on the surface of the cerebral cortex in fact stimulate neurons in the thalamus (through the cortico-thalamic pathways) is irrelevant for treatment, and it is technically easier to place stimulating electrodes on the cortex than on the auditory thalamus.

When interpreting the effect of electrical (or magnetic) stimulation, it is important to consider how electrical stimulation acts on neural activity. High frequency electrical stimulation can inactivate cells by constantly depolarizing the cells, which is normally the anticipated effect of electrical stimulation, but electrical stimulation is likely to also activate fiber tracts. Even the electrical current elicited by extracranial magnetic stimulation with single impulses can deactivate cells in the visual cortex [5]. This means that the same electrical stimulation may activate some parts of the nervous systems while inactivating other parts.

Phantom signs from amputations

The sensory abnormalities that often follow amputations of limbs may be regarded as examples of compensatory actions in response to deprivation of somatosensory or proprioceptive input from the amputated limb, including changed visual perception of a missing body part. These plastic changes include changed cortical representation (mapping) of the amputated limb and adjacent structures, and change in motor and sensory function. The awareness of one's own body is related to brain maps that are constantly updated based on input from multiple sensory systems, tactile and visual being the most important ones. Such updating of brain maps after amputation of a limb is involved in producing the phantom limb syndrome [90].

Studies of individuals who have had an upper limb amputated [90] found that almost all had an awareness of the amputated limb, and that awareness could be altered by tactile stimulation of the stump and to a lesser degree by visual input. Tactile stimulation of the stump, or of the face, gave a dual perception of the anatomical location of the stimulation in half of the studied individuals. This dual representation was strongest with eyes closed and visual input could override this dual perception [90], but the spontaneous awareness of the limb was not affected by visual input. The observation that cortical re-mapping occurs after amputation is supported by results from imaging studies in patients who experience referred phantom sensations such as often occurs in SCI [163].

Sensorimotor interactions

A few studies have shown that deprivation of motor function such as may occur after severance of motor nerves can cause cortical re-organization [48]. Such reorganization of motor areas most likely occurs after amputation of limbs, and because motor functions are closely linked to perception, this form of post injury reorganization may contribute to abnormal sensations that are experienced after limb amputation. Cortical representation can also be induced by changes in utilization of specific muscles [103] (see p. 285).

Phantom visual sensations

Phosphens is the term for phantom visual sensations that do not include specific patterns or meaningful pictures. The phantom eye syndrome that can occur, for example, after removal of an eye is characterized by visual sensations (and pain) [208]. The sensations were mostly in the form of flickering light or permanent light (phosphens). A few reports describe individuals who were seeing contours, objects or scenes. These sensations were mostly experienced in darkness and before falling asleep and some forms of light sensations (phosphens) can interfere with sleep. Black patches in the visual field (scotoma) are signs of disorders of the central visual nervous system.

Other phantom sensations

Phantom taste (phantageusia) [85] consisting of metallic taste often occurs after section of the chorda tympani. Other abnormal taste sensations may occur as a side effect of medications. Phantosmia (phantom smell perception) [76, 85] is usually unpleasant. Vertigo is a form of phantom sensation that is related to the vestibular system, but the vestibular system is normally not regarded as a sensory system because activation of the vestibular system that occurs under normal circumstances does not cause any conscious sensations (the vestibular system is discussed in Chapter 6).

Changes in processing of sensory information

Change in processing of sensory information can cause several symptoms and signs of disorders. Abnormal perception of sensory stimuli such as hyperacusis, distortion of sounds, inability or reduced ability to understand speech while being able to effectively "hear" the speech, and abnormal sensations such as metallic taste and hypersensitivity of light, are examples of symptoms and signs that are caused by abnormal processing of sensory input. Changes in processing of sensory information may include altered perception of strength such as hyperacusis, or over sensitivity to light. Impaired comprehension of speech and other sounds are typical age-related changes. Hyperpathia is a pain sensation that is caused by abnormalities in the processing of painful stimuli (see Chapter 4).

Changes in processing of sensory information may be caused by deprivation of input, overexposure, exposure to chemical agents or from morphological changes such as from injuries, tumors or age-related changes. Expression of neural plasticity, for instance caused by reduced input from sensory receptors, is a frequent cause of functional change in the nervous system that causes abnormal processing of sensory information and often increased sensitivity.

The impairment of temporal coherence of the neural activity in the auditory nerve such as may occur after injury to the nerve (including age-related changes), contributes to poor speech discrimination (see Chapter 2, p. 56). Reorganization of the auditory nervous system that is caused by expression of neural plasticity, may also contribute to the poor speech discrimination that accompanies high frequency hearing loss in some individuals.

Studies in animals have shown that deprivation of input to the auditory system can cause hypersensitivity [64]. Altered temporal integration such as may occur after overstimulation of the auditory system [224] or deprivation of input [63, 65] is an example of altered processing of sensory information. The physiological changes that cause such alterations may be altered balance between inhibition and excitation.

Abnormal sensations such as phantom sensations may be caused by re-routing of sensory information. Allodynia is an example of re-routing of somatosensory information to pain circuits (see p. 204). Cross modal interaction between the auditory and the somatosensory system [3, 25, 148, 222] is also an example of re-routing of information that is caused by expression of neural plasticity.

The functional changes that are related to abnormal sensory input (or deprivation of input) may involve changes in synaptic efficacy, or the elimination of synapses and axons. Hebb's principle states that morphological connections are established between neurons that are activated together ("neurons that fire together, wire together") [83]. The reverse of that hypothesis would imply that connections that are not used are eliminated (this may just be a version of the general rule of "use it or lose it") and that could perhaps explain some forms of age-related hearing loss. Changes in the GABA system that occur normally with age may be the cause of some of the observed changes in processing of sensory information.

Information may be re-routed in the CNS as a result of expression of neural plasticity. Such re-routing can occur through morphological changes such as sprouting of axons and dendrites, and through formation of new synapses. It may also occur without any morphological signs by change in synaptic threshold or efficacy. Changes in the function of synapses can make synapses that are normally not conducting, become conducting (unmasking of dormant synapses [230]). This may open new routes for information to take in the CNS. Changes in discharge pattern, such as from continuous firing to burst firing, can also cause functional re-routing, because it can open dormant synapses or close synapses that are normally conducting nerve impulses (see pp. 151, 200).

Little is known about the effect of re-routing of information as a source of symptoms and signs of disorders. There is some evidence that individuals with some forms of autism have an abnormal cross-modal interaction, and it has been shown that electrical stimulation of the median nerve affects the perception of loudness of sounds in some individuals with autism [159].

Abnormal cross-modal interaction

Several studies have demonstrated that cross-modal interactions occur between the somatosensory and the auditory systems in individuals with tinnitus [25–27, 148]. Such interaction is a sign of re-routing of information. Human studies have shown that interaction between the auditory and the somatosensory system occurs normally in children, but it does not normally occur in adults [148, 155].[14] This abnormal cross-modal interaction between the somatosensory and auditory systems that occurs in some patients with tinnitus was interpreted to indicate an abnormal involvement of the non-classical (extralemniscal) auditory pathways [148, 155]. Only non-classical sensory pathways receive input from more than one sensory system at subcortical levels, and the cells of the classical sensory pathways (up to the primary cerebral cortices) only respond to one sensory modality (see p. 72). The studies that showed the presence of cross-modal interaction between the auditory and somatosensory systems therefore support the hypothesis that the non-classical auditory pathways are involved in some forms of tinnitus. Imaging studies have shown a greater involvement of limbic structures in some patients with tinnitus [128], supporting the hypothesis of abnormal activation of non-classical auditory pathways.

> Animal experiments have demonstrated that cross-modal interaction between the auditory and the somatosensory systems occurs in some neurons in the external nucleus and dorsal cortex of the IC [3, 4, 220, 222], and in the cochlear nucleus [91, 201].

Anatomical connections between the somatosensory system of the head (trigeminal system) with the auditory system [202] may explain the beneficial effect on tinnitus from electrical stimulation of the skin [51, 97, 182, 193]. The SC, which is normally not regarded as a sensory nucleus, integrates sensory input at the subcortical level and more extensive integration of sensory information

---

[14] The subjects in these studies compared the loudness of the sounds during electrical stimulation with that without electrical stimulation. The sounds used were meaningless (40) pps clicks at 65 dB hearing level and presented to one ear at a time. The somatosensory system was stimulated by applying electrical impulses to the median nerve at the wrist through surface electrodes, at a strength that produced a strong tingling but no pain.

from different senses occurs in the association cortices [218]. However, the cross-modal interaction between sensory modalities that occurs in some patients with tinnitus is different from the interaction that occurs in the SC and from that which occurs in association cortices, because stimuli of one modality can modulate the sensation of another modality when presented simultaneously.

Electrical stimulation of the skin can also cause or increase tinnitus in some individuals [26, 27, 148]. The fact that electrical stimulation of the skin can have different effects on tinnitus [148] may be explained by the diversity in the pathophysiology of tinnitus, and it may explain why, for instance, TMJ disorders are often associated with tinnitus [166, 167]. TMJ disorders are likely to cause abnormal stimulation of the trigeminal sensory system.

Some observations indicate that stimulation of receptors of one sensory modality may be perceived as a different modality in patients with tinnitus. This is most apparent in patients who have tinnitus after injuries of their auditory nerve close to the brainstem; they report perceiving sounds from specific tactile stimulation. Møller and Møller (unpublished observation, 1982) noted one patient who reported that rubbing his back with a towel gave rise to a sensation of sound [145, 151]. The fact that some patients with tinnitus can change their tinnitus by voluntary muscle contractions (such as eye muscles and jaw muscles) [26, 27, 36], is a sign of an abnormal cross-modal interaction. Some patients report that they can alter their tinnitus by pressing on their cheek, mastoid, or any other spot in the head–neck region [124].

Interaction between the auditory, somatosensory and visual systems has been reported in animal studies in which it was shown that sound evoked activity in neurons in the thalamus could be affected both by visual and somatosensory stimulation [89]. The specific effect of visual input on tinnitus is unknown; however, sound can evoke phosphens in some individuals with optic nerve disorders [122, 171], thus, a sign of abnormal sensory cross-modal interaction between the visual and the auditory systems.

The role of non-classical ascending sensory pathways

The presence of cross-modal sensory interaction between sensory inputs in adults [25–27, 128, 148] that presumably occurs subcortically, have been interpreted as a sign of abnormal involvement of non-classical pathways. While it is known that the non-classical ascending auditory pathways receive input from both the auditory and somatosensory system (Fig. 3.1), the function of non-classical sensory pathways is poorly understood. It is known, however, that the non-classical auditory pathways have subcortical connections to the nuclei of the amygdala, via the dorsal-medial thalamus (see p. 81), and this means that the non-classical auditory pathways provide a subcortical route of auditory information to the limbic system [120] (Fig. 3.7). Such subcortical connections to the amygdala from the dorsal and medial thalamic nuclei of the non-classical auditory pathways [120] may explain why some patients with severe tinnitus experience fear from sounds (phonophobia) and it may explain the high incidence of depression in individuals with severe tinnitus.

References

1. Adlington, P. and J. Warrick, Stellate Ganglion Block in the Management of Tinnitus. *J. Laryngol. Otol.*, 1971. **85**: pp. 159–168.

2. Ahissar, E., R. Sosnik, and S. Haidarliu, Transformation from Temporal to Rate Coding in a Somatosensory Thalamocortical Pathway. *Nature*, 2000. **406**(6793): pp. 302–6.

3. Aitkin, L. M., *The Auditory Midbrain, Structure and Function in the Central Auditory Pathway*. 1986, Humana Press: Clifton, NJ.

4. Aitkin, L. M., L. Tran, and J. Syka, The Responses of Neurons in Subdivisions of the Inferior Colliculus of Cats to Tonal, Noise and Vocal Stimuli. *Exp. Brain Res.*, 1994. **98**: pp. 53–64.

5. Amassian, V. E., R. Q. Cracco, P. J. Maccabee, J. B. Cracco, A. Rudell, and L. Eberle, Suppression of Visual Perception by Magnetic Coil Stimulation of Human Occipital Cortex. *Electroenceph. Clin. Neurophysiol.*, 1989. **74**(6): pp. 458–62.

6. Andersen, R. G. and W. L. Meyerhoff, Otologic Pathology and Tinnitus, in *Tinnitus and Its Management*, J. G. Clark and P. Yanick, Editors. 1984, Charles C Thomas Publishers: Springfield, Ill.

7. Aran, J. M. and I. Cazals, Electrical Suppression of Tinnitus, in *Ciba Foundation Symposium 85*. 1981, Pitman Books Ltd: London. pp. 217–225.

8. Bach, S., M. F. Noreng, and N. U. Tjellden, Phantom Limb Pain in Amputees During the First 12 Months Following Limb Amputation, after Preoperative Lumbar Epidural Blockade. *Pain*, 1988. **33**: pp. 297–301.

9. Bartels, S., S. Ito, D. R. Trune, and A. L. Nuttall, Noise-Induced Hearing Loss: The Effect of Melanin in the Stria Vascularis. *Hear. Res.*, 2001. **154**: pp. 116–123.

10. Berlin, C. I., T. Morlet, and L. J. Hood, Auditory Neuropathy/Dyssynchrony: Its Diagnosis and Management. *Pediatric Clinics of North America*, 2003. **50**(2): pp. 331–40.

11. Blackburn, S., Hyperbilirubinemia and Neonatal Jaundice. *Neonatal Netw.*, 1995. **14**: pp. 15–25.

12. Bluestone, C. D., Otitis Media: A Spectrum of Diseases, in *Pediatric Otology and Neurotology*, A. K. Lalwani and K. M. Grundfast, Editors. 1998, Lippincott-Raven: Philadelphia. pp. 233–40.

13. Blum, P. S., L. D. Abraham, and S. Gilman, Vestibular, Auditory, and Somatic Input to the Posterior Thalamus of the Cat. *Exp. Brain Res*, 1979. **34**: pp. 1–9.

14. Bocca, E., Distorted Speech Tests, in *Sensory-Neural Hearing Processes and Disorders*, B. A. Graham, Editor. 1965, Little, Brown & Co: Boston.

15. Boivie, J., G. Grant, and H. Silfvenius, A Projection from the Nucleus Z to the Ventral Nuclear Complex of the Thalamus in the Cat. *Acta Physiol. Scand.*, 1970. **80**(4): pp. 11A.

16. Bonin Von, G. and P. Bailey, *The Neocortex of the Macaca Mulatia*. 1947, Urbana, IL: University of Illinois Press.

17. Borg, E. and A. R. Møller, Noise and Blood Pressure: Effects on Lifelong Exposure in the Rat. *Acta Physiol. Scand.*, 1978. **103**: pp. 340–42.

18. Borg, E., Noise Induced Hearing Loss in Rats with Renal Hypertension. *Hear. Res.*, 1982. **8**: pp. 93–99.

19. Borg, E., Noise Induced Hearing Loss in Normotensive and Spontaneously Hypertensive Rats. *Hear. Res.*, 1982. **8**: pp. 117–130.

20. Borsel Van, J., L. M. G. Curfs, and J. P. Fryns, Hyperacusis in Williams Syndrome: A Sample Survey Study. *Genetic Counseling*, 1997. **8**(2): pp. 121–126.

21. Brackmann, D. E., C. Shelton, and M. A. Arriaga, *Otologic Surgery*. Vol. 2nd ed. 2001, Philadelphia: W. B. Saunders Co.

22. Braun, C. M., M. Dumont, J. Duval, I. Hamel-Hebert, and L. Godbout, Brain Modules of Hallucination: An Analysis of Multiple Patients with Brain Lesions. *J Psychiatry Neurosci.*, 2003. **28**(6): pp. 432–49.

23. Brodal, P., *The Central Nervous System*. 1998, Oxford University Press: New York.

24. Burns, W. and D. W. Robinson, *Hearing and Noise in Industry*. 1970, Her Majesty's Stationery Office: London.

25. Cacace, A. T., T. J. Lovely, D. J. McFarland, S. M. Parnes, and D. F. Winter, Anomalous Cross-Modal Plasticity Following Posterior Fossa Surgery: Some Speculations on Gaze-Evoked Tinnitus. *Hear. Res.*, 1994. **81**: pp. 22–32.

26. Cacace, A. T., J. P. Cousins, S. M. Parnes, D. J. McFarland, D. Semenoff, T. Holmes, C. Davenport, K. Stegbauer, and T. J. Lovely, Cutaneous-Evoked Tinnitus. Ii: Review of Neuroanatomical, Physiological and Functional Imaging Studies. *Audiol. Neurotol.*, 1999. **4**(5): pp. 258–268.

27. Cacace, A. T., J. P. Cousins, S. M. Parnes, D. Semenoff, T. Holmes, D. J. McFarland, C. Davenport, K. Stegbauer, and T. J. Lovely, Cutaneous-Evoked Tinnitus. I: Phenomenology, Psychophysics and Functional Imaging. *Audiol. Neurotology*, 1999. **4**(5): pp. 247–257.

28. Cacace, A. T., Expanding the Biological Basis of Tinnitus: Crossmodal Origins and the Role of Neuroplasticity. *Hear. Res.*, 2003. **175**: pp. 112–132.

29. Calza, L., L. Giardino, M. Zanni, R. Galetti, P. Parchi, and G. Galetti, Involvement of Cholinergic and Gabaergic Systems in Vestibular Compensation, in *Vestibular Compensation: Facts, Theories and Clinical Perspectives*, M. Lacour, *et al.*, Editors. 1989, Elsevier: Paris. pp. 189–199.

30. Canlon, B., E. Borg, and A. Flock, Protection against Noise Trauma by Pre-Exposure to a Low Level Acoustic Stimulus. *Hear. Res.*, 1988. **34**: pp. 197–200.

31. Caspary, D. M., A. Raza, Lawhorn, B. A. Armour, J. Pippin, and S. P. Arneric, Immunocytochemical and Neurochemical Evidence for Age-Related Loss of GABA in the Inferior Colliculus: Implications for Neural Presbycusis. *J. Neurosci.*, 1990. **10**: pp. 2363–2372.

32. Caspary, D. M., J. C. Milbrandt, and R. H. Helfert, Central Auditory Aging: GABA Changes in the Inferior Colliculus. *Exp. Gerontol.*, 1995. **30**: pp. 349–360.

33. Caspary, D. M., T. M. Holder, L. F. Hughes, J. C. Milbrandt, R. M. McKernan, and D. K. Naritoku, Age-Related Changes in GABA$_A$ Receptor Subunit Composition and Function in Rat Auditory System. *Neuroscience*, 1999. **93**(1): pp. 307–312.

34. Cazals, Y., M. Negrevergne, and J. M. Aran, Electrical Stimulation of the Cochlea in Man: Hearing Induction and Tinnitus Suppression. *J. Am. Audiol. Soc.*, 1978. **3**: pp. 209–213.

35. Chowdhury, S. A. and N. Suga, Reorganization of the Frequency Map of the Auditory Cortex Evoked by Cortical Electrical Stimulation in the Big Brown Bat. *J. Neurophys.*, 2000. **83**(4): pp. 1856–63.

36. Coad, M. L., A. H. Lockwood, R. J. Salvi, and R. Burkhard, Characteristics of Patients with Gaze-Evoked Tinnitus. *Otol. Neurotol.*, 2001. **22**: pp. 650–4.

37. Colletti, V., F. G. Fiorino, L. Sacchetto, V. Miorelli, and C. M., Hearing Habilitation with Auditory Brainstem Implantation in Two Children with Cochlear Nerve Aplasia. *Int. J. Pediatric Otorhinolaryngol.*, 2001. **60**(2): pp. 99–111.

38. Conlon, B. J. and D. W. Smith, Attenuation of Neomycin Ototoxicity by Iron Chelation. *Laryngoscope*, 1998. **108**: pp. 284–7.

39. Conlon, B. J., J.-M. Aran, J.-P. Erre, and D. W. Smith, Attenuation of Aminoglycoside-Induced Cochlear Damage with the Metabolic Antioxidant a-Lipoic Acid. *Hear. Res.*, 1999. **128**: pp. 40–44.

40. Dancer, A. L., D. Henderson, R. J. Salvi, and R. P. Hamernik, *Noise Induced Hearing Loss*. 1990, Mosby Year Book: St. Louis.

41. De Ridder, D., G. De Mulder, V. Walsh, N. Muggleton, S. Sunaert, and A. Møller, Magnetic and Electrical Stimulation of the Auditory Cortex for Intractable Tinnitus. *J Neurosurg*, 2004. **100**(3): pp. 560–4.

42. Densert, B. and K. Sass, Control of Symptoms in Patients with Ménière's Disease Using Middle Ear Pressure Applications: Two Years Follow-Up. *Acta Otolaryng. (Stockh.)*, 2001. **121**: pp. 616–621.

43. Densert, O., Adrenergic Innervation in the Rabbit Cochlea. *Acta Otolaryngol. (Stockh.)*, 1974. **78**: pp. 345–356.

44. Diamond, I. T., The Subdivisions of Neocortex: A Proposal to Revise the Traditional View of Sensory, Motor, and Association Areas., in *Progress in Psychobiology and Physiological Psychology*, J. M. Sprague and A. N. Epstein, Editors. 1979, Academic Press: New York. pp. 2–44.

45. Diamond, M. E. and M. Armstrong-James, The Role of Parallel Sensory Pathways and Cortical Columns in Learning. *Concepts Neurosci.*, 1992. **3**: pp. 55–78.

46. Dinse, H. R., B. Godde, T. Hilger, G. Reuter, S. M. Cords, T. Lenarz, and W. Von Seelen, Optical Imaging of Cat Auditory Cortex Cochleotopic Selectivity Evoked by Acute Electrical Stimualtion of a Multi-Channel Cochlear Implant. *Eur. J. Neurosci*, 1997. **9**(9): pp. 113–9.

47. Dolan, T. R., H. W. Ades, G. Bredberg, and W. D. Neff, Inner Ear Damage and Hearing Loss after Exposure to Tones of High Intensity. *Acta Otolaryngol. (Stockholm)*, 1975. **80**: pp. 343–352.

48. Donoghue, J. P., S. Suner, and J. N. Sanes, Dynamic Organization of Primary Motor Cortex Output to Target Muscles in Adult Rats. Ii. Rapid Reorganization Following Motor Nerve Lesions. *Exp. Brain Res.*, 1990. **79**(3): pp. 492–503.

49. Eggermont, J. J., On the Pathophysiology of Tinnitus: A Review and a Peripheral Model. *Hear. Res.*, 1990. **48**: pp. 111–124.

50. Eggermont, J. J., Between Sound and Perception: Reviewing the Search for a Neural Code *Hear. Res.*, 2001. **157**: pp. 1–42.

51. Engelberg, M. and W. Bauer, Transcutaneous Electrical Stimulation for Tinnitus. *Laryngoscope*, 1985. **95**: pp. 1167–1173.

52. Evans, E. F. and T. A. Borerwe, Ototoxic Effects of Salicylate on the Responses of Single Cochlear Nerve Fibers and on Cochlear Potentials. *Br. J. Audiol.*, 1982. **16**: pp. 101–108.

53. Falck, B., N. A. Hillarp, G. Thieme, and A. Torp, Fluorescence of Catcholamines and Related Compound Condensed with Formaldehyde. *Brain Res. Bull.*, 1982. **9**: pp. 1–6.

54. Fitzgerald, D. C. and A. S. Mark, Sudden Hearing Loss: Frequency of Abnormal Findings on Contrast-Enhanced Mr Studies. *Am J Neuroradiol.*, 1998. **19**(8): pp. 1433–6.

55. Flor, H., T. Elbert, S. Knecht, C. Wienbruch, C. Pantev, N. Birbaumer, L. W., and E. Taub, Phantom-Limb Pain as a Perceptual Correlate of Cortical Reorganization Following Arm Amputation *Nature*, 1995. **375**(6531): pp. 482–4.

56. Forge, A. and J. Schacht, Aminoglycoside Antibiotics. *Audiol. Neurotol.*, 2000. **5**: pp. 3–22.

57. Fowler, E. P., The Illusion of Loudness of Tinnitus – Its Etiology and Treatment. *Ann. Otol. Laryngol.*, 1942. **52**: pp. 275–285.

58. French, J. D., M. Verzeano, and H. W. Magoun, An Extralemniscal Sensory System of the Brain. *AMA Arch. Neurol. Psychiat.*, 1953. **69**: pp. 505–519.

59. Fu, K. M., T. A. Johnston, A. S. Shah, L. Arnold, J. Smiley, T. A. Hackett, P. E. Garraghty, and C. E. Schroeder, Auditory Cortical Neurons Respond to Somatosensory Stimulation. *J. Neurosci.*, 2003. **23**(20): pp. 7510–5.

60. Galambos, R., R. Myers, and G. Sheatz, Extralemniscal Activation of Auditory Cortex in Cats. *Am. J. Physiol.*, 1961. **200**: pp. 23–28.

61. Gates, G. A., N. N. Couropmitree, and R. H. Myers, Genetic Associations in Age-Related Hearing Thresholds. *Arch. Otolaryngol. Head & Neck Surg.*, 1999. **125**(6): pp. 654–9.

62. Gejrot, T., Intravenous Xylocaine in the Treatment of Attacks of Ménière's Disease. *Acta Otolaryngol. (Stockh)*, 1963. **Suppl 188**: pp. 190–195.

63. Gerken, G. M., Temporal Summation of Pulsate Brain Stimulation in Normal and Deafened Cats. *J. Acoust. Soc. Am.*, 1979(66): pp. 728–734.

64. Gerken, G. M., S. S. Saunders, and R. E. Paul, Hypersensitivity to Electrical Stimulation of Auditory Nuclei Follows Hearing Loss in Cats. *Hear. Res.*, 1984. **13**: pp. 249–260.

65. Gerken, G. M., J. M. Solecki, and F. A. Boettcher, Temporal Integration of Electrical Stimulation of Auditory Nuclei in Normal Hearing and Hearing-Impaired Cat. *Hear. Res.*, 1991. **53**: pp. 101–112.

66. Gerken, G. M., P. S. Hesse, and J. J. Wiorkowski, Auditory Evoked Responses in Control Subjects and in Patients with Problem Tinnitus. *Hear. Res.*, 2001. **157**: pp. 52–64.

67. Giardino, L., M. Zanni, M. Fernandez, A. Battaglia, O. Pigntaro, and L. Calza, Plasticity of Gaba$_a$ System During Aging: Focus on Vestibular Compensation and Possible Pharmacological Intervention. *Brain Res.*, 2002. **929**: pp. 76–86.

68. Glasgold, A. and F. Altman, The Effect of Stapes Surgery on Tinnitus in Otosclerosis. *Laryngoscope*, 1966. **76**: pp. 1524–1532.

69. Glasscock, M. C., B. A. Thedinger, and P. A. Cueva, An Analysis of the Retrolabyrinthine Vs the Retrosigmoid Vestibular Nerve Section. *Otolaryngol. Head Neck Surg.*, 1991. **104**: pp. 88–95.

70. Godde, B., T. Berkefeld, M. David-Jurgens, and H. R. Dinse, Age-Related Changes in Primary Somatosensory Cortex of Rats: Evidence for Parallel Degenerative and Plastic-Adaptive Processes. *Neurosci. Biobehavioral Rev.*, 2002. **26**(7): pp. 743–52.

71. Goodale, M. A. and A. D. Milner, Separate Pathways for Perception and Action. *Trends Neurosci.*, 1992. **15**(1): pp. 20–25.

72. Goodwin, P. E. and P. M. Johnson, The Loudness of Tinnitus. *Acta Otolaryngol. (Stockh)*, 1980. **90**: pp. 353–359.

73. Gordon, G. and G. Grant, Dorsolateral Spinal Afferents to Some Medullary Sensory Nuclei. An Anatomical Study in the Cat. *Exp. Brain Res.*, 1982. **46**(1): pp. 12–23.

74. Graybiel, A. M., Some Fiber Pathways Related to the Posterior Thalamic Region in the Cat. *Brain Behavior Evol.*, 1972. **6**: pp. 363–393.

75. Gross, C. G., H. R. Rodman, P. M. Gochin, and M. W. Colombo, Inferior Temporal Cortex as a Pattern Recognition Device, in *Computational Learning and Cognition*, E. Baum, Editor. 1993, SIAM Press: Philadelphia.

76. Grouios, G., Phantom Smelling. *Percept Mot Skills.*, 2002. **94**(3): pp. 841–50.

77. Hackett, T. A., I. Stepniewska, and J. H. Kaas, Thalamocortical Connections of the Parabelt Auditory Cortex in Macaque Monkeys. *J. Comp. Neurol.*, 1998. **400**(2): pp. 271–86.

78. Halpern, M., The Organization and Function of the Vomeronasal System. *Ann. Rev. Neurosci.*, 1987. **10**: pp. 325–62.

79. Hamernik, R. P., D. Henderson, and R. J. Salvi, *New Perspectives on Noise-Induced Hearing Loss*. 1982, Raven Press: New York.

80. Harrison, J. M. and M. E. Howe, *Anatomy of the Descending Auditory System in Auditory System*. Handbook of Sensory Physiology, ed. W. D. Keidel and W. D. Neff. Vol. V/1. 1974, Springer Verlag: Berlin.

81. Hartmann, R., R. K. Shepherd, S. Heid, and R. Klinke, Response of the Primary Auditory Cortex to Electrical Stimulation of the Auditory Nerve in the Congenitally Deaf White Cat. *Hear Res.*, 1997. **112**: pp. 115–33.

82. Hawkins, J. E., Auditory Physiologic History: A Surface View, in *Physiology of the Ear*, A. F. Jahn and J. Santos-Sacchi, Editors. 1988, Raven Press: New York.

83. Hebb, D. O., *The Organization of Behavior*. 1949, Wiley: New York.

84. Heid, S., T. K. Jahn-Siebert, R. Klinke, R. Hartmann, and G. Langner, Afferent Projection Patterns in the Auditory Brainstem in Normal and Congenitally Deaf White Cats. *Hear. Res.*, 1997. **110**: pp. 191–199.

85. Henkin, R. I., L. M. Levy, and C. S. Lin, Taste and Smell Phantoms Revealed by Brain Functional Mri (FMRI). *J. Comput. Assist. Tomogr.*, 2000. **24**(1): pp. 106–23.

86. Herbert, H. and C. B. Saper, Organization of Medullary Adrenergic and Noradrenergic Projections to Periaqueductal Gray Matter in the Rat. *J. Comp. Neurol.*, 1992. **315**: pp. 34–52.

87. Hilbig, H., J. Holler, H. R. Dinse, and H. J. Bidmon, In Contrast to Neuronal Nos-I, the Inducible Nos-II Expression in Aging Brains Is Modified by Enriched Environmental Conditions. *Exp. & Toxicol. Pathol.*, 2002. **53**(6): pp. 427–31.

88. Hirose, K., D. M. Hockenbery, and E. W. Rubel, Reactive Oxygen Species in Chick Hair Cells after Gentamicin Exposure in Vitro. *Hear. Res.*, 1997. **104**: pp. 1–14.

89. Hotta, T. and K. Kameda, Interactions between Somatic and Visual or Auditory Responses in the Thalamus of the Cat. *Exp. Neurol.*, 1963. **8**: pp. 1–13.

90. Hunter, J. P., J. Katz, and K. D. Davis, The Effect of Tactile and Visual Sensory Inputs on Phantom Limb Awareness. *Brain*, 2003. **126**(3): pp. 579–89.

91. Itoh, K., H. Kamiya, A. Mitani, Y. Yasui, M. Takada, and N. Mizuno, Direct Projections from Dorsal Column Nuclei and the Spinal Trigeminal Nuclei to the Cochlear Nuclei in the Cat. *Brain Res.*, 1987. **400**: pp. 145–150.

92. Jastreboff, P. J., Phantom Auditory Perception (Tinnitus): Mechanisms of Generation and Perception. *Neurosci. Res.*, 1990. **8**: pp. 221–254.

93. Jastreboff, P. J. and M. M. Jastreboff, Tinnitus Retraining Therapy (TRT) as a Method for Treatment of Tinnitus and Hyperacusis Patients. *J. Am. Acad. Audiol.*, 2000. **11**(3): pp. 162–77.

94. Joachims, H. Z., J. Segal, A. Golz, A. Netzer, and D. Goldenberg, Antioxidants in Treatment of Idiopathic Sudden Hearing Loss. *Otol. Neurotol.*, 2003. **24**: pp. 572–5.

95. Johnson, L. R., L. E. Westrum, and M. A. Henry, Anatomic Organization of the Trigeminal System and the Effects of Deafferentation, in *Trigeminal Neuralgia*, G. H. Fromm and B. J. Sessle, Editors. 1991, Butterworth-Heinemann: Boston. pp. 27–69.

96. Johnsson, L. G. and H. L. Hawkins, Sensory and Neural Degeneration with Aging, as Seen in Microdissections of the Human Inner Ear. *Ann. Otol. Rhinol. Laryngol.*, 1972. **81**: pp. 179–193.

97. Kaada, B., S. Hognestad, and J. Havstad, Transcutaneous Nerve Stimulation (Tns) in Tinnitus. *Scand. Audiol. (Stockh)*, 1989. **18**: pp. 211–217.

98. Kaas, J. H., L. A. Krubitzer, Y. M. Chino, A. L. Langston, E. H. Polley, and N. Blair, Reorganization of Retinotopic Cortical Maps in Adult Mammals after Lesions of the Retina. *Science*, 1990. 229–232.

99. Kaltenbach, J. A. and C. E. Afman, Hyperactivity in the Dorsal Cochlear Nucleus after Intense Sound Exposure and Its Resemblance to Tone-Evoked Activity: A Physiological Model for Tinnitus. *Hear. Res.*, 2000. **140**: pp. 165–72.

100. Kauffman, T., H. Theoret, and A. Pascual-Leone, Braille Character Discrimination in Blindfolded Human Subjects. *NeuroReport*, 2002. **13**(5): pp. 571–4.

101. Kawamoto, K., S. Ishimoto, R. Minoda, D. E. Brough, and Y. Raphael, Math1 Gene Transfer Generates New Cochlear Hair Cells in Mature Guinea Pigs in Vivo. *J. Neurosci.*, 2003. **23**(11): pp. 4395–400.

102. Keay, K. A., C. I. Clement, A. Depaulis, and R. Bandler, Different Representations of Inescapable Noxious Stimuli in the Periaqueductal Gray and Upper Cervical Spinal Cord of Freely Moving Rats. *Neurosci Lett*, 2001. **313**(1–2): pp. 17–20.

103. Khaslavskaia, S., M. Ladouceur, and T. Sinkjaer, Increase in Tibialis Anterior Motor Cortex Excitability Following Repetitive Electrical Stimulation of the Common Peroneal Nerve. *Exp. Brain Res.*, 2002. **143**(3): pp. 309–315.

104. Kilgard, M. P. and M. M. Merzenich, Plasticity of Temporal Information Processing in the Primary Auditory Cortex. *Nature Neurosci.*, 1998. **1**: pp. 727–731.

105. Kilgard, M. P. and M. M. Merzenich, Cortical Map Reorganization Enabled by Nucleus Basalis Activity. *Science*, 1998. **279**: pp. 1714–1718.

106. Klein, A. J., B. L. Armstrong, M. K. Greer, and F. R. Brown, Hyperacusis and Otitis Media in Individuals with Williams Syndrome. *J. Speech Hear. Dis.*, 1990. **55**: pp. 339–344.

107. Klinke, R., R. Hartmann, S. Heid, J. Tillein, and A. Kral, Plastic Changes in the Auditory Cortex of Congenitally Deaf Cats Following Cochlear Implantation. *Audiol. Neurootol.*, 2001. **6**: pp. 203–206.

108. Kondo, A., J. Ishikawa, T. Yamasaki, and T. Konishi, Microvascular Decompression of Cranial Nerves, Particularly of the Seventh Cranial Nerve. *Neurol. Med. Chir. (Tokyo)*, 1980. **20**: pp. 739–751.

109. Koralek, K. A., K. F. Jensen, and H. P. Killackey, Evidence for Two Complementary Patterns of Thalamic Input to the Rat Somatosensory Cortex. *Brain Res.*, 1988. **463**(2): pp. 346–51.

110. Korsan-Bengtsen (Also Known as M. B. Møller), M., Distorted Speech Audiometry. *Acta Otolaryng. (Stockholm)*, 1973. **Suppl. 310**: pp. 1–75.

111. Kral, A., R. Hartmann, J. Tillrin, S. Heid, and R. Klinke, Congenital Auditory Deprivation Reduces Synaptic Activity within the Auditory Cortex in Layer Specific Manner. *Cerebral Cortex*, 2000. **10**: pp. 714–726.

112. Kral, A., R. Hartmann, J. Tillein, S. Heid, and R. Klinke, Delayed Maturation and Sensitive Periods in the Auditory Cortex. *Audiol. Neurootol.*, 2001. **6**(346–362).

113. Kral, A., R. Hartmann, J. Tillein, S. Heid, and R. Klinke, Hearing after Congenital Deafness: Central Auditory Plasticity and Sensory Deprivation. *Cereb. Cortex*, 2002. **12**: pp. 797–807.

114. Kvasnak, E., D. Suta, J. Popelar, and J. Syka, Neuronal Connections in the Medial Geniculate Body of the Guinea-Pig. *Exp. Brain Res.*, 2000. **132**: pp. 87–102.

115. Kwiat, G. C. and A. I. Basbaum, The Origin of Brainstem Noradrenergic and Serotonergic Projections to the Spinal Cord Dorsal Horn in the Rat. *Somatosensory and Motor Res.*, 1992. **9**: pp. 157–173.

116. Lamm, K., H. Lamm, and W. Arnold, Effect of Hyperbaric Oxygen Therapy in Comparison to Conventional or Placebo Therapy or No Treatment in Idiopathic

Sudden Hearing Loss, Acoustic Trauma, Noise-Induced Hearing Loss and Tinnitus. A Literature Survey. *Adv. Otorhinolaryngol.*, 1998. **54**: pp. 86–99.

117. Landgren, S. and H. Silfvenius, Nucleus Z, the Medullary Relay in the Projection Path to the Cerebral Cortex of Group I Muscle Afferents from the Cat's Hind Limb. *J. Physiol. (Lond)*, 1971. **218**: pp. 551–71.

118. Laurikainen, E. A., D. Kim, A. Didier, T. Ren, J. M. Miller, W. S. Quirk, and A. L. Nuttall, Stellate Ganglion Drives Sympathetic Regulation of Cochlear Blood Flow. *Hear. Res.*, 1993. **64**: pp. 199–204.

119. LeDoux, J. E., A. Sakaguchi, and D. J. Reis, Subcortical Efferent Projections of the Medial Geniculate Mediate Emotional Responses Conditioned by Acoustic Stimuli. *J. Neurosci.*, 1984. **4**: pp. 683–698.

120. Ledoux, J. E., Brain Mechanisms of Emotion and Emotional Learning. *Curr. Opin. Neurobiol.*, 1992. **2**: pp. 191–197.

121. Lenarz, T., Treatment of Tinnitus with Lidocaine and Tocainide. *Scand. Audiol. (Stockh)*, 1986. **26**: pp. 49–51.

122. Lessell, S. and M. M. Cohen, Phosphenes Induced by Sound. *Neurology*, 1979. **29**(11): pp. 1524–6.

123. Leventhal, A. G., J. Wang, M. Pu, Y. Zhou, and Y. Ma, GABA and Its Agonists Improved Visual Cortical Function in Senescent Monkeys. *Science*, 2003. **300**: pp. 812–815.

124. Levine, R. A., Somatic (Craniocervical) Tinnitus and the Dorsal Cochlear Nucleus Hypothesis. *Am. J. Otolaryngol.*, 1999. **20**(6): pp. 351–62.

125. Liberman, M. C. and N. Y. S. Kiang, Acoustic Trauma in Cats. *Acta Otolaryngol. (Stockh)*, 1978. **Suppl 358**: pp. 1–63.

126. Liberman, M. C., Chronic Changes in Acoustic Trauma: Serial-Section Reconstruction of Stereocilia and Cuticular Plates. *Hear. Res.*, 1987. **26**: pp. 65–88.

127. Lidén, G., *Audiology*. 1985, Almquist & Wiksell: Stockholm.

128. Lockwood, A., R. Salvi, M. Coad, M. Towsley, D. Wack, and B. Murphy, The Functional Neuroanatomy of Tinnitus. Evidence for Limbic System Links and Neural Plasticity. *Neurology*, 1998. **50**: pp. 114–120.

129. Lu, S. M. and R. C. Lin, Thalamic Afferents of the Rat Barrel Cortex: A Light- and Electron-Microscopic Study Using Phaseolus Vulgaris Leucoagglutinin as an Anterograde Tracer. *Somatosensory & Motor Research.*, 1993. **10**(1): pp. 1–16.

130. Lumb, B. M., Inescapable and Escapable Pain Is Represented in Distinct Hypothalamic-Midbrain Circuits: Specific Roles of Ad- and C-Nociceptors. *Exp. Physiol.*, 2002. **87**: pp. 281–86.

131. Maison, S. F. and M. C. Liberman, Predicting Vulnerability to Acoustic Injury with a Non-Invasive Assay of Olivocochlear Reflex Strength. *J. Neurosci.*, 2000. **20**: pp. 4701–4707.

132. Marczynski, T. J., J. Artwohl, and B. Marczynska, Chronic Administration of Flumazenil Increases Life Span and Protects Rats from Age-Related Loss of Cognitive Functions: A Benzodiazepine/Gabaergic Hypothesis of Brain Aging. *Neurobiology of Aging*, 1994. **15**(1): pp. 69–84.

133. Marczynski, T. J., GABAergic Deafferentation Hypothesis of Brain Aging and Alzheimer's Disease Revisited. *Brain Res Bull.*, 1998. **45**(4): pp. 341–79.

134. Martich-Kriss, V., S. S. Kollias, and W. S. Ball Jr., Mr Findings in Kernicterus. *Am. J. Neuroradiol.*, 1995. **16**: pp. 819–21.

135. Mattox, D. E. and F. B. Simmons, Natural History of Sudden Hearing Loss. *Otolaryngol. Head Neck Surg.*, 1977. **88**: pp. 111–3.

136. Maxwell, A. P., S. M. Mason, and G. M. O'Donoghue, Cochlear Nerve Aplasia: Its Importance in Cochlear Implantation. *Am. J. Otol.*, 1999. **20**(3): pp. 335–337.

137. McCormick, M. S. and J. N. Thomas, Mexiletine in the Relief of Tinnitus: A Report on a Sequential Double-Blind Crossover Trial. *Clin. Otolaryngol. & Allied Sci.*, 1981. **6**(4): pp. 255–8.

138. McDonald, A. J., Cortical Pathways to the Mammalian Amygdala. *Progr. Neurobiol.*, 1998. **55**(3): pp. 257–332.

139. Melding, P. S., R. J. Goodey, and P. R. Thorne, The Use of Lignocaine in the Diagnosis and Treatment of Tinnitus. *J. Laryngol. Otol.*, 1978. **92**: pp. 115–121.

140. Melzack, R., Phantom Limbs. *Sci. Am.*, 1992. **266**: pp. 120–126.

141. Merzenich, M. M., J. H. Kaas, J. Wall, R. J. Nelson, M. Sur, and D. Felleman, Topographic Reorganization of Somatosensory Cortical Areas 3b and 1 in Adult Monkeys Following Restricted Deafferentiation. *Neuroscience*, 1983. **8**(1): pp. 3–55.

142. Miller, J. M., C. S. Watson, and W. P. Covell, Deafening Effects of Noise on the Cat. *Acta Oto Laryng. Suppl.* 176, 1963: pp. 1–91.

143. Milner, A. D. and M. A. Goodale, Visual Pathways to Perception and Action. *Progr. Brain Res.*, 1993. **95**: pp. 317–37.

144. Mishkin, M., L. G. Ungerleider, and K. A. Macko, Object Vision and Spatial Vision: Two Cortical Pathways. *Trends Neurosci.*, 1983. **6**: pp. 415–417.

145. Møller, A. R. and M. B. Møller, Unpublished Observation. 1982.

146. Møller, A. R., Pathophysiology of Tinnitus. *Ann. Otol. Rhinol. Laryngol.*, 1984. **93**: pp. 39–44.

147. Møller, A. R., M. B. Møller, P. J. Jannetta, and H. D. Jho, Compound Action Potentials Recorded from the Exposed Eighth Nerve in Patients with Intractable Tinnitus. *Laryngoscope*, 1992. **102**: pp. 187–197.

148. Møller, A. R., M. B. Møller, and M. Yokota, Some Forms of Tinnitus May Involve the Extralemniscal Auditory Pathway. *Laryngoscope*, 1992. **102**: pp. 1165–1171.

149. Møller, A. R., Tinnitus, in *Neurotology*, R. K. Jackler and D. Brackmann, Editors. 1994, Mosby Year Book, Inc.: St. Louis.

150. Møller, A. R., *Intraoperative Neurophysiologic Monitoring*. 1995, Harwood Academic Publishers: Luxembourg.

151. Møller, A. R., Similarities between Chronic Pain and Tinnitus. *Am. J. Otol.*, 1997. **18**: pp. 577–585.

152. Møller, A. R., Vascular Compression of Cranial Nerves. I: History of the Microvascular Decompression Operation. *Neurol. Res.*, 1998. **20**: pp. 727–731.

153. Møller, A. R., Similarities between Severe Tinnitus and Chronic Pain. *J. Amer. Acad. Audiol.*, 2000. **11**: pp. 115–124.

154. Møller, A. R., *Hearing: Its Physiology and Pathophysiology*. 2000, Academic Press: San Diego.

155. Møller, A. R. and P. Rollins, The Non-Classical Auditory System Is Active in Children but Not in Adults. *Neurosci. Lett.*, 2002. **319**: pp. 41–44.

156. Møller, A. R., *Sensory Systems: Anatomy and Physiology*. 2003, Academic Press: Amsterdam.

157. Møller, A. R., Tinnitus, in *Neurotology*, R. K. Jackler and D. Brackmann, Editors. 2003. Mosby Year Book Inc.: St. Lauis.

158. Møller, A. R., Pathophysiology of Tinnitus, in *Otolaryngologic Clinics of North America*, A. Sismanis, Editor. 2003, W. B.Saunders: Amsterdam. pp. 249–266.

159. Møller, A. R. and J. K. Kern, Are the Non-Classical Auditory Pathways Involved in Autism and PDD? *Neurol. Res.* 2005. **27**

160. Møller, M. B., Hearing in 70 and 75 Year-Old People. Results from a Cross-Sectional and Longitudinal Population Study. *Am. J. Otolaryngol.*, 1981. **2**: pp. 22–29.

161. Møller, M. B., A. R. Møller, P. J. Jannetta, and H. D. Jho, Vascular Decompression Surgery for Severe Tinnitus: Selection Criteria and Results. *Laryngoscope*, 1993. **103**: pp. 421–427.

162. Møller, M. B., Audiological Evaluation *J. Clin. Neurophysiol.*, 1994. **11**: pp. 309–318.

163. Moore, C. I., C. E. Stern, C. Dunbar, S. K. Kostyk, A. Gehi, and S. Gorkin, Referred Phantom Sensations and Cortical Reorganization after Spinal Cord Injury in Humans. *Proc. Natl. Acad. Sci.*, 2000. **97**(26): pp. 14703–8.

164. Morest, D. K., M. D. Ard, and D. Yurgelun-Todd, Degeneration in the Central Auditory Pathways after Acoustic Deprivation or over-Stimulation in the Cat. *Anat. Rec.*, 1979. **193**: pp. 750.

165. Morest, D. K. and B. A. Bohne, Noise-Induced Degeneration in the Brain and Representation of Inner and Outer Hair Cells. *Hear. Res.*, 1983. **9**: pp. 145–152.

166. Morgan, D. H., Temporomandbular Joint Surgery. Correction of Pain, Tinnitus, and Vertigo. *Dental Radiography and Photography*, 1973. **46**(2): pp. 27–46.

167. Morgan, D. H., Tinnitus of Tmj Origin. *J. Craniomandibular Practice*, 1992. **10**(2): pp. 124–129.

168. Mountcastle, V. B., Neural Mechanisms in Somesthesia, in *Medical Physiology*, V. B. Mountcastle, Editor. 1974, St. Louis: Mosby.

169. Mühlnickel, W., E. T., E. Taub, and H. Flor, Reorganization of Auditory Cortex in Tinnitus. *Proc. Nat. Acad. Sci. USA*, 1998. **95**(17): pp. 10340–3.

170. Noikaido, A. M., E. H. Ellinwood Jr., D. G. Heatherly, and S. K. Gupta, Age-Related Increase in CNS Sensitivity to Benzodiazepines as Assessed by Task Difficulty. *Psychopharmacology*, 1990. **100**: pp. 90–97.

171. Page, N. G., J. P. Bolger, and M. D. Sanders, Auditory Evoked Phosphenes in Optic Nerve Disease. *J. Neurol. Neurosurg. Psych.*, 1982. **45**(1): pp. 7–12.

172. Passe, E. G., Sympathectomy in Relation to Ménière's Disease, Nerve Deafness and Tinnitus. A Report of 110 Cases. *Proc. Roy. Soc. Med.*, 1951. **44**: pp. 760–772.

173. Penfield, W. and E. Boldrey, Somatic Motor and Sensory Representation in the Cerebral Cortex of Man as Studied by Electrical Stimulation. *Brain*, 1937. **60**: pp. 389–443.

174. Pensak, M. L., M. E. Glasscock, A. F. Josey, C. G. Jackson, and A. J. Gulya, Sudden Hearing Loss and Cerebellopontine Angle Tumors. *Laryngoscope*, 1985. **95**(10): pp. 1188–93.

175. Pichler, M., Z. Wang, C. Grabner-Weiss, D. Reimer, S. Hering, M. Grabner, H. Glossmann, and J. Striessning, Block of P/Q-Type Calcium Channels by Therapeutic Concentrations of Aminoglycoside Antibiotics. *Biochemistry*, 1996. **35**: pp. 14659–14664.

176. Pierson, L. L., K. J. Gerhardt, G. P. Rodriguez, and R. B. Yanke, Relationship between Outer Ear Resonance and Permanent Noise-Induced Hearing Loss. *Am. J. Otolaryngol.*, 1994. **15**: pp. 37–40.

177. Pierson, M. G. and A. R. Møller, Prophylaxis of Kanamycin-Induced Ototoxitity by a Radioprotectant. *Hear. Res.*, 1981. **4**: pp. 79–87.

178. Plewnia, C., M. Bartels, and C. Gerlof, Transient Suppression of Tinnitus by Transcranial Magnetic Stimulation. *Ann. Neurol.*, 2003. **53**(2): pp. 263–266.

179. Portmann, G., The Saccus Endolymphaticus and an Operation for Draining the Same for the Relief of Vertigo. *J. Laryng. Otol.*, 1927. **42**: pp. 809.

180. Portmann, M., R. Dauman, and J. M. Aran, Audiometric and Electrophysiological Correlations in Sudden Deafness. *Acta Otolaryngol*, 1985. **99**(3–4): pp. 363–8.

181. Priuska, E. M. and J. Schacht, Formation of Free Radical by Gentamycin and Iron and Evidence for an Iron/Gentamycin Complex. *Biochem. Pharmacol.*, 1995. **50**: pp. 1749–52.

182. Rahko, T. and V. Kotti, Tinnitus Treatment by Transcutaneous Nerve Stimulation (TNS). *Acta Otolaryngol. (Stockh)*, 1997. **Suppl 529**: pp. 88–89.

183. Rauschecker, J. P., Auditory Cortical Plasticity: A Comparison with Other Sensory Systems. *Trends Neurosci.*, 1999. **22**: pp. 74–80.

184. Rauschecker, J. P. and B. Tian, Mechanisms and Streams for Processing of "What" and "Where" in Auditory Cortex. *Proc. Nat. Acad. Sci. USA*, 2000. **97**: pp. 11800–11806.

185. Reed, G. F., An Audiometric Study of 200 Cases of Subjective Tinnitus. *Arch. Otolaryngol.*, 1960. **71**: pp. 94–104.

186. Robertson, D. and D. R. Irvine, Plasticity of Frequency Organization in Auditory Cortex of Guinea Pigs with Partial Unilateral Deafness. *J. Comp. Neurol.*, 1989. **282**(3): pp. 456–471.

187. Robertson, D., B. M. Johnstone, and T. McGill, Effects of Loud Tones on the Inner Ear: A Combined Electrophysiological and Ultrastructural Study. *Hear. Res.*, 1990. **2**: pp. 39–53.

188. Rouiller, E. M., Functional Organization of the Auditory System, in *The Central Auditory System*, G. Ehret and R. Romand, Editors. 1997, Oxford University Press: New York. pp. 3–96.

189. Rubinstein, J. T., R. S. Tyler, A. Johnson, and C. J. Brown, Electrical Suppression of Tinnitus with High-Rate Pulse Trains. *Otology & Neurotology*, 2003. **24**: pp. 478–485.

190. Sakai, M. D. and N. Suga, Plasticity of the Cochleotopic (Frequency) Map in Specialized and Nonspecialized Cortices. *Proc. Nat. Acad. Sci. USA*, 2001. **98**(6): pp. 3507–3512.

191. Salt, A. N., Regulation of Endolymphatic Fluid Volume. *Ann N Y Acad Sci*, 2001. **942**: pp. 306–12.

192. Schleuning, A. J., Management of the Patient with Tinnitus. *Med. Clin. N. Am.*, 1991. **75**: pp. 1225–1237.

193. Schulman, A., J. Tonndorf, and B. Goldstein, Electrical Tinnitus Control. *Acta Otolaryngol. (Stockh)*, 1985. **99**: pp. 318–325.

194. Schwaber, M. K., Neuroplasticity of the Adult Primate Auditory Cortex Following Cochlear Hearing Loss. *Am. J. Otol.*, 1993. **14**(3): pp. 252–258.

195. Seligmann, H., L. Podoshin, J. Ben-David, M. Fradis, and G. M., Drug-Induced Tinnitus and Other Hearing Disorders. *Drug Safety*, 1996. **14**(3): pp. 198–212.

196. Sessle, B. J., Recent Development in Pain Research: Central Mechanism of Orofacial Pain and Its Control. *J. Endodon.*, 1986. **12**: pp. 435–444.

197. Sessle, B. J., Physiology of the Trigeminal System, in *Trigeminal Neuralgia*, G. H. Fromm and B. J. Sessle, Editors. 1991, Butterworth-Heinemann: Boston. pp. 71–104.

198. Sha, S. H. and J. Schacht, Stimulation of Free Radical Formation by Aminoglycoside Antibiotics. *Hear. Res.*, 1999. **128**: pp. 112–118.

199. Shambaugh, G. E., Surgery of the Endolymphatic Sac. *Arch. Otol.*, 1966. **83**: pp. 302.

200. Shepherd, G. M., *Neurobiology*. 3rd ed. 1994, Oxford University Press: New York.

201. Shore, S. E., D. A. Godfrey, R. H. Helfert, R. A. Altschuler, and S. C. Bledsoe, Connections between the Cochlear Nuclei in Guinea Pig. *Hear. Res.*, 1992. **62**(1): pp. 16–26.

202. Shore, S. E., Z. Vass, N. L. Wys, and R. A. Altschuler, Trigeminal Ganglion Innervates the Auditory Brainstem. *J Comp. Neurol.*, 2000. **419**(3): pp. 271–285.

203. Sie, K. C. Y. and E. W. Rubel, Rapid Changes in Protein Synthesis and Cell Size in the Cochlear Nucleus Following Eighth Nerve Activity Blockade and Cochlea Ablation. *J. Comp. Neurol.*, 1992. **320**: pp. 501–508.

204. Silverstein, H., H. Norrell, T. Haberkamp, and A. B. McDaniel, The Unrecognized Rotation of the Vestibular and Cochlear Nerves from the Labyrinth to the Brain Stem: Its Implications to Surgery of the Eighth Cranial Nerve. *Otolaryngol Head Neck Surg*, 1986. **95**: pp. 543–549.

205. Silverstein, H., J. Arruda, S. I. Rosenberg, D. Deems, and T. O. Hester, Direct Round Window Membrane Application of Gentamicin in the Treatment of Ménière's Disease. *Otolaryngol. Head & Neck Surg.*, 1999. **120**(5): pp. 649–55.

206. Simpson, J. J. and E. Davies, Recent Advances in the Pharmacological Treatment of Tinnitus. *Trends Pharmacol. Sci.*, 1999. **20**: pp. 12–18.

207. Song, B. B., S. H. Sha, and J. Schacht, Iron Chelators Protect from Aminoglycoside-Induced Cochleo- and Vestibulotoxicity in Guinea Pig. *Free Rad. Biol. Med.*, 1998. **25**: pp. 189–195.

208. Soros, P., O. Vo, I. W. Husstedt, S. Evers, and H. Gerding, Phantom Eye Syndrome: Its Prevalence, Phenomenology, and Putative Mechanisms. *Neurology*, 2003. **60**(9): pp. 1542–3.

209. Spangler, K. M., N. B. Cant, C. K. Henkel, G. R. Farley, and W. B. Warr, Descending Projections from the Superior Olivary Complex to the Cochlear Nucleus of the Cat. *J. Comp. Neurol.*, 1987. **259**: pp. 452–465.

210. Spencer, R. F., W. T. Shaia, A. T. Gleason, A. Sismanis, and S. M. Shapiro, Changes in Calcium-Binding Protein Expression in the Auditory Brainstem Nuclei of the Jaundiced Gunn Rat. *Hear. Res.*, 2002. **171**: pp. 129–141.

211. Spoendlin, H., Structural Basis of Peripheral Frequency Analysis, in *Frequency Analysis and Periodicity Detection in Hearing*, R. Plomp and G. F. Smoorenburg, Editors. 1970, A. W. Sijthoff: Leiden. pp. 2–36.

212. Spoendlin, H., Anatomical Changes Following Noise Exposure, in *Effects of Noise on Hearing*, D. Henderson, *et al.*, Editors. 1976, Raven Press: New York.

213. Spoendlin, H. and A. Schrott, Analysis of the Human Auditory Nerve. *Hear. Res.*, 1989. **43**: pp. 25–38.

214. Spoor, A., Presbycusis Values in Relation to Noise Induced Hearing Loss. *Int. Audiol.*, 1967. **6**: pp. 48–57.

215. Starr, A., T. W. Picton, Y. Sininger, L. J. Hood, and C. I. Berlin, Auditory Neuropathy. *Brain*, 1996. **119**: pp. 741–53.

216. Starzl, T. E. and H. W. Magoun, Organization of the Diffuse Thalamic Projection System. *J. Neurophysiol*, 1951. **14**: pp. 133–146.

217. Starzl, T. E. and D. G. Witlock, Diffuse Thalamic Projection System in the Monkey. *J. Neurophysiol.*, 1952. **15**: pp. 449–468.

218. Stein, B. E., M. W. Wallace, T. R. Stanford, and W. Jiang, Cortex Governs Multisensory Integration in the Midbrain. *Neuroscientist*, 2002. **8**(4): pp. 306–14.

219. Syka, J., N. Rybalko, and J. Popelar, Enhancement of the Auditory Cortex Evoked Responses in Awake Guinea Pigs after Noise Exposure. *Hear. Res.*, 1994. **78**: pp. 158–168.

220. Syka, J., J. Popelar, and E. Kvasnak, Response Properties of Neurons in the Central Nucleus and External and Dorsal Cortices of the Inferior Colliculus in Guinea Pig. *Exp. Brain Res.*, 2000. **133**: pp. 254–266.

221. Syka, J., Plastic Changes in the Central Auditory System after Hearing Loss, Restoration of Function, and During Learning. *Physiol Rev*, 2002. **82**(3): pp. 601–36.

222. Szczepaniak, W. S. and A. R. Møller, Interaction between Auditory and Somatosensory Systems: A Study of Evoked Potentials in the Inferior Colliculus. *Electroencephologr. Clin. Neurophysiol.*, 1993. **88**: pp. 508–515.

223. Szczepaniak, W. S. and A. R. Møller, Effects of (-)-Baclofen, Clonazepam, and Diazepam on Tone Exposure-Induced Hyperexcitability of the Inferior Colliculus in the Rat: Possible Therapeutic Implications for Pharmacological Management of Tinnitus and Hyperacusis. *Hear. Res.*, 1996. **97**: pp. 46–53.

224. Szczepaniak, W. S. and A. R. Møller, Evidence of Neuronal Plasticity within the Inferior Colliculus after Noise Exposure: A Study of Evoked Potentials in the Rat. *Electroenceph. Clin. Neurophysiol.*, 1996. **100**: pp. 158–164.

225. Terayama, Y., Y. Ishibe, and J. Matsushima, Rapidly Progressive Sensorineural Hearing Loss. *Acta Oto Laryng Suppl 456*, 1988: pp. 43–48.

226. Turner, J. G. and J. F. Willott, Exposure to an Augmented Acoustic Environment Alters Auditory Function in Hearing-Impaired DBA/2j Mice. *Hear. Res.*, 1998. **118**: pp. 101–113.

227. Ungerleider, L. G. and J. V. Haxby, "What" and "Where" in the Human Brain. *Curr. Opin. Neurobiol.*, 1994. **4**: pp. 157–165.

228. Vernon, J., The Loudness of Tinnitus. *Hear Speech Action*, 1976. **44**: pp. 17–19.

229. Wahlig, J. B., A. M. Kaufmann, J. Balzer, T. J. Lovely, and P. J. Jannetta, Intraoperative Loss of Auditory Function Relieved by Microvascular Decompression of the Cochlear Nerve. *Can J Neurol Sci.*, 1999. **26**(1): pp. 44–7.

230. Wall, P. D., The Presence of Ineffective Synapses and Circumstances Which Unmask Them. *Phil. Trans. Royal Soc. (Lond.)*, 1977. **278**: pp. 361–372.

231. Warr, W. B., Organization of Olivocochlear Systems in Mammals, in *The Mammalian Auditory Pathway: Neuroanatomy*, D. B. Webster, A. N. Popper, and R. R. Fay, Editors. 1992, Springer-Verlag: New York.

232. Warren, E. H. and M. C. Liberman, Effects of Contralateral Sound on Auditory-Nerve Responses. I. Contributions of Cochlear Efferents. *Hear. Res.*, 1989. **37**: pp. 89–104.

233. Warrick, J. W., Stellate Ganglion Block in the Treatment of Ménière's Disease and in the Symptomatic Relief of Tinnitus. *Br. J. Otol.*, 1969. **41**: pp. 699–702.

234. Whitaker, S., Idiopathic Sudden Hearing Loss. *Am. J. Otol.*, 1980. **1**: pp. 180–3.

235. Willott, J. F. and S. M. Lu, Noise Induced Hearing Loss Can Alter Neural Coding and Increase Excitability in the Central Nervous System. *Science*, 1981. **16**: pp. 1331–1332.

236. Willott, J. F., *Neurogerontology*. 1999, Springer Publishing Company: New York.

237. Willott, J. F., J. G. Turner, and V. S. Sundin, Effects of Exposure to an Augmented Acoustic Environment on Auditory Function in Mice: Roles of Hearing Loss and Age During Treatment. *Hear. Res.*, 2000. **142**: pp. 79–88.

238. Willott, J. F., T. H. Chisolm, and J. J. Lister, Modulation of Presbycusis: Current Status and Future Directions. *Audiol. Neurotol.*, 2001. **6**: pp. 231–249.

239. Winer, J. A., D. T. Larue, J. J. Diehl, and B. J. Hefti, Auditory Cortical Projections to the Cat Inferior Colliculus. *J. Comp. Neurol.*, 1998. **400**(2): pp. 147–74.

240. Winer, J. A., J. J. Diehl, and D. T. Larue, Projections of Auditory Cortex to the Medial Geniculate Body of the Cat. *J. Comp. Neurol.*, 2001. **430**(1): pp. 27–55.

241. Wladislavorsky-Wasserman, P., G. W. Facer, B. Mokri, and L. T. Kurland, Ménière's Disease: A 30 Year Epidemiologic and Clinical Study in Rochester, MN, 1951–1980. *Laryngoscope*, 1984. **94**: pp. 1098–1102.

242. Wu, W. J., S. H. Sha, J. D. McLaren, K. Kawamoto, Y. Raphael, and J. Schacht, Aminoglycoside Ototoxicity in Adult CBA, C57BL and BALB Mice and the Sprague-Dawley Rat. *Hear. Res.*, 2001. **158**: pp. 165–178.

243. Wu, W. J., S. H. Sha, and J. Schacht, Recent Advances in Understanding Aminoglycoside Ototoxicity and Its Prevention. *Audiol. Neurootol.*, 2002. **7**(171–4).

244. Yoshida, M., A. Rabin, and A. Anderson, Monosynaptic Inhibition of Pallidal Neurons by Axon Collaterals of Caudatonigral Fibers. *Exp. Brain Res*, 1972. **15**: pp. 33–347.

245. Yoshida, N. and M. C. Liberman, Sound Conditioning Reduces Noise-Induced Permanent Threshold Shift in Mice. *Hear. Res.*, 2000. **148**: pp. 213–219.

4

Pain

Introduction

Pain has many forms. It can be a warning of bodily injury that is important for avoiding injuries and therefore important for survival. Pain that is not caused by acute injuries can be a nuisance to a person or it can alter a person's entire life and affect his or her relatives in a major way.

Pain is purely subjective and it is often interpreted in an emotional context.[1] There are great individual differences in the way pain is perceived. The reaction to pain often varies from time to time within the same individual. Pain that persists for a long time reduces the quality of life, a factor that unfortunately has not attracted the attention of the medical community that it deserves. Pain can be the cause of suicide, thus an extreme indication of its effect on the quality of life. Quality of life considerations are important in medical treatment (or lack of treatment), and likewise play an important role in pain management.

The intensity of pain is difficult to measure, and it is difficult to objectively assess the degree of pain that a certain individual may experience. An individual's perception of pain depends on a combination of factors such as the individual's emotional state, the circumstances under which the pain was acquired, and whether it is perceived as a threatening signal. The perception of pain is affected by factors such as arousal, attention, distraction and/or expectation.

Pain is more related to suffering than to any other descriptions, but the degree of suffering varies between individuals and within a given individual.

---

[1] International Association for the Study of Pain (IASP) definition of pain: An unpleasant sensory and emotional experience associated with tissue damage or potential damage or described in such terms.

Factors such as helplessness and expectation are important for the perception of the degree of pain. There are few, if any, objective tests available for assessing the severity of pain. What matters for an individual person, as well as for the physician who treats the person, is the person's perception of the severity of the pain. The perception of pain depends on whether it is under the control of the individual (escapable) or not (inescapable). Visceral pain is often perceived to be more severe than pain that originates from the surface of the body.

It has been said that the only pain that is tolerable is someone's else's pain.[2]

Pain is different from many disorders in that it seldom exhibits any detectable morphological or chemical abnormalities. That means that the physician is often left to treat pain disorders based on the patient's description alone. Compounding this dilemma is the fact that the anatomical location to which pain is referred, may be different from the actual anatomical location of the physiological abnormalities that cause the pain.

Pain plays an important role in medicine, and is the most common reason for visits to the emergency room. Yet, the efforts to treat patients experiencing pain, and the basic research that is devoted to pain, is much less than what one would regard to be justified by the degree of suffering and the number of people who are affected by pain. Pain is in many ways an enigma, available treatments are often ineffective, and some treatments cause severe side effects.

Historically, pain was regarded as being caused by neural activity in the central nervous system (CNS) that was elicited by stimulation of pain receptors and transmitted in distinct pathways through the CNS. We now know that pain signals undergo far more complex processing in ascending and descending pathways than earlier assumed. It is now established knowledge that expression of neural plasticity[3] (see Chapter 1) plays an important role in many forms of pain. Pain that is caused by activation of nociceptors is subjected to change through expression of neural plasticity in the neural circuits that transmit and process pain signals and pain can be caused by neural activity that is generated in the CNS without any peripheral input.

Recent studies have targeted abnormal function of sensory and pain systems that often accompany severe chronic pain. We are beginning to understand some of the mechanisms that are responsible for abnormal sensations such as allodynia (pain from normally innocuous stimulation) or hyperpathia (exaggerated and prolonged response to stimulation of nociceptors). Such recent advances in

---

[2] René Leriche, French surgeon, 1879–1955

[3] Neural plasticity: Capability of the nervous system to be formed and molded in response to external or internal (body) factors. It consists of changes in synaptic efficacy, formation of new synapses or elimination of synapses; axonal sprouting or elimination of axons. Neural plasticity has many similarities with learning.

our knowledge about pain emphasize the great complexities of pain, especially pain that is not caused by stimulation of specific pain receptors.

Pain is a more complex sensation than other somatosensory sensations, yet it is usually not included in textbook descriptions of sensory systems. The sensation and perception of pain is much more variable than that of ordinary sensory stimuli. The diversity of the expression of pain and its cause is a severe obstacle for effective diagnosis and treatment. Current physician training is often inadequate and falls short of the goal of effective treatment and care for patients with severe pain.

If the saying "that possession of knowledge is power" then it is this author's hope that knowledge will provide the power to relieve people from their suffering of pain.

In this chapter, we will mainly focus upon pain conditions in which neural plasticity is involved in one way or another. The chapter begins with a description of different forms of pain and various specific ways of classifying pain conditions. Next, is a description of the anatomical and physiological basis for pain caused by stimulation of pain receptors; provided as a basis for understanding the pathophysiology of more complex forms of pain that are discussed in the remaining part of the chapter.

4.1   Different forms of pain

4.1.1   Classification of pain

Several different classifications of pain have been proposed. One such classification relates to the way pain is elicited and it divides pain into two large groups, namely:

1. Pain caused by stimulation of specific receptors known as nociceptors.
2. Pain that is not caused by stimulation of nociceptors and which often is referred to as central neuropathic pain.

Each of these two groups has several sub categories [211] (Fig. 4.1). Acute pain is elicited by activation of pain receptors in normal tissue, and that is known as physiological pain [34]. Pathophysiological pain, or clinical pain [19], is pain elicited by inflammatory processes and which is associated with peripheral and central sensitization. Central (neuropathic) pain includes pain caused by lesions or dysfunction in the CNS [13, 124].

It is generally difficult to distinguish between central and peripheral neuropathic pain. For example, post-herpetic neuralgia is both central and peripheral. The term central pain is usually used to describe post stroke or thalamic pain but all pain may have a central component.

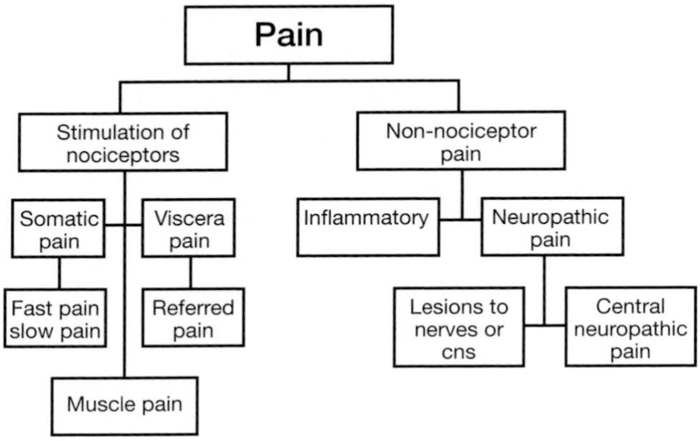

Pain

Stimulation of nociceptors

Non-nociceptor pain

Somatic pain

Viscera pain

Inflammatory

Neuropathic pain

Fast pain slow pain

Referred pain

Lesions to nerves or cns

Central neuropathic pain

Muscle pain

Fig. 4.1 An example of classification of different forms of pain [211].

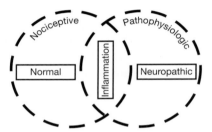

Fig. 4.2 A classification of pain that defines two main overlapping groups of pain namely: 1. Nociceptive pain that can occur as a normal condition and as a result of inflammatory processes; 2. Pathophysiological pain that includes neuropathic pain and pain caused by inflammatory processes [42].

Other investigators [13, 42] have defined three main types of pain namely:

1. Physiologic
2. Inflammatory and
3. Neuropathic pain.

Physiologic pain is the result of normal stimulation of nociceptors; inflammatory pain is caused by varying kinds of inflammation, of different kinds and by tissue damage (Fig. 4.2). Nociceptive pain and pathophysiological pain overlap, in that nociceptive pain includes both the normal condition of stimulation of nociceptors, and inflammatory pain. Inflammatory pain may be classified as a type of pathophysiologic pain together with neuropathic pain [42].

While inflammatory pain is caused by activation of pain receptors the tissue is not normal and therefore the pain is regarded as being pathophysiological

[13]. Neuropathic pain[4] is not caused by activation of specific pain receptors, but instead is caused by abnormal neural activity. Neuropathic pain is defined as pain caused by lesions to the nervous system such as to nerves [42] or to the CNS (central pain[5]). Lesions to the CNS that cause central pain include trauma, strokes and other causes of ischemia (insufficient blood supply to local regions of the CNS) [13, 124].

Central neuropathic pain[6] is not directly caused by or related to stimulation of pain receptors nor to verifiable lesions of nerves. Neither is it directly related to tissue damage nor altered chemical states of the body — but central pain is caused by abnormal neural activity in the CNS that may be caused by functional re-organization of the nervous system. The re-organization may have a wide range of causes. The re-organization may be elicited through expression of neural plasticity that is caused by activation of pain receptors. The term *central neuropathic pain* is used to distinguish this type of pain from other forms of pain caused by morphologically verifiable lesions of nerves and the CNS [210]. Central neuropathic pain is similar to other "phantom" sensations such as those from amputated limbs, paresthesia and tinnitus, which are caused by the expression of neural plasticity [79, 120].

These different categories of pain may interact with each other and, in particular, central neuropathic pain may be initiated by any one of the other types of pain.

In yet another classification, different forms of pain are divided according to what is believed to have caused the pain and its pathophysiology [210]. One such classification has five groups:

1. Pain caused by stimulation of somatic or visceral nociceptors
2. Neuralgia (severe pain in the course or distribution of peripheral or cranial nerves)
3. Muscle pain[7]
4. Neuropathic pain[8]
5. Pain caused by injuries to CNS structures.

---

[4] Neuropathic pain: The use of the term neuropathic pain is usually restricted to pain from peripheral and cranial nerves, although the term relates to pain from the nervous system in general.

[5] Central pain is pain caused by a lesion or dysfunction in the CNS [124] by the IASP.

[6] Central neuropathic pain is a subgroup of central pain that is caused by abnormal activity in the CNS that is a result of functional changes in the CNS.

[7] Muscle contractions can cause pain and a specific form of muscle pain is known as myofascial pain, referring to the involvement of both muscles and fascia.

[8] Theoretically, neuropathic pain is pain of the nervous system, but neurologists mostly use the term neuropathic pain for pain that is related to peripheral nerves and cranial nerves.

Pain may also be classified into acute and chronic pain [32, 110, 124]. The distinction between acute and chronic pain is arbitrary, but most authors (and the IASP) regard pain that lasts more than 6 months as chronic pain. Chronic pain may be caused by chronic diseases such as rheumatoid arthritis, but chronic pain is often not directly related to stimulation of pain receptors from tissue damage or altered chemical states of the body, but rather caused by re-organization of the CNS (central neuropathic pain). Often chronic pain is caused by a combination of these two causes.

Pain that is elicited by activation of pain receptors (physiological pain) is essential for maintaining a normal life, but it is difficult to understand what the advantages to the organism are from central neuropathic pain. While absence of the sensation of pain causes early deaths because of unnoticed injuries and lack of awareness of dangerous situations, central neuropathic pain is a serious and frequent condition that causes tremendous sufferings without any obvious advantages to the individual.

Pain may cause many different reactions and activate other parts of the nervous system such as the autonomic nervous system. Pain can often cause emotional (affective) reactions such as anger and fear, anxiety and depression, which can be related to an abnormal activation of limbic structures, especially the amygdala but also the cingulate gyrus [64, 105] and the periaqueductal gray (PAG) [88, 134]. This activation of the amygdala may occur through cortical routes from the dorsal thalamus [102], see [131]. Chronic pain is often accompanied by allodynia (pain from normally innocuous stimulation) or hyperpathia and hyperalgesia) (exaggerated and prolonged response to stimulation of nociceptors).

While pain that is caused by activation of nociceptors may not be regarded as a disorder of the nervous system, central neuropathic pain is definitely in the field of neurological disorders and discussion of this type of pain therefore belongs to the topic of this book. Acute pain is interesting from the view of this book because it often is a precursor to central neuropathic pain and because understanding of the anatomical and physiological basis for acute pain is essential for understanding the basis of other forms of pain.

The fact that neural activity elicited by stimulation of nociceptors can reach limbic structures through subcortical routes and cause uncontrollable emotional reactions is another reason to consider acute pain in the context of pathologies of the nervous system. We will therefore first discuss the anatomy and physiology of systems that process acute pain. Later in this chapter, we will devote considerable attention to the pathophysiology of other forms of pain, such as pain where neural plasticity plays an important role. Later in the chapter, we will discuss some treatments for pain and their mechanisms of action, as well as their side effects.

4.1.2   Causes of pain

Pain can have different causes and pain can be associated with many different body systems. The causes of *somatic* pain are different from that of *visceral* pain, which is more complex and often accompanied by *referred* pain. Additionally, pain from muscles and pain that is generated in the nervous system form separate groups:

1. Somatic pain
2. Visceral pain
3. Muscle pain
4. Nervous system pain

Some forms of pain have multiple causes, and it is often difficult to properly identify the anatomical location of the physiological abnormality that causes the pain. Expression of neural plasticity is involved in many forms of pain.

Somatic pain

Tissue damage, such as that caused by injuries from accidents, is a common cause of acute pain. Most forms of postoperative pain are from tissue damage caused by the surgical procedure. Ischemia can cause pain by stimulation of specific pain receptors, and is probably the cause of an aspect of muscle pain that occurs after strong and strenuous exercise (see p. 171). Inflammation of the skin, joints and muscles are also common causes of pain. Teeth are especially prone to produce pain, and this pain is often poorly defined (lacking the fast phase, see p. 193) and therefore perceived as aching. Muscle and joint pain such as in rheumatoid arthritis, are common causes of chronic pain.

Acute or chronic back pain is a typical example of a pain condition with complex causes [110]. Back pain is the most common medical complaint in industrial countries. Back or leg pain is often associated with mechanical (structural) spine abnormalities – such as bulging or herniated vertebral disks – and is often believed to be the cause of the common low back pain. The common low back pain is a typical example of a pain disorder that has many different forms and where the cause often is unknown. While compression of spinal nerve roots can cause back pain, not all back pain is caused by compression of spinal nerve roots [110, 201] and much is musculoskeletal in origin. In fact, similar abnormalities of vertebral discs that are observed in patients with back pain also occur in asymptomatic individuals [69]. Such a paradox occurs in other situations, such as in connection with vascular contact (compression) of cranial nerves [128] (see pp. 333, 334). Various kinds of spondylitic[9] diseases can cause back pain [201].

---

[9] Spondylitis: Inflammation of vertebra.

Spinal stenosis[10] is a frequent cause of back pain, but again the abnormalities that are revealed from MRI or CT scans are poorly correlated with the pain that the patients actually experience [110].

> The economic costs associated with back pain and traumatic nerve injuries are enormous, and it is a frequent cause of disability and early retirement for individuals. However, the difficulty in establishing a causal relationship between morphological changes and the perceived pain is a problem that has many aspects. Insurance problems are one such aspect, and the lack of detectable abnormalities may set the credibility of the patients in question and thereby prevent adequate treatment.

Pain associated with cancer is common, but it is normally caused by processes that are secondary to the cancers such as from expansion of structures that are invaded by tumors, obstruction of canals, inflammatory processes, thromboses, etc. [27]. Pain associated with cancer can also be caused by diagnostic and therapeutic intervention such as surgical operations and chemotherapy [28].

It has been shown that specific cells in the thalamus are involved in pain from ischemia of the heart [141]. Often ischemia of the heart occurs without specific pain sensations. The sensation from myocardial infarction is instead often limited to a general feeling of being unwell, and it may be associated with other diffuse symptoms such as nausea [135].

> In many cases, myocardial infarction does not present with any pain symptoms, but rather gives diffuse symptoms such as feeling ill, nausea etc. In a large population study (Framingham study) it was found that as many as 25% of the incidences of myocardial infarction were unrecognized by the individuals, and in one half of these the episodes were truly silent [85, 149].

Visceral pain

Visceral pain is caused by activation of visceral afferents in the viscera including the heart and carried to the spinal cord. Stretching of smooth muscles and ischemia are common causes of visceral pain from the gut. Cutting, crushing and burning of the bowel does not evoke pain but distension of muscles and hollow organs, stretching of organs, ischemia and necrosis generate pain. Chemical irritation of the gut can result in pain as can inflammation. It is debated whether there are specific pain receptors in the viscera and there is evidence that visceral pain is caused by activation of non-specific wide dynamic range receptors rather than specific nociceptors [24, 155].

---

[10] Spinal stenosis: Decrease in size of spinal foramina with subsequent compression of spinal nerves.

Visceral pain is not perceived in the same way as somatic pain, the location of the pain is less specific than somatic pain [32] and it often has an emotional component being inescapable [11]. Pain that originates in the viscera and the heart is often referred to locations on the surface of the body [32, 34, 149, 161] and such pain is known as referred pain.

Referred pain is an example of redirected (misdirected) spatial pain information [34]. Pain from the heart such as may occur in myocardial infarction is caused by ischemia, but the pain is not always localized to the heart [32] but, instead, referred to a different location on the body, most often the surface of the body [32, 149, 161]. The locations of such referral pain vary among individuals. Generally, pain from the heart is referred to the left arm, jaw and epigastrium; whereas pain from the gall bladder is often referred to right shoulder, hip and knee. Pain from organs in the pelvis is referred to dermatomes of T_{12}-L_1 (and perhaps L_2 and L_3), often bilaterally.

No secondary neuron in the spinal cord receives only visceral input and there are many fewer visceral afferents than somatic afferents [24]. These facts are most likely the reason why pain from viscera is poorly localized.

Muscle pain

Muscle pain is manifested in two main forms: pain that is associated with muscle contractions; and pain that occurs independently of muscle contractions. Naturally, muscle spasm and excessive exercise may cause pain in muscles from exhaustion, but many forms of muscle pain are not related to muscle contractions; in fact, several disorders with muscle referred pain are not associated with any detectable muscle pathologies. To complicate this issue, the description that patients provide of such pain varies greatly [139].

The term myalgia is used to describe muscle pain of many etiologies, including some that have cerebral involvement such as encephalomyelitis and chronic fatigue syndrome[11] (fibromyalgia).

Myofascial pain is a poorly defined syndrome that has few objective signs, and the diagnosis must be made based on the patient's history and the presence of trigger zones. Both muscles and fascia are assumed to be involved. Reduced range of motion, local pain and muscle tenderness are common symptoms that occur together with pain in the myofascial pain syndrome. The cause is uncertain but may be inflammatory; however, some investigators believe that it is psychosomatic. The myofascial pain syndrome is often associated with trigger

---

[11] Chronic fatigue syndrome is an ill-defined disorder that is more likely a group of disorders that involve many unknown factors together with stress, boredom, unsatisfying work or home conditions, etc.

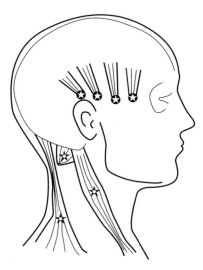

Fig. 4.3 Tension type headaches often involve trigger zones in the temporalis muscle (⊙), in suboccipital, sternocleidomastoid, and upper trapezius muscles (✭), from where pain attacks can be elicited. (Based on Simons and Mense 1998 [173].)

points from where pain attacks can be elicited (see p. 196). Referred pain is common in disorders of myofascial pain [71].

Pain from the nervous system

Neuropathic pain theoretically includes all forms of pain from the nervous system caused by morphological changes in the nervous system, or by functional changes such as those that result from expression of neural plasticity. Neurologists, however, usually only use the term neuropathic pain to describe pain that is associated with nerves. We will use the term central neuropathic pain to describe pain that is generated by abnormal activity in the CNS without input from nociceptors.

Pain associated with nerves is common, and the causes can be compression, trauma or inflammation. Compression and trauma (including surgically induced trauma) usually affect a single nerve, as do some forms of viral-induced inflammation. Many nerves can be affected such as in diabetes and alcohol-related neuropathies (see Chapter 2). Age-related changes may also cause pain that is related to nerves. Pain from the CNS may be caused by trauma or ischemia such as from strokes (infarcts or bleeding). Since subdural bleedings do not usually produce pain, pain that occurs together with intracranial bleeding (approximately 15% of all strokes are hemorrhagic) may be caused by the accompanying vasospasm.

Central neuropathic pain is fundamentally different from pain that is caused by stimulation of nociceptors, and its neural substrate is probably different from that of nociceptor elicited pain.

While plastic changes (expression of neural plasticity, see Chapter 1) in the nervous system undoubtedly play a role in most pain conditions, they play a dominating role in central neuropathic pain [210, 211]. Consequently, MRI and conventional neurophysiologic tests do not reveal any noticeable abnormalities in patients with central neuropathic pain. The patient's description of the symptoms is the only assessable measure of central neuropathic pain.

Phantom pain is a typical form of central neuropathic pain, where the sensation of pain is referred to a different location of the body than that where the neural activity that causes the pain is generated. Phantom pain is similar to other phantom sensations such as some forms of tinnitus [79, 80, 129] (see pp. 124, 340). Phantom pain is often accompanied by somatic sensations such as tingling [120]. Phantom limb sensations, consisting of pain, paresthesia and other abnormal sensations, are the clearest examples of sensations that are caused by abnormal neural activity in the CNS. The existence of phantom sensations clearly demonstrates that sensations can be generated in the CNS without peripheral stimulation and perceived as originating from a peripheral location [79].

> It has been hypothesized that the phantom limb syndrome occurring after amputation of a limb, is related to overstimulation that occurs during the surgical operation to amputate the limb. Some studies have shown that the risk of phantom limb symptoms can be reduced by applying local anesthetics to the peripheral nerve before surgery [4]. However, other studies have set that in doubt [118]. Pre-emptive analgesia may work better for surgery on extremities compared with surgery to viscera. Similar pre-treatment by epidural anesthesia has been tried for reduction of postoperative pain [202]. The efficiency of this treatment would support the hypothesis that neural plasticity is an important factor in such manifestations of pain.

Itch sensation

Itch has many similarities with pain and it may fit the IASP definition for pain. It is believed that similar (but not the same) receptors are involved in creating sensation of itch as those that mediate sensation of pain [168]. Itch can be caused by substances that are applied on, or into, the skin, and which elicit secretion of histamine that sensitize nerve fibers. That form of itch typically occurs from insect bites. Itch sensation can also be caused by CNS activity that occurs without stimulation of sensory receptors.

4.1.3   Assessment of pain intensity

The measurement of pain in a clinical setting is a difficult task because of its subjective nature, but is crucial in clinical management. In the office setting, it is common to ask patients to grade their current pain level on a 0–10 scale with 0 representing no pain and 10 the worst pain they have ever experienced, in order to provide a rough index of the severity of pain. In addition to this subjective rating, the examiner assesses the effect that the pain has had on limiting the patient's activities under the assumption that more severe pain tends to be associated with greater reductions in physical activities. The clinician also evaluates the psychological effects of pain including depression in order to obtain a better picture of the severity and the effects of the patient's pain.

In order to improve the reliability of pain estimates over time in a single patient, and to compare pain levels in different patients, a number of "quantitative" scales have been developed. For the rating of pain there are many common instruments. The patient may indicate pain levels on a Likert scale [67] of pain intensity; or may use a visual instrument such as Wong-Baker FACES scale in which the patient selects from a set of facial caricatures showing various levels of pain that most closely describes what they are feeling. In addition, there are a number of scales that assess quality of life and the impact of pain, such as the SF-36 and the Sickness Impact Profile (SIP) [15]. Other scales have been specifically designed to measure the severity of specific types of pain such as cancer pain, arthritis pain, back pain, etc. The advantage of using these semi-quantitative scales is that clinical testing has been performed to demonstrate the reliability of these scales and their correlation with clinical responses to therapy.

In patients that have difficulty communicating, other measurements such as autonomic function, blood pressure, restlessness, and agitation can also be used as indices of pain. For instance, it is common for anesthesiologists to use acute elevations in the patient's blood pressure as an indicator that the patient may be experiencing pain and hence require appropriate anesthesia.

4.2   Organization of normal pain systems

This section describes the anatomical and physiological bases for nociceptor mediated pain. While the systems that mediate pain elicited by stimulation of nociceptors have similarities with the somatosensory system, we prefer to regard it as a separate subsystem of the somatosensory system. In this book, we will regard the system that mediates and processes somatic pain from stimulation of nociceptors as the *non-classical* somatosensory system (also known as the anteriorlateral system). We will stress the difference between the anatomical connections and functional connections, and we will emphasize the role of neural plasticity as a cause of the variability of the neural connections and the subsequent variability in processing of pain stimuli.

4.2.1   Nociceptor pain

The anatomy of pain systems is more complex than that of the classical sensory systems (for a description of classical sensory systems, see Møller, 2003 [131]) and the pain pathways connect to more parts of the CNS than the sensory systems. The anatomical basis for pain elicited by stimulation of nociceptors has been studied extensively in animals and much of our knowledge therefore, is based on the anatomy of animals. Fewer studies have been done in humans and such studies have revealed varying degrees of difference between the neuroanatomy of humans and that of animals. It is therefore important to be aware of the source of information that is to be applied to humans.

Nociceptors

While sensory receptors sense innocuous stimuli, pain receptors (nociceptors) sense noxious stimuli. Pain receptors are located in the skin, muscles, joints, tendons and internal (visceral) organs. The coverings of peripheral nerves have pain receptors, but the brain itself and the spinal cord do not have pain receptors. The dura mater and certain cerebral vessels have nociceptors. Temperature receptors that respond to heat and cold are regarded as nociceptors because they mediate a noxious stimulation, while warmth and cool receptors belong to sensory receptors because these temperatures are regarded as innocuous stimuli. For more detailed descriptions of the function of pain receptors, see Møller, 2003 [131].

Innervation of pain receptors

The fibers that innervate nociceptors have smaller diameters than those that innervate sensory receptors that respond to innocuous stimulation and proprioceptors. Some pain fibers belong to the Aδ group (diameter 1–5 μm and conduction velocity of 6–30 m/sec) and other groups are unmyelinated (C fibers, diameter, 0.2–2 μm; conduction velocity 0.5–1 m/sec) (Fig. 4.4). (Aβ fibers innervate mainly sensory receptors that respond to innocuous stimulation, and proprioceptors. Aβ fibers have conduction velocities from 40 to 60 m/sec and diameters of 8–12 μm. Aα fibers are the fastest conducting nerve fibers and mainly innervate muscles.)

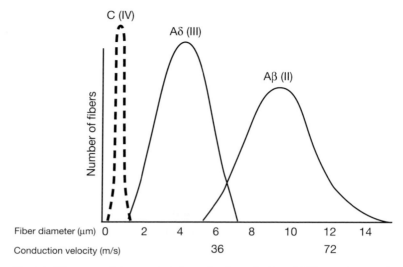

Fig. 4.4 Diameter of the axons and conduction velocity of different classes of nerve fibers.

A recent study [190] showed that the conduction velocity of C-fibers in the spinothalamic tract (STT) in humans was 2.9 +/− 0.8 m/sec, while the conduction velocity of the peripheral path of C fibers are 1.2+/−0.2 and 1.1+/− 0.1 for the upper and lower limbs respectively. Another study [74] found the average conduction velocity of Aδ was 15.6 m/s. Microneurography has shown a range of conduction velocities from 5 to 30 m/s for Aδ fibers [194].

The difference in diameter between fibers conducting pain and other sensations is important clinically. During the process of nerve block, a local anesthetic such as Lidocaine, Procaine, or Bupivicaine is placed near a nerve, and diffusion carries the local anesthetic toward the nerve. These agents block sodium channels and hence the active process of impulse propagation. Smaller diameter fibers have shorter space constants and hence shorter distances over which the impulse can propagate passively. Thus, pain fibers (Aδ and C fibers) are affected before larger fibers carrying motor, sensory and proprioceptive information.

4.2.2   Visceral pain

Stretching of viscera and smooth muscles elicits sensations of pain whereas, for instance, cutting with a sharp knife or burning does not elicit any pain sensation. Not all activation of pain receptors in visceral organs reaches consciousness; only activation of pain receptors in the peritoneum and abdominal wall normally reach consciousness.

Most visceral nociceptors are free nerve endings that are chemoreceptors or stretch receptors [24]. The chemoreceptors are sensitive to substances from inflammation or ischemia and are thus regarded as being nociceptors. Other receptors in the viscera are mechanoreceptors (stretch receptors), and they can respond to innocuous stimulation but they can convey sensation of pain if strongly stimulated. Some of the mechanoreceptors in visceral organs are Pacinian corpuscles, but their exact anatomical role and functions are not yet fully known [17]. Activation of these receptors is perceived as deep touch.

4.2.3   Central pain pathways

Pain pathways are usually regarded as belonging to the somatosensory system [131], but the CNS pathways of pain (the anteriorlateral system) has both similarities and differences with the part of the somatosensory system that mediates innocuous sensations. In this book we regard the pain pathways to be the non-classical somatosensory pathways. Like sensory systems, central pain pathways consist of ascending and descending pathways. The ascending pathways communicate information from the periphery to central structures that provide the conscious reactions to pain stimuli, as well as unconscious reactions. The descending pathways communicate information from central structures to neurons along the ascending pathways, including the dorsal horn of the spinal cord and sensory nuclei of the brainstem (mainly the trigeminal nucleus). The descending pathways can modulate the neural traffic in these ascending pathways. In addition to these ascending and descending pathways, the autonomic nervous system plays a role in the processing of pain information in the spinal cord. The sympathetic nervous system can modulate the sensitivity of nociceptors (mainly sensitize), and it can affect the synaptic threshold and synaptic efficacy of neurons in the spinal cord. Diffusion of neuroactive substances in the gray matter of the spinal cord can affect spinal cord synaptic transmission of pain. (For information about the pharmacology of the dorsal horn, see [213, 214].)

Neural circuitry in the spinal cord

Pain fibers that enter the spinal cord in dorsal roots make synaptic contact with cells in the dorsal horn (Fig. 4.5), and most of the axons of these cells cross the midline at the segmental level and ascend in the anteriorlateral tracts [17]. Most C fibers terminate mainly on cells in lamina II[12] of the dorsal horn (Fig. 4.5). The short axons of these cells make synaptic contact with cells in lamina I. (Laminas I and II is also known as the substantia gelatinosa.) Aδ fibers

---

[12] Rexed's classification [157].

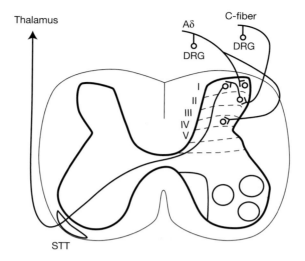

Fig. 4.5 Illustration of the termination of Aδ fibers and C fibers in the dorsal horn. DRG: Dorsal root ganglia. Lamina I and II are also known as substantia gelatinosa.

terminate on cells in layer I and collateral fibers of these Aδ fibers terminate in lamina IV and V of the dorsal horn [17]. Some of the interneurons in lamina I send collaterals (secondary branches) to segments above and below their own segment traveling in the tract of Lissauer (dorsolateral fasciculus), which give rise to fibers of the anteriorlateral tract [17] (Fig. 4.6). Some cells are modality specific and others are polymodal [37], meaning that they receive input from nociceptors that respond to different modalities of noxious stimuli.

Input from large diameter (Aβ) fibers that innervate sensory receptors that respond to innocuous stimuli in the skin muscles and joints converge on cells in lamina III, IV and V [37] (Fig. 4.7). Since the input from these Aβ fibers is inhibitory on the cells that respond to noxious stimulation, innocuous sensory input can modulate (inhibit) conduction of pain impulses in the dorsal horn (see p. 181). Neurons in lamina I and in lamina V send axons that cross the midline and ascend in the STT (Fig. 4.7).

When circuitry of the spinal cord is illustrated as it is in Figs. 4.5–4.7, it must be remembered that such description is highly simplified. It shows mainly connections from receptors to the spinal cord and from the spinal cord to supraspinal structures and it omits most of the internal connections in the spinal cord. Each cell has many inputs and in fact most of the synaptic connections to cells in the spinal horns originate in other cells in the spinal horn of the same or other segments of the spinal cord. This internal circuitry is very important for processing of pain information but its anatomy and physiology

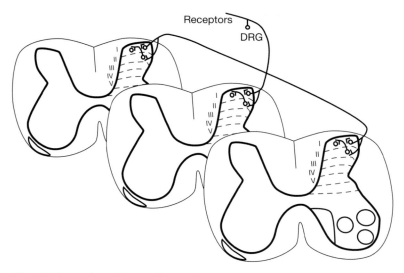

Fig. 4.6 Illustration of how collateral interneurons in lamina I terminate in spinal segments above and below the segment where their innervation enters (tract of Lissauer)

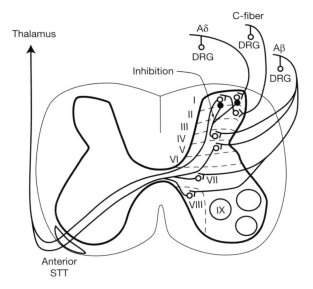

Fig. 4.7 Schematic illustration of the connections through which innocuous sensory input mediated by large myelinated (Aβ) fibers can inhibit pain neurons in lamina I that receive noxious input from Aδ fibers and C fibers via interneurons and which give rise to axons of the STT.

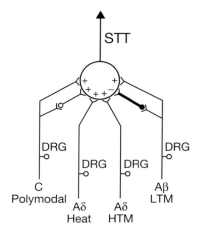

Fig. 4.8 Schematic drawing of a WDR neuron showing the different kinds of inputs that converge on a WDR neuron. LTM: Low threshold mechanoreceptors; HTM: High threshold mechanoreceptors. (Adapted from Price [147].)

is poorly understood with a few exceptions such as the inter-segmental connections illustrated in Fig. 4.6.

Wide dynamic range neurons

Some of the neurons in lamina IV–V are known as the wide dynamic range (WDR) neurons [17]. WDR neurons receive input from several types of receptors including high and low threshold mechanoreceptors through Aδ and Aβ fibers, heat receptors (Aδ fibers) and polymodal receptors that are innervated by C fibers and responding to different kinds of noxious stimulation (Fig. 4.8) [172]. The axons of the WDR neurons cross the midline and ascend in the anterior STT (see p. 168). The WDR neurons are important for mediating pain signals. Due to their involvement in the generation of central neuropathic pain, and their ability to change the way they respond as an expression of neural plasticity, WDR neurons have received significant attention [146].

Trigeminal system

The nerve fibers that innervate pain receptors in the skin of the face and inside the mouth, including the teeth, travel mainly in the fifth and ninth cranial nerves, and make synaptic contact with cells in the nucleus of the trigeminal nerve (Fig. 4.9). The axons of these cells cross the midline and ascend to the thalamus. The sensory fibers of the trigeminal nerve that mediate innocuous stimulation enter the most rostral parts of the nucleus; whereas pain fibers enter the more caudal parts of the nucleus, which extend into the upper part of the spinal cord (Fig. 4.9).

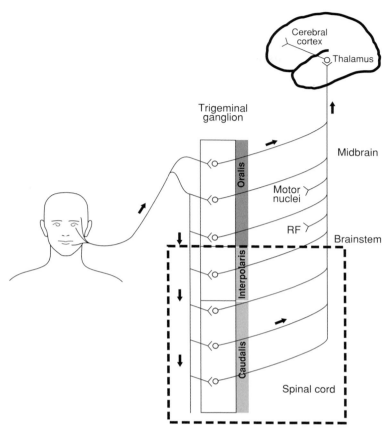

Fig. 4.9 Pain pathways from the head of the trigeminal nucleus (indicated by dashed rectangle). RF: Reticular formation. (Adapted from Sessle, 1986 [169].)

Visceral pain

The nerve fibers that innervate nociceptors in visceral organs in the lower abdomen including the reproductive organs (visceral afferents) follow sympathetic nerves and enter the spinal cord as dorsal root fibers in the T_{12}-L_4 dorsal roots (Fig. 4.10). Pain fibers from visceral organs send collaterals to several segments of the spinal cord, therefore complicating a determination of exactly where the pain originates. At each segment of the spinal cord visceral pain fibers make collaterals that terminate on the same cells in lamina I of the dorsal horn that receive input from pain receptors in the skin (through Aδ fibers). Other collaterals of the visceral pain fibers terminate on cells in the intermediolateral column of the spinal horn [17]. These cells connect to sympathetic efferents and to motoneurons that innervate skeletal muscles. The intermediolateral column is only present from T_{12} to L_2 [17].

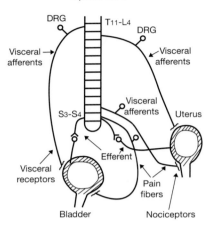

Fig. 4.10 Visceral afferent innervation in the lower body and motor (efferent) innervation. The afferent pathways of visceral nociceptors in the bladder, and those of the neck of the bladder (including the prostate gland and the uterus) are shown together with motor innervation of the bladder and the uterus.

There is one exception to this pattern of innervation of visceral nociceptors, however, namely the nociceptive innervation of the neck of the bladder, the prostate, the cervix of the uterus and the distal rectum. The fibers of these nociceptors travel together with parasympathetic pelvic nerves and enter the spinal cord as sacral spinal dorsal nerves (S_2-S_4) [17] (Fig. 4.10).

4.2.4   Ascending pathways from the spinal cord

The ascending pain pathways are the anterior lateral tracts consisting of the STT, the spinoreticular tract and the spinomesencephalic tracts. The STT, which is regarded as the most important of the anterior lateral tracts, consists of a lateral and a medial part, the functions of which differ. The STT and the spinomesencephalic tracts mainly are crossed pathways while the spinoreticular tract is bilateral.

The spinothalamic tract

The fibers of the STT in humans originate mostly in interneurons in lamina I and V ([17], Kuric 1949, cited by Craig and Dostrovsky 1999 [37]) but additionally the axons of WDR neurons in deeper layers of the spinal horn contribute. These axons cross the midline at the segmental level and ascend as the STT towards the thalamus (Fig. 4.11).

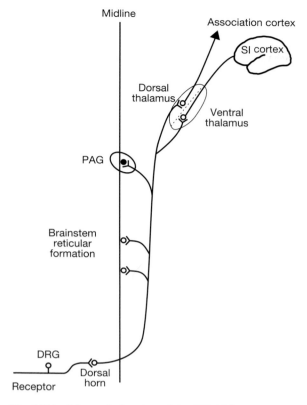

Fig. 4.11A Schematic drawing of the STT. Main connections from dorsal root fibers to the dorsal and ventral thalamic nuclei and somatosensory cortices. Note the collaterals from the spinothalamic tract to the brainstem reticular formation and the periaqueductal gray (PAG).

The STT ascends in two fiber tracts; the dorsal and ventral portions that ascend as the lateral and anterior funiculi of the spinal cord, respectively. Some fibers of the anterior STT originate in the WDR neurons in lamina IV and V of the spinal cord. These WDR neurons (Fig. 4.8) receive input from both mechanoreceptors and nociceptors in the skin. The cells of lamina VII and VIII that send fibers in the anterior STT are polysensory and therefore more complex than cells in other lamina of the spinal cord (Fig. 4.7). These cells have polysynaptic innervation by converging sensory fibers that respond to both innocuous and noxious stimuli. Some of these cells probably also integrate motor and sensory information [37].

The targets of the anterior STT are the lateral, medial and intermediate parts of the ventral thalamus (ventral posterior lateral (VPL), the ventral posterior medial (VPM), ventral posterior inferior (VPI) nuclei and several nuclei in the

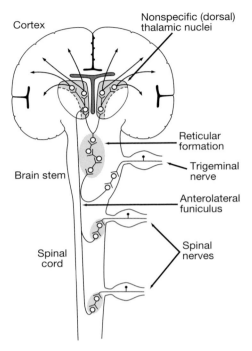

Fig. 4.11B Anatomical location of the components of the spinothalamic tract including the trigeminal system [131].

medio-dorsal thalamus (Figs. 4.11A & B) [37]. The anterior portion of the STT gives off collateral fibers to several structures in the brainstem (Fig. 4.12). The neurons of the VPL and VPI project to the primary somatosensory cortex (SI), and this pathway is likely responsible for the fast phase of pain (see p. 186) that is clearly localized. The dorsomedial thalamic neurons connect to neurons in the reticular formation and in the PAG[13].

The fibers of the lateral part of the STT mainly originate in cells in lamina I of the dorsal horn, and project to the medial and posterior thalamus. The axons of these cells project to the insula and to some extent to area 3a of the SI [37] (Fig. 4.13). Activity in unmyelinated C fibers reaches both SI and SII on the contralateral side, and SII on the ipsilateral side (Fig. 4.14) [84]. The fact that pure C fiber activation reaches the SI cortex may imply that activation of C fibers may produce a sensation of pressure or touch, in addition to a sensation of pain.

---

[13] The PAG (also known as the central gray) surrounds the aqueduct interconnecting the third and fourth ventricle. It is involved in (suppression of) pain and it has many other functions. The PAG connects to the amygdala, hypothalamus, thalamus, locus coeruleus and other structures.

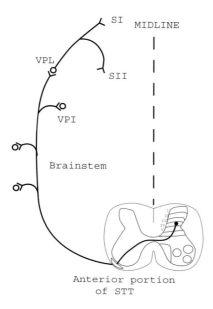

Fig. 4.12 Ascending projections of the anterior portion of the STT from neurons in lamina IV–V of the spinal horn. VPI: Ventral posterior inferior (nuclei of thalamus); VPL: Ventral posterior lateral (nuclei of thalamus); SI: Primary somatosensory cortex; SII: Secondary somatosensory cortex [37].

A recent study [74] showed that the Aδ fibers of the STT, which mediate a sharp pricking sensation, mainly project bilaterally to SII cortices with a simultaneous projection to the contralateral SI in only some (5 of 18) of the individuals tested (Fig. 4.14). The arrival of activity at the ipsilateral SII was later (18 ms) than at the contralateral SII. This indicates that the pathways to SII neurons could involve fibers of the corpus callosum or a slower pathway from the thalamus.

Other ascending tracts

Of the other ascending tracts of the anterior lateral system, the spinoreticular tract (Fig. 4.15) is largely bilateral and its main target is the reticular formation of the brainstem. The main target of the spinomesencephalic tract (Fig. 4.16) is the PAG. This means that only the STT (Fig. 4.11) has connections to the ventral thalamus and, from there, fibers connect to the SI.

Figure 4.17 shows a simplified summary diagram of the ascending central portions of pain pathways, emphasizing that stimulation of nociceptors produces two kinds of information, namely objective ("what") and spatial ("where") information. Figure 4.17 also shows some of the regions of the brain that can be reached by neural activity that is elicited by painful stimuli. The

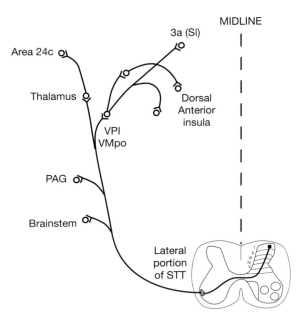

Fig. 4.13 Projections of the lateral portion of the STT from cells in lamina I of the dorsal horn. VPI: Ventral posterior inferior (nuclei of thalamus); VMpo: Ventromedial posterior oralis (nuclei of thalamus); SI: Primary somatosensory cortex [37].

nuclei of the ventral thalamus also receive input from the somatosensory system via the medial lemniscus, providing spatial information regarding skin stimulation.

It should be remembered that the fibers of all the anterior lateral tracts collateralize at many locations along their ascending paths. Many of these collaterals terminate in the reticular formation of the brainstem, thus affecting wakefulness.

Ascending for visceral pain pathways

The visceral afferents of the cranial nerves terminate in the solitary nucleus, and those entering the spinal cord through dorsal roots ascend in the spinothalamic and the spinoreticular tracts [17]. Visceral afferents participate in autonomic reflexes such as the vomiting reflex generated from irritation of the gastric mucosa (as well as the vestibular system). Similarly, the emptying reflexes of the bladder and the rectum are mediated by stretch receptors, the afferents of which enter the spinal cord at S_3-S_4 [17] (Fig. 4.10). Since these reflexes can be suppressed voluntarily, their pathways must receive input from high

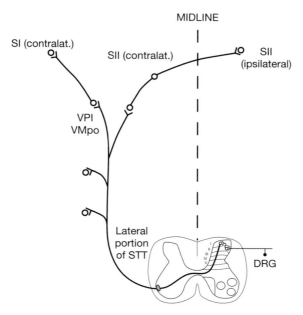

Fig. 4.14 Schematic illustration of the projection of unmyelinated C fibers. Notice that the projection to SII is bilateral but only the SI area receives input from C fibers [84].

CNS centers. This is contrary to many other autonomic reflexes that cannot be modulated voluntarily.

It is important to keep in mind that most of the knowledge about these ascending pain pathways was obtained using anatomical methods of investigation. Much less is known about the functional importance of specific tracts, which depends on the efficacy of the synapses with which they terminate on their target cells including those of the cerebral cortex. The synaptic efficacy is subjected to changes through the expression of neural plasticity that can be initiated by many factors (see Chapter 1). Neural connections (sprouting and elimination of axons and synapses) may also occur because of expression of neural plasticity.

Differences between nociceptive and visceral pain circuits

Pain impulses from lamina I and II of the dorsal horn can take two different paths to the midbrain pain circuits [111]. Visceral pain and other forms of pain that are not under the control of the individual seem mostly to project to the ventrolateral parts of the PAG, whereas brief pain that is caused by stimulation of superficially located pain receptors mostly project to the dorsolateral and

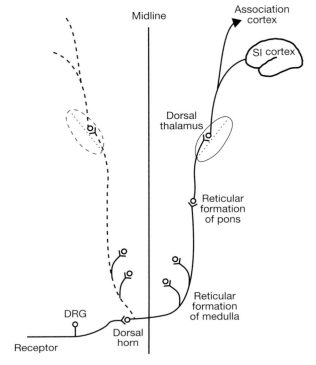

Fig. 4.15 Spinoreticular tract [131].

lateral parts of the PAG. While the dorsolateral and lateral parts of the PAG mediate reduced responsiveness to noxious signals, excitation of the sympathetic nervous system and increased motor activity (fight-or-flight response) the neurons in the ventrolateral column of the PAG coordinate instead inhibit sympathetic activity and decrease motor activity [134]. The reaction to pain stimuli that activate ventrolateral parts of the PAG is associated with recuperation such as after intense exercise or in connection with chronic pain that are perceived to be an inescapable stress [87, 88]. Inescapable pain is also related to depression or depression-like symptoms, and it activates the hypothalamo-pituitary-adrenal axis [11].

It has been suggested that the separation of pain circuits in the PAG may be related to the types of fibers that provide the input to these two parts of the PAG. Visceral pain fibers [155] are mainly C fibers whereas superficial pain to a greater extent is mediated by Aδ fibers. The pain sensations mediated by Aδ fibers (pricking pain) is bearable, whereas that mediated by C fibers is less bearable.

The ventral PAG receives more input from the anterior hypothalamus than the dorsolateral and lateral parts of the PAG. Considering the extensive input to the

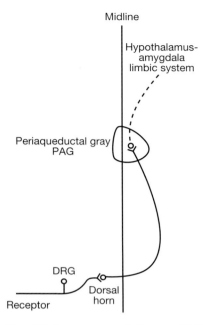

Midline

Hypothalamus-
amygdala
limbic system

Periaqueductal gray
PAG

DRG

Dorsal
horn

Receptor

Fig. 4.16 Spinomesencephalic tract [131].

hypothalamus from spinal pain circuits, these hypothalamic-PAG connections are likely to be important for the reactions to pain stimuli. There are also here ample possibilities of influence of expression of neural plasticity through the hypothalamic-PAG circuit.

4.2.5   *Descending pathways*

There are at least three separate descending systems that can modulate the transmission of pain signals, and which originate in supraspinal structures. Primarily this modulation occurs by influencing neurons in lamina I and II of the dorsal horn. Two of these pathways involve the PAG and connect to dorsal horn neurons through at least one interneuron in the rostral ventromedial medulla (RVM) (Fig. 4.18), and in the dorsolateral pontomesencephalic tegmentum (DLTP) (Fig. 4.19) [49]. The vagus nerve may also be regarded as a descending pathway that can modulate pain [54, 90].

Rostral ventromedial medulla pathway

The nuclei of the RVM include the nucleus raphe magnus and some parts of the reticular formation. The connections from the RVM mainly target neurons in lamina I and II of the dorsal horn [6] (neurons in lamina I and II mainly receive input from nociceptors, see p. 163) (Figs. 4.5 and 4.7).

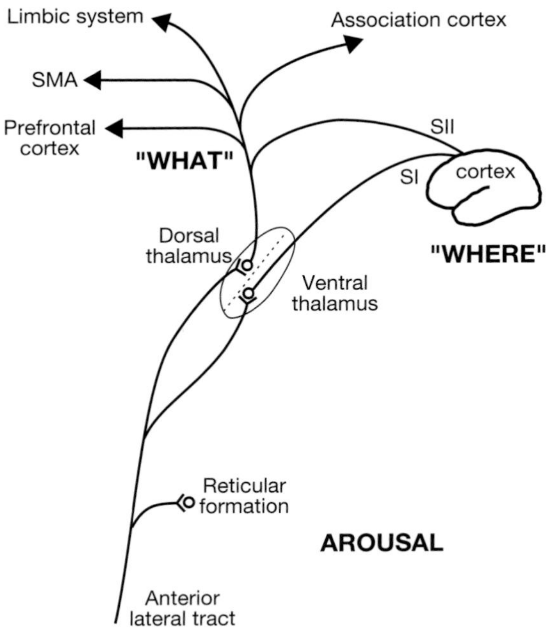

Fig. 4.17 Simplified diagram of pathways involved in mediating the sensation of nociceptor pain. Central pain pathways project to primary cortices conveying spatial ("where") information. Objective ("what") information can reach many different parts of the CNS such as the prefrontal cortex, supplementary motor area (SMA) and the amygdala. Information that travels in the anterior lateral pathways can also reach the reticular formation and thereby contribute to arousal [131].

Periaqueductal gray pathway

The PAG, in addition to receiving ascending input from pain receptors (see p. 172) through the mesencephalic system (Fig. 4.16), also receives input from the frontal lobe via the hypothalamus, and from the amygdala. Several brainstem structures, such as nucleus cuneiformis, the pontomedular reticular formation, locus coeruleus and other catecholaminergic nuclei, also provide input to the PAG [66].

Dorsolateral pontomesencephalic tegmentum pathways

The dorsolateral pontomesencephalic tegmentum pathways (DLPT) connect the PAG with dorsal horn neurons through interneurons located in the dorsolateral tegmentum (Fig. 4.19). This pathway projects to dorsal horn neurons and exerts mainly excitatory influence on dorsal horn pain neurons.

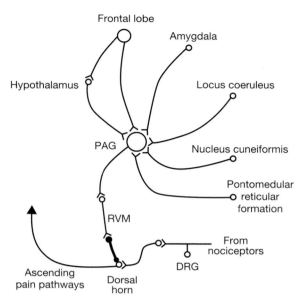

Fig. 4.18 Input to the PAG and pathways through which modulation of transmission of pain signals by the PAG can occur through the RVM pathway.

NA-Serotonin pathway

As shown above, ascending pain activity can be modulated in the spinal cord by input from the DLTP and RVM systems (Figs. 4.18, 4.19). A third system that can modulate the ascending activity that is activated by stimulation of noci-ceptors, is a norepinephrine-serotonin (NA[14]-serotonin) pathway that originates in the brainstem reticular formation. Fibers of this pathway also communicate motor signals (p. 263) (Fig. 4.20), and it is at times described as a separate NA-Serotonin pathway. Other descriptions may combine the NA-serotonin pathway together with the reticulospinal (motor) pathways (see p. 182).

The descending pathways that terminate in pain neurons in the dorsal horn are mainly inhibitory, thus suppressive of pain, but they can also have excitatory effect.

4.2.6   The vagus nerve

The vagus nerve is not normally included in descending pain pathways, but recent studies have shown its importance for pain control. The anatomy of

---

[14] NA (Norepinephrine) is a catecholamine, as is epinephrine and dopamine, common neural transmitters that are often associated with "stress".

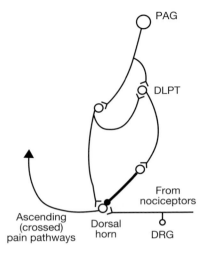

Fig. 4.19 Schematic diagram showing the dorsolateral pontomesencephalic tegmentum pathway (DLTP).

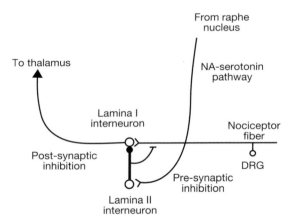

Fig. 4.20 Schematic diagram showing the descending pathways from raphe nucleus (NA-serotonin pathway) that terminate on pain neurons in the dorsal horn [34].

the vagus nerve is complex and it has both descending and ascending sensory fibers and pain fibers, in addition to its major content of parasympathetic fibers that innervate the lower body. Parts of the vagus nerve have been shown to be involved in pain and pain control. There is evidence that the vagus nerve carries information from pain receptors in various parts of the body and connects to STT afferents in the cervical spinal cord [9, 51]. Vagal afferents project to neurons that can exert both inhibitory and excitatory influence on nociceptive processing in the spinal cord, via bulbospinal pathways [9, 154]. It is believed that activation of

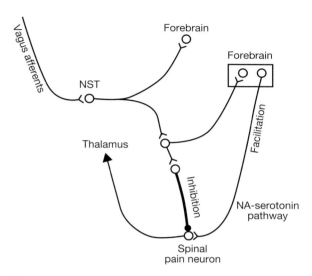

Fig. 4.21 Schematic illustration of the innervation by the vagus nerve of organs in the lower abdomen involving the NST showing how these connections can have inhibitory influence on spinal pain neurons and how they connect with neurons in the forebrain.

vagus afferents produces vague sensations such as feeling ill rather than distinct pain sensations.

The vagus nerve projects to neurons in the nucleus of the solitary tract (NST) (secondary neurons) (Fig. 4.21), and these NST neurons connect to neurons in many brainstem nuclei including those that are important for peripheral control of pain through the locus coeruleus-nucleus raphe magnus system (NA-serotonin system, see Fig. 4.23) [9, 54]. Facilitatory influence on spinal cord pain neurons are probably mediated through a longer and more complex route from NST through the forebrain to the dorsal horn neurons, probably involving the RVM system of ON and OFF cells (Fig. 4.16) [9]. These pathways may mediate the suppression of pain from electrical stimulation of the vagus nerve that has been observed [90]. The vagus nerve also seems to be involved in mediating the analgesic effect of opioids, and vagotomy decreases the analgesic effect of systemically administered morphine [54, 154]. The vagus nerve innervates many organs and, for example, the pain reduction from stimulation of the vagina as shown in animal experiments [39] and in humans [204], may be mediated by the vagus nerve. Electrical stimulation of the vagus nerve suppresses experimental pain [90] and electrical stimulation of the vagus nerve is in clinical use for treatment of pain [54] (and depression and epilepsy).

4.2.7   Cortical pain circuits

Pain pathways project to several cortical regions through dorsal and ventral routes. The STT and the spinoreticular pathways project to the somatosensory cortex similar to that of the somatosensory system (see p. 85).

The involvement of limbic structures, especially the cingulate gyrus, is supported by the beneficial effect of cingulotomy [64]. The fact that recordings from subdural electrodes placed over the cingulate gyrus in humans show responses to experimentally induced painful stimulation of the skin [105] indicates that nociceptive input reaches the anterior cingulate gyrus (Brodmann's area 24). The involvement of the cingulate cortex can explain the emotional components of pain especially central neuropathic pain.

4.3   Physiology of nociceptor pain

Perception of acute pain typically has two phases, one sharp perception that occurs with a short delay, and a diffuse and burning second sensation that occurs later (Fig. 4.22). The sharp perception is closely referred to the location of the stimulus on the body surface, whereas the location of the later phase of pain is less well defined. The sharp initial phase of pain sensation is mediated by small myelinated (Aδ) fibers, and the sensation of burning pain is mediated by (unmyelinated) C fibers. Interruption of the myelinated fibers causes pain perception that lacks the first phase, and conduction block of the C fibers eliminates the burning phase of the pain (Fig. 4.22).[15]

The sensitivity of nociceptors can be modulated (increased, peripheral sensitization) by liberation of norepinephrine from sympathetic nerve endings that are located near the receptors. Propagation of neural activity in pain fibers in the opposite direction to which it normally travels (antidromic activation) can cause release of substance P (SP) at the peripheral termination of the fibers, and this may cause release of histamine that can cause edema and pain. That process is unlikely to occur normally, but it may play a role in certain pathological situations.

4.3.1   Spinal cord processing of pain signals

Pain signals that enter the spinal cord are processed in a complex network of neurons in the dorsal horn of the spinal cord. Pain from the face, mouth and throat, which is mediated by the trigeminal and glossopharyngeal nerves,

---

[15] Compression of a mixed nerve first affects large fibers causing numbness with preserved pain sensation, while (light) local anesthetics affect unmyelinated fibers more than myelinated fibers causing interruption of pain transmission with preserved sensation of touch.

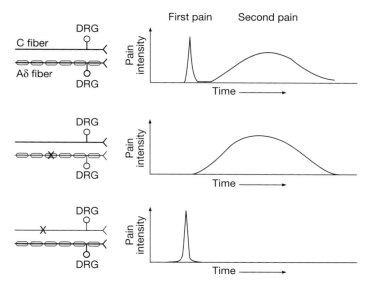

Fig. 4.22 Stimulation of nociceptors causes an initial fast, and a later slow component of pain sensation. The pain signals that cause these two different types of sensation are carried in two different types of nerve fibers (Aδ and C fibers) [131].

is processed in similar networks in the sensory nucleus of the trigeminal nerve in the brainstem and upper spinal cord.

The network of neurons in the dorsal horn that are involved in transmission of pain signals to supraspinal structures is complex, and the processing that occurs in these neurons is incompletely understood. It is known, however, that interneurons in the dorsal horn and the trigeminal nucleus play an important role in the modulation of transmission of pain impulses because they receive inhibitory as well as excitatory input from supraspinal sources (see pp. 181, 182). Input from sensory receptors in the skin can modulate the transmission of pain signals in the dorsal horn of the spinal cord and in the trigeminal nucleus. The function of these interneurons is affected by chemicals such as SP and other potent neuroactive substances (such as norepinephrine and serotonin) that reach these interneurons through diffusion in the gray matter of the spinal cord or the trigeminal nucleus.

Peripheral control of pain

Activity in large fibers (Aβ) that innervate low threshold sensory receptors in the skin exert an inhibitory influence (through an inhibitory interneuron) on the cells in lamina I and II of the dorsal horn of the spinal cord that processes pain information (Fig. 4.7). Activity in collaterals of large diameter (Aβ) sensory fibers also provides inhibitory influence on WDR neurons in the dorsal horn, likely via an inhibitory interneuron. Decreasing or elimination of the normal spontaneous input from large (Aβ) fibers may therefore increase the pain from stimulation of pain receptors, and in some situations it can even cause sensation of pain without stimulation of the specific pain receptors in the skin.

> Blowing air on a spot that has been hurt by heat is a natural way of accomplishing inhibition of pain pathways from stimulation of sensory receptors in the skin and activating Aβ fiber. Transdermal electric nerve stimulation (TENS) [205], using low intensity and high frequency electrical impulses, likely alleviate acute pain in a similar way. Loss of input from Aβ fibers can occur, for example, in connection with skin lesions from trauma or from surgical treatment, where the outer layers of the skin are removed (for example for removal of tattoos). Electrical stimulation (TENS) can provide inhibitory input from Aβ fibers to pain circuits in the dorsal horn, and thereby alleviate such pain. TENS is also beneficial on long term treatment of pain through expression of neural plasticity (see p. 164).

Central control of pain

The processing of pain signals in the spinal cord is under considerable control from supraspinal structures. This is a normal function that is important for the control of pain, and it offers a way to reduce nociceptor pain. The central influence on the transmission and processing of pain signals in the spinal cord is much more extensive than the processing of innocuous sensory information. Several different supraspinal structures exert strong control of pain transmission at the segmental level of the spinal cord (Figs. 4.18, 4.19). Similar control of pain transmission occurs in the trigeminal nucleus.

The PAG is an important source of descending activity that can modulate transmission of pain signals that are elicited by activation of nociceptors. Descending activity from the PAG can modulate transmission of pain impulses at spinal segmental level (or brainstem level) [49, 206] through the pathways described in Figs. 4.18 and 4.19. Descending monoaminergic (serotonin and norepinephrine) connections from the reticular formation to the dorsal horn (Fig. 4.20) may suppress pain impulses in the dorsal horn, and thus prevent pain impulses from reaching higher CNS structures [34].

The PAG receives its input from the frontal lobe, the limbic system and the forebrain, and there is direct connection from the medial prefrontal and insular cortex to the PAG [5]. The amygdala provides input to the PAG [2] as well as the hypothalamus [49, 156] (Fig. 4.23). The hypothalamus is important in connection with pain, and it has been shown that electrical stimulation or infusion of opioids (natural morphine or synthetic morphine-like substances) in specific parts

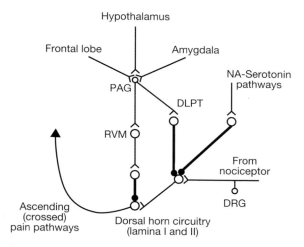

Fig. 4.23 Summary of the three different descending spinal tracts to cells in lamina I and II of the dorsal horn (RVM, DLPT and NA-Serotonin pathways), showing the sources of input to the PAG.

of the hypothalamus can produce analgesia. Electrical stimulation of prefrontal cortex can also alleviate pain (see p. 222).

There are a few direct connections between neurons of the PAG and dorsal horn neurons, but the neurons of the RVM act as interneurons between the PAG and the neurons in the dorsal horn of the spinal cord (Fig. 4.23). PAG cells that activate interneurons in the RVM can influence interneurons in lamina II of the dorsal horn, and thereby control the flow of neural activity that is elicited by noxious stimulation. Endogenous opioids (endorphins and enkephalins) act on local circuits in the RVM [113], and electrical stimulation of the RVM nuclei or injection of opioids in these structures produces analgesia and inhibits the response of dorsal horn neurons from stimulation of nociceptors [49].

Electrical stimulation of the nucleus coneiformis, which is one of the components of the DLPT, inhibits dorsal horn pain neurons. The nuclei of the DLPT have reciprocal connections with the PAG, and RVM influences neurons in lamina I of the dorsal horn (Fig. 4.24). The DLPT neurons have two-way communication with the PAG and the RVM, in addition to projecting to pain cells in the dorsal horn (Fig. 4.24).

The DLPT neurons that project to the RVM are noradrenergic, and the locus coeruleus neurons supply noradrenaline-containing neurons that project to cells in the dorsal horn [100]. The noradrenergic neurons in the DLPT relay information from neurons in the RVM to the spinal cord, and electrical stimulation of the RVM release noradrenaline in the spinal gray matter to an extent that it becomes detectable in the spinal cord fluid [61].

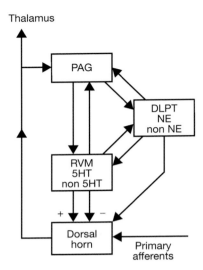

Thalamus

Fig. 4.24 Schematic illustration of the two-way connections between PAG, DLPT and RVM and their connections to the dorsal horn. (Adapted from Fields and Basbaum, 1999 [49].)

Animal experiments have shown that electrical stimulation of the DLPT, the RVM, or the locus coeruleus, can block input from nociceptors including abolition of the withdrawal reflex. Other studies have shown that electrical stimulation of the DLPT can relieve chronic pain in humans [65, 217].

Nociceptive cells in the dorsal horn receive two kinds of input from the RVM, namely excitatory input from RVM cells (on-cells) that are inhibited by morphine, and inhibitory input from RVM (off-cells) that are excited by morphine (Fig. 4.25). Inhibition of the on-cell reduces nociceptive transmission in the dorsal horn of the spinal cord and inhibition of off-cells increases nociceptive transmission [49].

Reduction of suppression of the dorsal horn nociceptor neurons may play a role in promoting expression of neural plasticity that can lead to the development of central neuropathic pain (see p. 200). It is interesting that a gamma amino butyric acid type A receptor (GABA$_A$) antagonist, bicuculine, has antinociceptive effects similar to morphine when injected into either the PAG or the RVM [160]. The fact that GABA$_A$ receptor antagonists have a similar effect as opioids means that GABA$_A$ receptor agonists, such as benzodiazepines, may have the opposite effect as opioids, thus, an anti-analgesic effect. The reason for that effect is that GABAergic activation reduces the inhibitory influence on dorsal horn pain cells that the cells normally receive from RVM neurons. This means that benzodiazepines that are GABA$_A$ agonists may increase pain by reducing the

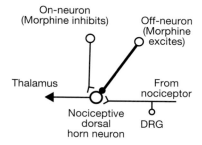

Fig. 4.25 Illustration of the dual inputs to dorsal horn cells from the RVM that provides the effect of "on" and "off" neurons on transmission of pain signals in the dorsal horn.

normal inhibitory influence on nociceptor neurons from input from the RVM. For example, this would indicate that the pain might increase from administration of benzodiazepines for individuals with back pain that arises from irritation of dorsal roots of the spinal cord. This would be contradictory to the common treatment of low back pain, which often includes the administration of diazepam for muscle relaxation, because muscle spasm contributes to low back pain. Benzodiazepines of one kind or another are commonly used as sleep agents because of their minimal (known) side effects including a low risk of suicide. The implication that administration of benzodiazepines can aggravate pain, because benzodiazepines decrease both the opioid induced and the normal suppression of pain in the dorsal horn, is rarely considered in the clinical environment.

Some investigators perceive this complex descending system that controls transmission of nociceptive information in the spinal cord, as a part of a negative feed-back system that may be activated by noxious stimulation, and exert an inhibitory effect on some forms of nociceptive input [7]. This would be similar to lateral inhibition that increases contrast in sensory systems [131], and it may explain why pain can inhibit pain. It is well known that pain in one part of the body can suppress pain in another part of the body [55] and the saying that one can only have pain in one place at a time is generally true, although it may mean that the CNS focuses on the worst pain. If that pain is gone, the next worst pain becomes "the worst pain". These observations emphasize that the perception of pain is different from the perception of innocuous sensory stimulation.

Role of the sympathetic nervous system

The PAG-RVM-DLPT pathways to the dorsal horn (Fig. 4.24) (and the NA-serotonin pathways, Fig. 4.20) are believed to deliver the inhibitory influence on spinal cord neurons that mediate the well-known stress-induced analgesia that occurs through activation of the sympathetic nervous system. Electrical stimulation of all three structures provides inhibition to nociceptive neurons in the dorsal horn [49, 100]. The opposite effect of activation of the sympathetic nervous system occurs because sympathetic activity causes liberation of norepinephrine near pain receptors, increasing their sensitivity and thereby increasing the effect of noxious stimulation, see [131]. This effect may counteract the above-mentioned effect on spinal cord neurons that causes stress-induced analgesia.

The sympathetic nervous system can thus exert control of pain in two ways: (1): by affecting the sensitivity of nociceptors (see p. 201) and (2): by affecting transmission of pain signals in the dorsal horn (see p. 174). The effect on receptors increases their sensitivity to noxious stimuli and the sympathetic effect on dorsal horn neurons suppresses transmission of nociceptor-mediated neural activity. That is the basis for the stress-induced analgesia. The sympathetic nervous system can affect the excitability of α motoneurons and that may cause painful muscle activity.

4.3.2   *Supraspinal processing of pain*

Pain that is mediated by myelinated (Aδ) fibers is processed in a different way from pain that is mediated by unmyelinated fibers (C fibers). The "fast pain" (Fig. 4.22) can reach the SI via the STT, which projects to the ventral thalamus (Fig. 4.11). The ascending pathways for the "slow" pain are presumed to use the dorsal thalamus, which project to subcortical and cortical structures (Fig. 4.26). Neurons in the dorsal thalamus project to the association cortices bypassing the SI and these neurons project to many parts of the CNS, such as limbic structures (the amygdala and hypothalamus), the PAG, and the brainstem reticular formation. The fact that these connections are subcortical means that they mediate information that is under little, or no, conscious control. The input to amygdala mediates various poorly defined qualities of pain sensations such as suffering, agonizing, etc. In the macaque monkey, there is a distinct nucleus in the posterior thalamus the neurons of which receive input from STT fibers that originate in lamina I of the spinal cord [36]. A nearly identical nucleus was found in the human thalamus that is involved in pain and temperature.

> The role of the thalamic nuclei in transmission and processing of pain impulses is being studied intensively now because of the therapeutic opportunities that have presented themselves by the introduction of stereotactic techniques for making lesions in specific deep brain structures. These techniques are now routinely used for control of severe pain

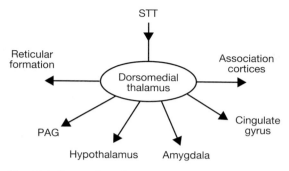

Fig. 4.26 Connections from neurons in the dorsomedial thalamus that are activated by STT fibers that originate in neurons in lamina I of the dorsal horn.

(see p. 222). The more recent introduction of deep brain stimulation (DBS)[16] has provided further methods to control severe pain [218, 219] and it has provided opportunities for research on pain [12, 103]. Such research has already provided much valuable information regarding the normal function of pain pathways and other somatosensory pathways [53, 72].

The fact that pain impulses reach several structures in the brain such as the somatosensory cortex, the prefrontal cortex, and structures of the limbic system, and that descending activity in these high CNS structures can modulate transmission of pain impulses in the spinal cord and the trigeminal nucleus, may explain how psychological factors can modulate the sensation of pain.

4.4   Pathophysiology of pain

Few pain disorders are caused by a single factor and often many factors act simultaneously, making treatment and diagnosis difficult. Changes of the function of receptors (peripheral sensitization) and changes in the function of the CNS (central sensitization and re-routing of information) are important factors in different forms of pain. Injuries such as trauma and ischemia can cause changes in the function of the CNS through expression of neural plasticity, which is an important factor in many forms of pain.

---

[16] DBS was introduced as a (reversible) substitute for ablation and other destructive procedures. However, electrical stimulation can cause two opposite effects: either inactivation by constant depolarization of neurons, or activation by causing cells or fibers to fire. Which of these two effects is achieved depends on the stimulus rate and the intensity (DBS is also discussed in Chapter 5 on movement disorders).

4.4.1   *Pathology of nociceptors*

Nociceptors that normally respond to noxious stimuli and produce the sensation of acute pain may under pathological conditions respond differently. Nociceptors may be sensitized by repeated activation or from sympathetic stimulation causing norepinephrine to be liberated by sympathetic nerve fibers that terminate near the receptors.

4.4.2   *Pathology of nerves*

Neurologists usually restrict the use of the term neuropathy to disorders of nerves and they distinguish between mononeuropathies [116] that affect one peripheral nerve and polyneuropathies that affect several nerves [167]. The terms mono- and polyneuropathy are used to describe the symptoms and are not related to the causes of the pain. Mononeuropathy may be caused by trauma to a peripheral nerve. Polyneuropathy frequently occurs in association with diabetes and age-related changes [151]. Pain from nerves can also be caused by inflammation or entrapment of nerves or nerve roots such as the dorsal spinal roots, but in many cases, the cause is unknown. Viral infections like those caused by strains of the herpes virus can cause painful conditions specifically in the radiation of single or multiple nerves (shingles, Ramsey-Hunt syndrome etc.). Pathologies of nerves such as from inflammation or ischemia can cause central pain through expression of neural plasticity that has been elicited by the abnormal function of the injured nerves and that pain often adds to the pain caused directly by the pathologies of nerves.

There are two ways that mechanical irritation (compression) of peripheral and cranial nerves can cause pain, namely stimulating of nociceptors in the *nervi nervorum* and by a nerve acting as a mechanoreceptor generating nerve impulses (becoming impulse generators). This may occur either spontaneously or in response to mechanical stimulation. Normally, peripheral nerves have a low degree of sensitivity to mechanical stimulation but injuries and other pathologies may change the membranes of axons so that they become mechanosensitive. Changes in the function of axons of peripheral nerves due to injuries, may make them sensitive to stretching or compression by changing the membrane of the axon, making it sensitive to deformation similar to that which occurs normally in Pacinian corpuscles.

Many studies have shown that nerve injury, neuroma formation, and nerve fiber degeneration, can cause spontaneous discharges in nerve fibers proximal to the injury level [197]. Such pathologies may cause pain because the generated neural activity is interpreted in the same way as activity that is caused by stimulation of nociceptors, thus generating a painful sensation.

The perception that is caused by abnormal neural activity, or activity from mechanical stimulation of slightly injured nerves, depends on which fibers are affected. Injury of large myelinated somatosensory fibers (Aβ fibers) typically causes paresthesia described as tingling, or "pins and needles" sensations. Mechanical stimulation of slightly injured nerves can cause pain when C fibers or Aβ fibers are activated. The nature of the pain depends on the kind of fibers that are activated. Activating C fibers is more likely to cause a burning sensation that is diffusely localized, while activating Aβ fibers is more likely to cause stinging and well localized pain.

The finding that the covering of peripheral nerves contains pain receptors (*Nervi nervorum*)[17] [182] has provided an explanation for some forms of acute pain from mechanical stimulation of peripheral nerves. Stimulation of these receptors may explain at least some of the instances of pain caused by compression, irritation, or injury to peripheral nerves. Whether or not the activation of the nociceptors in the sheaths of the nerve is regarded to be normal or pathological is a matter of opinion.

Mononeuropathies

Mononeuropathies that cause pain can be caused by traumatic injuries, compression, inflammation (such as viral), complex factors involving the CNS, and unknown factors.

Trigeminal neuralgia[18] (TGN) (or tic douloureux) is a typical mononeuropathy with a complex pathophysiology, involving the CNS. Although complex, TGN can be successfully treated by surgical operations aimed at the nerve root (such as microvascular decompression, partial sectioning[19] of the nerve root), and by medicine such as carbamazepine. TGN is one of only a few pain disorders that is well defined, and for which several effective and well-defined treatments are in use. TGN is discussed in further detail in Chapter 6 (p. 337).

Nerve compression and entrapment

Compression of nerves or nerve roots can cause mononeuropathies and cause pain, numbness and paresthesia. There are many forms of compression (or entrapment) of peripheral nerves that can cause pain. For example, the carpal tunnel syndrome and ulnar nerve entrapment are common causes of pain.

---

[17] Nervi nervorum: nerves that innervate the sheaths of nerve trunks.

[18] The term neuralgia is used to describe severe and sharp shooting pain that is perceived in the distribution of a nerve.

[19] Partial (or total) section of any nerve root involves high risks of severe complications such as anesthesia dolorosa and it is therefore rarely performed any more.

Compression of spinal nerve roots from trauma to vertebral disks, has been implicated in back pain.

Many incidences of pain to upper extremities often occur coincident with different forms of nerve compression related to the spine [110] and to joints [177], but like those of the lower back [110] and legs the causal relationship is often not obvious [177]. Carpal tunnel syndrome is a common nerve entrapment disorder, which is the second most common industrial injury in the USA [177]; it is believed to be caused by entrapment of the median nerve or pressure on the nerve [116, 177]. The carpal tunnel syndrome may occur without any detectable morphological signs of nerve entrapment or any other detectable morphological abnormalities. The pain (and tingling) can often be relieved by surgically decompressing the nerve, but the symptoms can also be relieved by splinting, cortisone injections, massage, and immersion of the hand in water. Resting the limb or change of activities can also relieve the symptoms. Like many other pain conditions, the pain from carpal tunnel syndrome is worsened by psychosocial factors such as boredom, stress, job dissatisfaction, monotonous routines, and insecurity. The fact that treatments that do not relieve the presumed entrapment are effective points to a central cause of at least some of the symptoms. While there may be some correlation between morphological findings (entrapments) and the perceived pain, it is unknown how frequent these morphological signs are in non-symptomatic individuals (cf. the common back pain, p. 155).

Ulnar nerve entrapment is the second most common entrapment neuropathy [116, 177] with symptoms of numbness and tingling in the distribution on the hand of the ulnar nerve (the fifth digit and the lateral aspect of the fourth). Other peripheral nerves such as the sciatic and common peroneal nerves are subject to similar entrapment (for an overview of mononeuropathies see [116]).

Compression of spinal roots has been associated with pain and neurological deficits in connection with the common back pain [201], but the pathophysiology of the common back pain is more complex and it is poorly understood [110]. Abnormalities and compression of nerve roots occur in only a few of the patients with back and leg pain [110]. It is possible that a morphological event such as nerve root compression from a vertebral disk rupture etc. may cause the initial pain. In some individuals, this event may activate neural plasticity causing changes in the CNS, which in turn cause changes in neural function, thus generating the sensation of pain. Back pain is often associated with muscle contractions (spasms), which can produce pain. The muscle contractions in these disorders are usually tonic and not easily observed. The clinical experience that back pain often can be treated successfully by benzodiazepine supports the hypothesis that the pain is related to muscle contraction or that the pain has a supraspinal origin. The general lack of objective signs of back pain has suggested that the pain in some cases has psychiatric causes [110], a not uncommon conclusion when detectable abnormalities are absent.

A more benign form of compression of peripheral nerves occurs when the sciatic nerve is compressed when sitting with crossed legs, or when resting the upper parts of the legs on a hard surface. Such compression interferes with the axoplasmatic flow in the axons, and causes ischemia which may be the cause of the specific sensations that are associated with acute compression of large peripheral nerves [98].

Viral infection (Herpes)

The herpes zoster virus resides in the ganglia of most individuals without producing any symptoms but occasionally it may cause pain and eruption of vesicles on the skin over some part of one, or more than one, dermatome. The pain is severe and may persist for a long time after the vesicular rash fades. Immediate treatment with antiviral agents such as acyclovir or famvir helps reduce the duration of the rash and the incidence of subsequent chronic pain. Herpes zoster oticus involves the eighth cranial nerve and is known as the Ramsey-Hunt syndrome. Medications such as gabapentin, or tricyclic antidepressants may be helpful for persistent pain. Opioids or local nerve blocks may be helpful in more difficult to control cases. Herpes simplex is the cause of blisters and sores most commonly occurring around the mouth, nose and genitals.

Deafferentiation pain

It is well known that lack of or reduction of normal sensory input can cause plastic changes in the function of the CNS. An extremely severe form of central neuropathic pain is anesthesia dolorosa, which is characterized by constant severe burning pain and reduced or absent sensation to innocuous stimulation. Anesthesia dolorosa occurs in connection with deafferentiation through injury to nerves and it often affects the face [115] but it can occur in other parts of the body [142]. Anesthesia dolorosa from injury to the trigeminal nerve is a rare variant of face pain that may occur as a complication to partial section of the trigeminal nerve for treatment of TGN [115]. It may occur from surgical sectioning of peripheral nerves or spinal nerve roots [142], although it has been claimed that anesthesia dolorosa is specific to the trigeminal system [184]. No known treatment is effective to treat that form of pain, although DBS recently has been found beneficial [171].

Polyneuropathies

Polyneuropathies are disorders that involve more than one peripheral nerve. They are typically divided into two groups, axonal polyneuropathies in which the main pathology is loss of axons and demyelinating polyneuropathies and in which the primary pathology is loss of myelin. The most common causes of axonal polyneuropathies are metabolic such as diabetic neuropathy. Alcohol (vitamin B_1 deficiency), solvents, heavy metals, B_{12} deficiency, autoimmune processes such as lupus and many drugs including chemotherapeutic agents such as vincristine and cis-platinum can cause polyneuropathy, sometimes producing pain. The pain is typically symmetrical (bilateral), affecting mainly sensory nerve fibers of small diameters and burning in nature. Distal fibers are most often affected more severely than proximal fibers. This means that pain first occurs in the feet in many of these disorders. It is important to note that the main clinical techniques used to determine the presence of neuropathy, the electromyographic (EMG) and nerve conduction studies, are only sensitive to injury to large fibers and hence may not reflect injury to small fibers conducting pain impulses. Other techniques such as the measurement of the sympathetic sweat reflex, sweating rates, and variations in heart rate with deep breathing may be helpful. The involvement of neural plasticity in these disorders is unknown but long-term pain of whatever cause often becomes accompanied by a component of the pain that is caused by expression of neural plasticity. Demyelinating neuropathies such as the Guillain-Barré syndrome are much less likely to be associated with pain than the axonal neuropathies because of the sparing of the unmyelinated C fibers.

4.4.3   Muscle pain

Pain from muscles may be caused by stimulation of nociceptors, but many forms of muscle pain such as myofascial pain and fibromyalgia have a complex pathophysiology, most of which is unknown. There is considerable evidence that altered function of CNS structures is involved in producing the pain that is associated with that form of muscle pain. Proprioceptors, such as tendon organs and receptors in joints, ligaments and muscle spindles, may be involved in causing pain from excessive muscle contractions. The output of proprioceptors may cause pain by activating neural circuits that are normally not activated by proprioceptors, thus similar to the cross-modal interaction that occurs in neuropathic pain causing allodynia (see p. 199). Local processes in the spinal cord that affect muscle tone can also affect the sensation of pain from muscles.

Studies have shown that there are specific nociceptors throughout muscles that may mediate pain [92, 139]. These nociceptors are free nerve endings that are mostly located near muscle endplates (endplate zones). They are innervated by Aδ fibers like the nociceptors found in the skin and they may play a role in causing pain from excessive muscle contractions [57]. Several kinds of noxious stimuli such as chemicals and mechanical stimulation can activate the same nociceptors [57, 221], which are also sensitive to endogenous substances, such as those released during inflammatory processes and injury. Exposure to chemical and mechanical stimuli can sensitize these receptors. Animal experiments have shown that serotonin combined with bradykinin [122] can cause muscle hyperalgesia from mechanical stimuli (pressure) [57]. The peripheral sensitization of muscle nociceptors is rapidly followed by changes in the function of dorsal horn neurons, similar to that which occurs in acute myositis.[20]

Exercise pain

The acute pain from excessive exercise is probably a result of compromised blood supply caused by increased intramuscular pressure. This type of pain disappears normally within seconds after stopping the exercise, and it leaves no long-term effects. Ischemic pain is assumed to be caused by toxic metabolites, but the role of lactic acid has been eliminated as a cause of such pain, while histamine, acetylcholine, serotonin, bradykinin, potassium and adenosine are suspected of being involved in causing muscle pain [57, 139]. Muscle pain that occurs many hours after unaccustomed exercise is mainly caused by lengthening of the active muscle by external force (mechanical factors) rather than metabolic factors and it is associated with damage to the muscles involved [139].

Muscle tension as a cause of pain

Muscle tension plays an important role as a cause of pain. Abnormally increased muscle tone can be caused either by changes in the viscoelastic properties of muscles or by contractile activity mediated by the motor nerve and the motoneurons (Fig. 4.27).

Myalgia (pain from muscles) can have many causes, and it may be difficult to differentiate it from pain that originates from other tissues such as joints, tendons, ligaments and bones. For example, headache that is caused by contraction of neck muscles may not be easily distinguished from pain from other causes. The muscle contractions that cause or contribute to severe pain are often tonic and therefore not as easy to detect as tremor or spasm. Painful muscle contractions may be associated with EMG activity, which is a sign that the contractions are caused by alpha motoneuron activity, but muscle contractions may

---

[20] Myositis: Inflammation of muscles

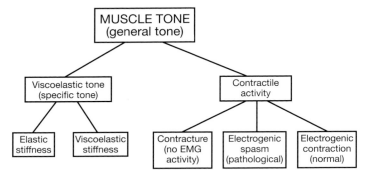

Fig. 4.27 Relationship between terms commonly used to characterize muscle tension: tone, stiffness, contracture, and spasm [173].

also result from chemical causes such as changes in the extracellular fluid or electrolytic imbalance [101].

There are three different forms of contractile activation of muscles: (1) electrogenic stiffness caused by activation of motoneurons and neuromuscular endplates (have observable EMG activity); (2) electrogenic spasm (pathological and involuntary electrogenic contraction); and (3) contracture (occurring within the muscle fibers independent of EMG activity) [173].

The tension or the tonus of a muscle depends both on the activation of the contractile apparatus and on the basic viscoelastic properties of the muscle tissue. Only the first mentioned form of activation is associated with EMG activity; the other form of contraction causes increased mechanical stiffness of the muscles that is not induced by activity in the motor nerve that innervates the muscle in question. Muscle contraction can therefore occur without any measurable electrophysiological signs, a factor that has clinical diagnostic importance. Such increased mechanical stiffness can be determined by physical examination and can be measured quantitatively as a resistance against a slowly applied force.

Words like muscle tone and muscle tension are sometimes used synonymously, but some authors [173] define muscle tone to mean only viscoelastic changes in a muscle that occur in absence of contractile neural activity.

The resting muscle tone has been assumed to be caused by low rate of firing of motor nerves thus caused by activity of alpha motoneurons. However, this assumption seems to rest on a misconception according to Simons and Mense [173] who described methods to measure muscle tone mechanically, and credited Walsh 1992 [200] for clarifying the misconception that muscle tone was normally caused by electrical activation of the contractile apparatus of muscles.

Increased muscle activity (spasm) contributes to such forms of pain as back pain and tension headache. The form of spasm of muscles that causes pain is usually tonic contractions. Hyperactivity of alpha motoneurons from increased excitatory input or decreased inhibitory input of segmental or supraspinal origin may cause spasm (see Chapter 5).

Input from the sympathetic nervous system increases alpha motoneuron excitability and since pain increases sympathetic activity, a vicious circle may be created, which can increase or maintain pain after the original cause of the pain has been eliminated. For example, if we assume that back pain is initiated by a transient compression or injury to a dorsal root, then the initial pain may cause increased sympathetic activity that further increases the activity of alpha motoneurons causing pain. This pain may be self-sustained and therefore continue after the injury of the dorsal root has healed. This process can only be interrupted if the pain is totally eliminated for some time, and it may explain the common experience that pain must be totally eliminated in order to achieve a long-term pain relief. Incomplete relief of acute pain may facilitate pain by further activating the sympathetic nervous system.

One likely pathway for maintaining pain from muscle contractions consists of neurons in the dorsal horn (or trigeminal nucleus) that receive input from nociceptors in muscles and which activate sensory cortical neurons through a thalamic pathway. These neurons in the sensory cortex then activate neurons in several regions of the brain such as limbic structures and SMA, the neurons of which can activate neurons in the motor cortex, and subsequently α motoneurons, completing a circle that can maintain muscle contractions [195]. Interrupting that vicious circle at any point can relieve the pain. Inducing pareses of the afflicted muscle for instance by Botulinum toxin is one way of doing that [50, 108, 145]. The finding that the effect of Botulinum treatment increased gradually over a 60-day observation period supports the hypothesis that neural plasticity of proprioception is involved.

It has been debated whether tension headache is a form of myofascial spasm [195]. The involvement of temporomandibular joint disorders, or a combination of that and some other factors, have been suspected in what is often called tension headaches. Anyhow, despite the frequency and the socioeconomic consequences of tension headaches [81], little is known about the pathophysiology of the disorder, and consequently search of treatments has been of an empirical nature [40].

Muscle pain may be caused by neural activity that does not reach the SI and it is therefore not distinctly located on the body, but instead presents as a diffuse sensation of a dull aching and unpleasant pain sensation. Referred pain patterns and trigger points are important factors in distinguishing headache caused by muscle activity [75, 173] from other causes of headaches.

Some components of the common back pain are often caused by muscle spasm [110], and the common low back pain therefore often responds favorably to treatment with benzodiazepines (GABA$_A$ receptor agonists), which cause muscle relaxation because of their action on the CNS. The efficiency of treatment of muscle spasm with benzodiazepines further supports the hypothesis that central structures are involved in such forms of muscle pain. Benzodiazepines mainly affect supraspinal input to motor circuits. Other methods of muscle relaxation are effective; even such simple actions as taking a deep breath can often reduce muscle tension and thereby pain.

Massage [152] or application of heat is efficient as treatment for muscle spasm because it stimulates receptors in the muscles. The massage of the tendons that activate the Golgi tendon organs is especially effective in reducing muscle spasm because of the inhibitory influence from these receptors on alpha motoneurons [35]. Golgi tendon receptors sense the tension of muscles and provide inhibitory input to alpha motoneurons.

The term muscle spasm is usually used to describe involuntary muscle contractions that are accompanied by EMG activity. Examples of pain from involuntary muscle contractions are spasmodic torticollis, trismus, stiff-man syndrome and nocturnal leg cramps, but even tension headaches belong to this group of disorders. Trismus is involuntary closing of the jaw due to tonic spasm of muscles of mastication. Spasmodic torticollis [144] was discussed in the chapter on movement disorders. It is a source of pain because of the persistent muscle contractions. Nocturnal leg cramps that involve mainly contraction of the gastrocnemius muscle are painful.

> The "stiff-man" syndrome is a rare condition that is characterized by slowly progressive stiffness of axial and proximal leg muscles and occasional painful muscle spasms. It is a disorder of spinal or brainstem origin [101] and is characterized by antibodies to glutamic acid decarboxylase (GAD) in a majority of patients. Involuntary muscle contractions that cause pain are often loosely described as cramp, contracture, spasm, or tetanus without making precise reference to the accurate definitions of these terms [71, 139].

Myofascial pain

Myofascial pain is closely related to painful muscle contractions (muscle spasm). Myofascial pain is a complex disorder, the pathophysiology of which is poorly understood. The presence of trigger points is typical for the disease and much research has been devoted to studies of the basis for such trigger points. Some studies have indicated that the trigger points represent a spinal reflex [62, 70, 71, 73] (Fig. 4.28).

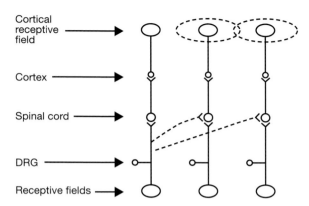

Fig. 4.28 Hypothesis about expansion of receptive field and creation of trigger points by unmasking of dormant synapses. Adapted from Hong and Simons (1998) [71].

Other investigators have hypothesized that the trigger points are regions of a muscle with a "local twitch response" (LTR) associated with loci of high sensitivity that have developed as a result of minor injuries. It has been shown that such "latent trigger points" [192] occur in 50% of asymptomatic individuals [73, 176]. These loci can be concerted into active trigger points by some external event, which cause them to aggregate and sensitize their nociceptors. Leakage of calcium and other substances may activate nearby muscle fibers resulting in the formation of a taut band. The EMG activity that can be recorded from these "taut bands" is very localized and is not caused by endplate potentials [73]. It has therefore been hypothesized that the EMG activity at the trigger points is caused by contractions of intrafusal muscles caused by sympathetic activity [73] (Fig. 4.29). That means that the LTR may be a polysynaptic reflex [73].

Fibromyalgia

Fibromyalgia [8, 179, 180] presents with a wealth of more or less diffuse symptoms, one being chronic and widespread muscle pain. Fibromyalgia has therefore been regarded as a muscle disorder (and therefore the name) but little evidence of abnormalities (pathologies) of muscles has been found despite great efforts to find such abnormalities [179, 180]. Criteria for what should be called fibromyalgia have been proposed but it seems clear that the disorder called fibromyalgia is not a single entity but rather a complex basket of pathologies. The symptoms may differ from person to person and from time to time. While the main symptoms of fibromyalgia are muscle pain, depression is an important

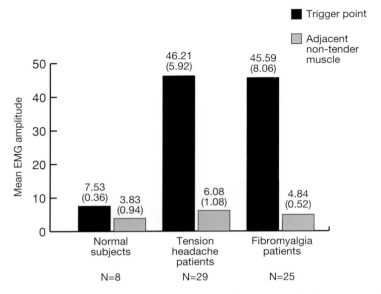

Fig. 4.29 Mean EMG amplitudes (and standard error) recorded from a muscle at a trigger point and at an adjacent non-tender muscle. Data from [73].

component as is fatigue [8, 198]. Recent studies indicate that the disorder is better characterized as a complex pain syndrome [8].

The pathophysiology of fibromyalgia has been debated and the view of which mechanisms are involved has changed over time. The lack of detectable pathologies in muscles has turned the attention to the CNS as the location of the abnormalities that causes the symptoms of fibromyalgia, and fibromyalgia is no longer regarded as a disorder of muscles. There is considerable evidence that neural plasticity is involved in creating the complex symptoms of fibromyalgia [8]. This view is supported by the fact that pain management aiming at central pain using psychotherapy, exercise and psychoactive drugs are effective means of treatment for this disorder. Plastic changes in the CNS could explain the altered pain processing such as central sensitization of pain processing that is now believed to be the main cause of the symptoms and signs of fibromyalgia [8, 14]. This, together with abnormal function of peripheral pain mechanisms, may explain the many, sometimes confusing, symptoms of fibromyalgia.

> We mentioned trigger zones in connection with trigeminal neuralgia (Chapter 6). Fibromyalgia and the myofascial pain syndrome often have trigger points from which pain attacks can be elicited [16, 70, 71, 73, 191]. Myofascial trigger points are described as being sensitive spots on a muscle where a palpable "taut" band of muscle fibers can be identified [70, 71]. These trigger points can be identified by finger palpation. Trigger

points can be located not only at the place to which the pain is referred but also to locations that are distant to that of the perceived pain. Studies have shown that various kinds of treatment directed to such trigger points can alleviate the pain [70].

4.4.4   *Pain not caused by (known) stimulation of nociceptors*

Pain may be caused by injuries to CNS structures that do not contain specific nociceptors. Lesions of the nervous system including lesions of peripheral nerves or disorders of the CNS, such as strokes, can cause neuropathic pain. It is not known, however, why lesions to the nervous system in some patients cause pain while similar lesions in other patients do not cause such conditions [210].

CNS pain

CNS pain is of two main kinds: one that is related to morphological changes such as trauma and strokes, and one that is related to functional changes such as those induced by expression of neural plasticity.

Injuries to the CNS such as those arising from trauma or ischemia can give pain but little is known about how such pain is related to the insult in question. Strokes and injury from trauma can cause pain depending on which regions of the brain are affected. Tissue damage and ischemia are assumed to cause the pain. A specific kind of pain is related to injuries of the thalamus (thalamic pain) (Dejerine-Roussy syndrome) [36, 68, 136]. It is noteworthy that lesions to specific structures of the thalamus can cause relief of pain. Nerve injuries may be associated with transsynaptic degeneration of cell bodies in the dorsal horn [183], and sprouting of A fibers to superficial lamina of the dorsal horn [209], which may cause pain sensations and pain from innocuous stimulation ("allodynia").

Migraine and cluster headache are other forms of pain that are caused by pathologies of the brain [40]. Migraine involves the trigeminovascular system and sensitization of nociceptors in the meninges as well as in the trigeminal nucleus are involved [14]. Migraine is often accompanied by allodynia indicating involvement of expression of neural plasticity [18]. Mild increase in blood pressure can aggravate the pain in migraine because of sensitization of peripheral nociceptors that innervate intracranial blood vessels and the meninges. Sensitization of second order neurons in the spinal cord on which input from intracranial structures and from skin in the ophthalmic skin converge may explain the allodynia that often accompanies migraine attacks and the referred pain in the periorbital region [18]. Allodynia outside the area of referred pain may be explained by sensitization of third order trigemino-vascular neurons that receive input from the head and the upper limb in addition to input from intracranial structures.

Cluster headache is a cousin to migraine and it often responds to the same treatments as are effective for migraine. The development of drugs in the family of triptans (e.g. Sumatriptan), which are selective 5-HT1B/1D receptor agonists, were great improvements in the treatment of migraine and cluster headache. Non-specific pain relieving drugs [40] and some unconventional treatment, such as application of capsaicin in the nose [52], have been shown to be beneficial. Cluster headache and migraine are complex disorders with symptoms other than pain, such as tearing and stuffy nose on one side. Recent studies seem to support the hypothesis that vascular pathologies are involved in causing the symptoms of migraine, in that it has been shown that individuals with migraine have a higher incidence of strokes than individuals without migraine headaches [97].

The pathophysiology of pain that is related to insult to the CNS such as strokes, other forms of ischemia or iatrogenic lesions, is poorly understood. It is interesting that lesions to the thalamus can give specific pain syndromes (thalamic pain [36]), while lesions in other parts of the thalamus are effective in treating pain [218]. Paradoxically, strokes that affect specific parts of the thalamus produce pain and analgesia and loss of temperature sensation at the same time [36].

Central neuropathic pain

Pain can be caused by expression of neural plasticity that causes generation of activity in neural circuits in the CNS causing the sensation of pain (central neuropathic pain). Central neuropathic pain causes more suffering than acute pain that is caused by stimulation of nociceptors, and it is more difficult to diagnose and treat this form of pain.

Central neuropathic pain is not caused by stimulation of nociceptors but instead such pain is caused by neural activity that is generated in the CNS but referred to a peripheral location. Central neuropathic pain, or stimulus independent pain, is fundamentally different from pain that is caused by stimulation of nociceptors and the neural substrate is different in these two types of pain. Central neuropathic pain is referred to specific regions of the body, although these regions may not contribute to the generation of the sensation of pain [149]. Phantom limb sensations consisting of pain, paresthesia and other abnormal sensations are the clearest examples of sensations that are caused by abnormal neural activity in the CNS while the sensations are referred to specific peripheral location.

The regions to which the pain is referred can vary over time, and they often extend with time, and there is therefore a form of lateral spread of activation of nerve cells in the CNS [71] (increased receptive fields, Fig. 4.28).

The symptoms of central neuropathic pain are persistent pain, changes in processing of nociceptor elicited pain (hyperpathia and altered temporal integration), re-direction of sensory information (allodynia) and affective symptoms. Central neuropathic pain affects many individuals, and it can have many different causes. Central neuropathic pain can be initiated by many causes, and pain that is initiated by the same insult can have widely different expressions in different individuals [178]. The degree and character of pain may vary over time, and it may be affected by many factors such as the emotional state of the patient. Acute pain is a frequent precursor of central neuropathic pain, and central neuropathic pain, or stimulus independent pain, may persist after healing of the trauma that caused acute pain.

Despite much research, the pathophysiology of this kind of pain is incompletely understood, but it is generally assumed that altered processing of nociceptive information at the segmental and at supraspinal levels are involved [210, 211] and both peripheral and central sensitization are most likely also involved in creating the symptoms of central neuropathic pain [14, 112].

Devor [41] described the characteristics of three different types of central neuropathic pain ("pathophysiological" pain), i.e. pain that is not caused by stimulation of nociceptors:

1. Increased sensitivity of nociceptors (peripheral sensitization).
2. Peripheral nerves acting as impulse generators.
3. Increased "gain" in central pain circuits (central sensitization).

In addition to these three typical characteristics of neuropathic pain, cross modal interaction (allodynia) and changes in processing (hyperpathia) are often present.

These changes in the function of the pain circuits in the CNS are caused by expression of neural plasticity. Changes can occur in the processing in the dorsal horn of the spinal cord and the trigeminal nucleus [207, 211] or in structures that are more central. Central sensitization and peripheral sensitization of pain receptors play important roles in creating central neuropathic pain [14, 208, 211]. Peripheral sensitization of receptors can be caused by secretion of noradrenaline near receptors, and central sensitization of pain circuits may occur in the dorsal horn of the spinal cord (and of the CN V nucleus) and at supraspinal levels.

Deprivation of input is a strong mediator of neural plasticity and it can be a cause of central neuropathic pain. Central neuropathic pain may be initiated by painful lesions of peripheral nerves from activation of receptors in the nervi nervorum [60]. Pain and tingling caused by mechanical compression of injured nerves is also often caused by complex processes involving changes in the function of the CNS that are brought about by expression of neural plasticity. There is considerable evidence that pain from injuries to peripheral nerves is especially powerful in initiating changes in the function of specific structures in the CNS through the expression of neural plasticity. That form of central neuropathic pain typically persists beyond healing of the original lesion and therefore any intervention at the original lesion carries no benefit to the patient. Other forms of pain that are caused by stimulation of nociceptors and have lasted a long time often include a component of central neuropathic pain. Central neuropathic pain may occur without any known cause.

Central neuropathic pain causes enormous suffering and it is a challenge to the physician with regard to both its diagnosis and its treatment, which is generally unsatisfactory. Identifying the cause of central pain is less important for the management of the pain than is the case for pain that is evoked by stimulation of pain receptors.

Deprivation of input or overstimulation can cause such plastic changes of the nervous system (see Chapter 1). Central neuropathic pain may occur as a sequel to acute somatic pain, and it often persists long after healing of the initial pathology. Deafferentiation pain and phantom limb pain are other examples of central neuropathic pain. A component of central neuropathic pain is often a component of pain that is caused by stimulation of nociceptors, when it has persisted over a long period of time.

There is no doubt that pain elicited by stimulation of nociceptors serves the organism, and the absence of pain from stimulation of nociceptors has disastrous consequences but the benefit from central neuropathic pain is not obvious. In fact, it is difficult to find any advantage to the organism from central neuropathic pain but it is easy to find disadvantages to an individual person from central neuropathic pain, which can ruin a person's life, cause affective disorders and result in suicide.

Reorganization of central pain pathways

The pathways that are involved in severe central neuropathic pain are complex and poorly understood. At least parts of these pathways are probably the same as those mediating pain from stimulation of nociceptors (Fig. 4.11). The organization of these pathways is dynamic and involves a high degree of parallel processing, including connections with autonomic systems and limbic structures. Affective symptoms such as depression often accompany severe pain, and these symptoms may be explained by the establishment of new connections in the pain pathways in the brain or spinal cord or by amplifying existing pathways. The medial portion of the thalamus is likely to be involved providing subcortical connections to limbic structures such as the amygdala nuclei [102], the SMA, and prefrontal cortex (Fig. 4.17). In these respects, central neuropathic pain has many similarities with other hyperactive sensory disorders such as tinnitus [19, 127, 129] (p. 113).

The role of the dorsal horn (and the trigeminal nucleus)   Like other CNS structures the neural circuits in the dorsal horn that are involved in processing noxious stimuli are plastic, and reorganization of these circuits play important roles in central neuropathic pain. Changes in processing in the dorsal horn can explain many of the characteristic features of central neuropathic pain. The changes in the function and the organization of the dorsal horn neural circuits can be caused by both external and internal factors that can cause expression of neural plasticity.

Evidence has been presented that the processing of pain signals in the dorsal horn of the spinal cord (and the trigeminal nucleus) can operate in four main states [46]:

State 1 is the normal state, where stimuli that activate low-threshold mechanoreceptors produce innocuous sensations such as that of touch, vibration, pressure, warmth or coolness. In this mode of function, activation of high threshold receptors produces localized pain sensations that are distinctly different from innocuous stimulations. The sensation of this kind of pain is not accompanied by any noticeable emotional engagement.

State 2 represents a functional re-organization of the dorsal horn (and the trigeminal sensory nucleus). This state is characterized by suppression of transmission of somatosensory information, and the ability of high intensity stimuli to evoke a sensation of pain is reduced in this state. The decrease in sensory transmission is caused by inhibitory influence on neurons in the dorsal horn. The source of the inhibition can be peripheral such as from activation of $A\beta$ fibers, or supraspinal such as a part of "flight or fight" reactions mediated by the NA-serotonin descending pathways (p. 178, Fig. 4.20). It is believed that these are the mechanisms through which stimulation of skin receptors, hypnosis, placebo, suggestions, distraction and cognition affect (suppress) the perception of painful stimuli. Pharmacological agents such as opioids, alpha-adrenergic agents and $GABA_A$ antagonists (bicuculine) can promote the expression of state 2 of the function of dorsal horn pain circuits.

State 3 represents an increased excitability of dorsal horn sensory cells facilitating or sensitizing their response to sensory stimuli. The cause is assumed to be a combination of increased excitatory synaptic transmission and decreased inhibition. The result is that stimulation of sensory receptors elicit larger than normal postsynaptic activity. In this mode of function, low intensity input, that is normally innocuous, generates a sensation of pain (allodynia) and exaggerated pain experience that outlasts the duration of noxious stimulation (hyperpathia).

Hyperpathia is caused by central sensitization. Mononeuropathies may promote the changes that occur in stage 3 [212], and the extension of existing nociceptive receptive fields of dorsal horn neurons may occur through activation of ineffective (dormant) synapses [71] (Fig. 4.28).

State 4 represents an anatomical re-organization with changes in morphology including deaths of cells, degeneration or atrophy of synapses, creation of new synapses and modification of the contacts between cells and synapses. Aβ fibers that normally terminate in layers III–V of the horns of the spinal cord may invade the territorium of C fibers (lamina II) and there make synaptic contact with cells that are innervated by C fibers [46]. That may explain why normally innocuous stimulation can be perceived as painful (allodynia).

In summary, changes in the mode of processing in the dorsal horn (and the nucleus of CN V) are characterized by change in sensitivity, change in the way stimuli are processed and change in the anatomical location where information is processed. Mode 1 is the normal state of the function of the dorsal horn of the spinal cord (and the trigeminal nucleus). Mode 2 represents a decreased gain regarding noxious stimulation. Mode 3 represents a transient and functional increased gain. Finally, mode 4 is a (anatomically) permanent state of increased pain and redirection of information. Change from mode 1 to mode 2 or 3 represent expression of neural plasticity that involves change in synaptic efficacy. Change to mode 4 is different because it involves structural (morphological) changes. The changes in mode 4 are therefore more difficult to reverse than the changes that occur in stage 2 and 3.

Change in neural processing

Central neuropathic pain is associated with several forms of changes in neural processing of pain. One such change is the "wind-up" phenomenon through which noxious stimuli can cause increased pain sensation when repeated at short intervals. Other forms of abnormal processing are allodynia and hyperpathia. Hyperpathia is a sign of changes in the processing of painful stimuli, whereas allodynia is a sign of re-routing of information (cross modal interaction, see p. 13).

Increase in sensitivity to pain The sensation of pain from stimulation of nociceptors is not as constant as the sensation of sensory stimuli such as touch, sound and light. Various factors can affect the sensation of pain and the perceived strength of stimulation of nociceptors by the same physical stimulation can change. Sensitization may occur at the receptor level (peripheral sensitization) or in the CNS (central sensitization) [14, 22, 207]. Decreased pain sensitivity can occur as a result of peripheral or supraspinal influence on neurons in the

Increased activity

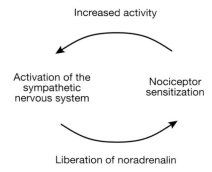

Activation of the
sympathetic
nervous system

Nociceptor
sensitization

Liberation of noradrenalin

Fig. 4.30 Vicious circle from activation of the sympathetic nervous system that serves as a basis for RSD (CRPS I).

dorsal horn of the spinal cord or in the trigeminal nucleus. Sensitization of the peripheral pain circuits, as well as central neurons, is important for generating many forms of pain [14, 30, 93, 153, 162, 193].

Peripheral sensitization Substances that are released during inflammatory processes and injury can sensitize the nociceptors, and serotonin can cause hyperalgesia to mechanical stimuli when combined with bradykinin [57, 122]. Repeated stimulation may cause increased sensitivity of nociceptors (autosensitization), and thereby cause an exaggerated response to painful stimuli. Sensitization of nociceptors may occur because of liberation of noradrenaline from sympathetic nerve fibers caused by activation of the sympathetic nervous system. This process produces positive feedback of pain evoked neural activity and it can create a vicious circle (Fig. 4.30), which in its severe form causes reflex sympathetic dystrophy (RSD) [20]. (RSD is now known as complex regional pain syndrome (CRPS type I) [166]. RSD has also been known as causalgia, now known as CRPS Type II [166].)

Central sensitization Hyperpathia is a sign of central sensitization such as occurs in state 3 of Doubell's classification of different states in which the dorsal horn can operate [46]. The "wind-up" phenomenon is related to central sensitization and it is assumed to develop when C fibers discharge in response to sustained stimuli at a high frequency [14]. This causes the WDR neurons to increase their response progressively after each stimulus. Central sensitization may also cause hyperpathia, which may have survival importance because it prevents manipulation of injured tissue but, in many situations, hyperpathia provides no obvious benefit to the organism. Hyperpathia may be regarded as a pathology in itself that adds to the suffering of neuropathic pain. The pathophysiology of hyperpathia is unknown but clinical experience shows that it can be alleviated by antidepressive drugs that affect serotonin receptors and that indicate that serotonin may play a role in causing hyperpathia (clinically amitriptylin and nortriptylin have been found to be the most effective antidepressive drugs in treating hyperpathia).

The regions of the body to which pain is referred often extend with time, thus a form of lateral spread of activation. It has been suggested that a peripheral nerve trunk is capable of sustaining a "flare" response similar to that observed in injured skin and other tissue [223] and thus cause an extension of the region from which pain sensation originates. Peptidergic fibers (nervi nervorum) that contain SP, calcitonin and other peptides may be involved in the creation of sustained neural activation that causes pain sensation to persist beyond the duration of the tissue damage.

Such changes are signs of central sensitization of excitatory synapses or depression of inhibition [211]. Stimulation of nociceptors, for example by inflammation or by peripheral nerve injuries, may cause such sensitization. There is considerable evidence that the WDR neurons play an important role in central sensitization by increased sensitivity to C fiber input. This occurs through the expression of neural plasticity, causing increased efficacy of excitatory synapses or by decreased efficacy of inhibitory synapses [211] (Fig. 4.31). Diffusion of SP in the spinal horn may change the function of WDR neurons so that they become hyperactive. Animal studies and studies in humans have supported the hypothesis of neural sensitization causing the development of hyperalgesia [1, 8].

Sustained and transient activation of C fiber nociceptors can induce central sensitization involving NMDA receptors [14, 20, 181]. Central sensitization may last as long as several weeks after it has been induced and the stimuli that caused the expression of neural plasticity has been terminated.

The threshold of WDR neurons may be further lowered by prostaglandins and nitric oxide synthesis. Excitotoxity and other effects of glutamate that may follow can cause permanent damage to cells that are involved in signaling pain such as those of the dorsal horn and the trigeminal nucleus. Activation of the NMDA receptor is permissive for the release of SP in the dorsal horn [107].

These changes in the function of WDR neurons are caused by expression of neural plasticity induced by lowered inhibitory input from large myelinated (A) fibers or increased C fiber input such as may occur in mononeuropathies [212] (Fig. 4.31). That would explain why mononeuropathies are associated with changes in the firing pattern of WDR neurons. One such change in the function of WDR neurons includes an increase of the maximal firing rate of WDR neurons and that may open normally inefficient synapses of the target neurons. Increased discharge rate or abnormal neural activity such as burst activity that replaces

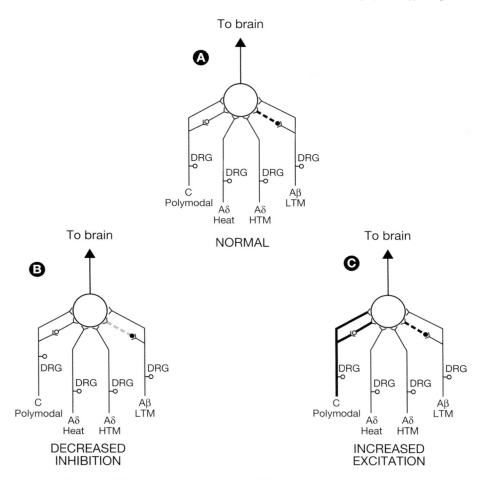

Fig. 4.31 WDR neurons showing three different states:

A: Normal situation

B: Decreased inhibitory input from LTM receptors through Aβ

C: Increased excitatory input from polymodal receptors through C fibers.

(Adapted from [147].)

a "smooth" train of nerve impulses may cause re-routing of pain signals (see Chapter 1, p. 29). This may be the basis for establishing functional connections between somatosensory circuits and pain circuits [29] and such abnormalities in the function of WDR neurons may therefore explain the cross modal interaction that is expressed as allodynia.

The N-methyl-D-aspartate (NMDA) receptors and neurokinin receptors are involved in central neuropathic pain [208] (see Chapter 1), and that has suggested that NMDA receptor antagonists such as the experimental drug

MK 801, would be effective in the treatment of central neuropathic pain. So far, however, attempts to modulate or affect the effect of glutamate that is found throughout the CNS has had little success. The NMDA receptor antagonist MK 801 has been available for many years, but the success in using it in treatment of pain has not materialized. Ketamine, another NMDA receptor antagonist, administered intravenously, has been shown to have some beneficial effect on such pain [179, 180]. However, these drugs have considerable side effects (in the form of psychiatric symptoms) that have prevented their introduction in clinical medicine. The abundance of glutamate and the presence of glutamate receptors in so many CNS systems have so far prevented development of practically useful drugs that manipulate glutamate or its receptors in a way that can be used to safely treat such specific medical conditions as pain.

Decrease in pain sensitivity Sympathetic input to the spinal cord (and trigeminal nucleus) can cause a decrease in sensitivity to pain. The NA-serotonin pathway provides inhibitory influence on pain circuits in the spinal cord (Fig. 4.20, p. 177). Failure of the normal control of pain by the descending PAG-RVM – DLPT pathways may increase pain sensation.

The output of the RVM has inhibitory influence on nociceptor neurons in the dorsal horn of the spinal cord (and the trigeminal nucleus) and GABA is the inhibitory transmitter substance to interneurons in the descending pathway of the RVM from the PAG (p. 226). It has been shown that a GABA$_A$ antagonist (bicuculine) administered to the RVM has a similar effect on pain transmission in the spinal cord as opioids. The reason is that bicuculine decreases GABAergic inhibition in the PAG-RVM pathway thus facilitating the transmission of signals in that pathway and subsequently increase its (inhibitory) influence on pain neurons in the dorsal horn of the spinal cord (Figs. 4.19, 4.23). This means that GABA$_A$ receptor agonists such as benzodiazepines may reduce the suppression of pain signals that is normally provided by the PAG – RVM pathway, resulting in less inhibitory influence on dorsal horn pain neurons. Administration of GABA$_A$ receptor agonists such as benzodiazepines may therefore increase pain from nociceptor stimulations.

Administration of GABA$_A$ agonists such as the benzodiazepines is often used in treatment of back pain because benzodiazepines (such as Valium) provide central muscle relaxation, which reduces the pain that is caused by muscle spasm. This beneficial effect, however, may be counteracted by the reduction in the suppressive effect of pain transmission in the dorsal horn that is normally provided by the PAG-RVM pathway. Most of the sleep medications that are used now are of the benzodiazepine family and they may in fact increase pain because of their suppressive effect on the PAG-RVM pathways that normally suppress transmission of pain signals in the spinal cord (and the trigeminal nucleus).

The DLPT circuits mediate influence on dorsal horn pain neurons in a similar way as the RVM circuits. Electrical stimulation of the DLPT has been shown to decrease chronic pain [217]. Both RVM and DLTP circuits have reciprocal connection between PAG neurons and the dorsal horn (Figs. 4.18, 4.19, 4.23), which is the neural substrate for complex control systems of pain. These circuits are dynamic and expression of neural plasticity can modify their function.

The "wind up" phenomenon and temporal integration

The "wind up" phenomenon is characterized by an increase in the sensation of pain when painful stimuli are repeated. This is a form of changed temporal integration[21] that changes the perception of pain caused by repetitive stimulation of nociceptors. Abnormal temporal integration including the wind up phenomenon are signs of change in neural processing that also include central sensitization (see Chapter 1) of excitatory synapses or depression of inhibition synapses [211]. Prolonged pain may lead to increased response of WDR neurons to C fiber input, causing the "wind up" phenomenon [14, 121, 187, 208]. Stimulation of nociceptors, for example by inflammation or peripheral nerve injuries, may cause such sensitization through expression of neural plasticity. One of the glutamate receptors, the NMDA receptor, may be involved in generating the wind up phenomenon [44] as indicated by the fact that administration of the experimental drug MK 801, an antagonist to NMDA receptors, abolished the wind up in spinal nociceptive neurons [43] (Fig. 4.32). (Ketamine may have a similar effect.)

> Other studies have shown that changes in processing of pain signals in the CNS after nerve injuries cause measurable changes in temporal integration of painful stimuli such as can be demonstrated by electrical stimulation of the skin [130] (Fig. 4.33). In individuals without pain, the threshold for pain sensation in response to stimulation with trains of electrical impulses decreases exponentially with increased repetition rate of the stimulus impulses (Fig. 4.33A) thus an indication of temporal integration. The threshold of sensation (tingling) is nearly independent on the rate of the stimulus impulses (Fig. 4.33A) indicating little or no temporal integration. Patients with neuropathic pain have altered temporal integration of painful stimuli [130] (Fig. 4.33B). Normally, the pain threshold to electrical stimulation of the skin is much higher than the threshold for detecting the stimulation and the threshold for pain normally decreases when the rate of the stimulation impulses is increased

---

[21] Temporal integration, in sensory systems, means that the sensation of a stimulus is affected by the past history of stimulation and that the threshold of a stimulus that is preceded by a similar stimulus is lower than when presented alone. Temporal summation is a property that is opposite to adaptation, and which is commonly present in sensory systems.

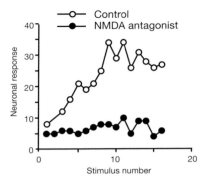

Fig. 4.32 Indications that the "wind up" is NMDA mediated. Response with and without an NMDA antagonist. (Data from [44].)

while the threshold to detection of the stimulation is nearly independent on the rate of stimulation (Fig. 4.33A). In individuals with neuropathic pain, the pain threshold is lower than normal, and it does not decrease when the stimulus rate is increased (interval between stimulus impulses is decreased) (Fig. 4.33B). Abnormal temporal integration is a sign of involvement of the CNS in pain, and testing of temporal integration in the way illustrated in Fig. 4.33 could serve as a diagnostic tool for neuropathic pain (physiologic or inflammatory pain). The hypothesis that carpal tunnel syndrome may involve changes in central processing is supported by the observation in a patient who developed carpal tunnel syndrome during a study of temporal integration of painful stimuli [130]. In the beginning of the study, this individual served as a normal subject in the above-mentioned study of temporal integration in patients with central neuropathic pain. During the course of the study, this individual developed symptoms of the carpal tunnel syndrome and at the same time the temporal integration of painful stimuli changed (Fig. 4.34) to resemble that of patients with central pain symptoms from upper limbs (Fig. 4.33B).

Hyperalgesia

Hyperalgesia[22] may be caused by peripheral or central sensitization (see pp. 201, 204). It can be initiated by trauma such as burns to the skin. It occurs not only in the affected region but also in a region that is adjacent to that which is traumatized (Fig. 4.35). The extension of the affected area of the skin is a result of spread of activation in the dorsal horn, thus probably a result of unmasking of dormant synapses [196]. (Recall that dorsal root fibers send collaterals to many neurons that are not normally activated because the synapses are ineffective.)

---

[22] Hyperalgesia: Extreme sensitivity to painful stimuli.

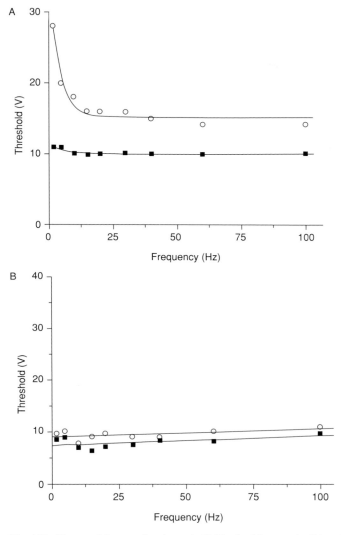

Fig. 4.33 Temporal integration in an individual without pain (A) and a patient with upper limb pain (B). The threshold of sensation (detection) (filled squares) and pain (open circles) in responses to electrical stimulation with impulses applied to the skin of the forearm is shown as a function of the frequency of the impulses. (Reprinted from A. R. Møller and T. Pinkerton. *Neurol. Res.* Vol. 19, 481–488; 1997, with permission [130].)

Hyperpathia

Hyperpathia[23] typically occurs after a period of severe pain. Hyperpathia is a clear sign of change in the central processing of painful stimuli but little is

---

[23] Hyperpathia: an exaggerated reaction to pain with a sensation that lasts beyond the stimulation that caused the pain.

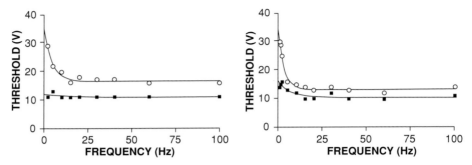

Fig. 4.34 Temporal integration of sensation and pain in response to electrical stimulation applied to the skin of the forearm (as in Fig. 4.33) in an individual who developed pain from carpal tunnel syndrome after being tested as an individual without pain. The results shown in the two graphs were obtained before (A) and after (B) the individual experienced chronic pain (7-month interval). (Reprinted from A. R. Møller and T. Pinkenton, *Neurol. Res.* vol. 19, 481–488; 1997, with permission [130].)

known about the physiological basis for such changes. The fact that hyperpathia can be treated successfully by tricyclic antidepressant medications suggest that abnormalities in serotonin pathways may be involved.

Abnormal cross-modal interaction

Abnormal cross modal interaction occurs when stimulation of one sensory system produces a sensation of another sensory modality [131] (see also Chapter 1, p. 14). When stimulation of mechanoreceptors that normally produces a sensation of light touch gives rise to a sensation of pain, it is a sign of an abnormal cross-modal interaction. When stimulation of skin receptors causes a sensation of sound it is likewise caused by rerouting of information from somatosensory receptors somewhere in the nervous system. Cross-modal interaction is a result of re-routing of sensory (or pain) information, which occurs because of expression of neural plasticity.

Allodynia

The sensation of pain from normally innocuous sensory stimulation (allodynia) that often accompanies central neuropathic pain is a sign that abnormal connections between the somatosensory system and pain circuits have been established. Such re-routing of information is the basis for the observed cross-modal interactions. Increased efficacy and lowered threshold of normally inefficient (dormant) synapses can cause such re-routing of information. Unmasking of inefficient synapses [196] may occur as a result of expression of neural plasticity and it can establish new functional connections in the spinal cord and the brainstem through which sensory systems can activate pain circuits. Change

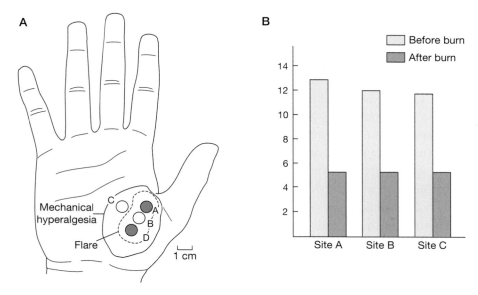

Fig. 4.35 Hyperalgesia from experimentally induced burns to the skin (53 degree C for 30 sec).
A. Mechanical hyperalgesia was recorded at 3 sites (A, B and C).
B. Threshold to pain before and after the burns at the three sites.
Adapted from Raja *et al.* 1984 [153].

in the input to a neuron from low impulse frequency to a high impulse frequency is another way in which a target neuron can respond to input from sources that normally do not elicit any response. High firing rates (short interval between incoming impulses) can create excitatory postsynaptic potentials (EPSPs) of sufficient amplitude to reach the threshold of a target neuron that cannot be activated by input of lower discharge rates (see Chapter 1, Fig. 7.4). Change from continuous firing to burst firing can make it possible to activate a target neuron even though the average firing rate is unchanged. Changes in firing pattern of neurons can occur through expression of neural plasticity or from various forms of insults to nerves (see Chapter 3).

There is evidence that new connections may be created through sprouting of axons and some studies have indicated that A fibers in the dorsal horn may sprout into the territorium of C fibers in the dorsal horn (lamina II) that normally process pain impulses [94, 95, 209].

Substance P (SP) is involved in generating neural activity in the dorsal horn that can be interpreted as pain. SP is an important nociceptive neural transmitter that can lower the threshold of synapses whereby it can unmask normally silent synapses. If SP is liberated into the gray matter of the spinal cord or the brainstem it can affect the transmission of pain signals by increasing the sensitivity of second order neurons [3, 8, 29, 164], and promote unmasking of dormant synapses.

Affective disorders caused by pain

Central neuropathic pain is often accompanied by more or less pronounced mood (affective) symptoms that in some individuals may attain the magnitude of clinical depression. One reason for this may be found in altered connections from pain circuits to the amygdala. The amygdala nuclei normally receive sensory input through association cortices via ventral thalamic nuclei and primary sensory cortices ("the high route" [102]). Activity in the dorsal or medial thalamic nuclei can also reach the lateral nucleus of the amygdala directly through a subcortical route (the "low route") [45, 102] (see p. 81), which may conduct sensory and pain information to the lateral nucleus of the amygdala and subsequently to the basolateral and central nuclei of the amygdala. From there, information can reach autonomic, behavioral, endocrine centers, and the nucleus basalis [117] (see also [131]). Activity from nucleus basalis promotes neural plasticity in the cerebral cortex and provides arousal of primary and secondary sensory cortical areas [89] (see also [131]).

Information that reaches the amygdala through the "high route" is highly processed by the cerebral cortex and subjected to modulation and control from many sources, but the information that reaches the amygdala nuclei from the dorsal thalamus is less processed and under less cerebral control. Neural activity in hyperactive disorders such as central neuropathic pain and tinnitus may be routed through the medial and dorsal thalamic nuclei and reach limbic structures directly through a subcortical route. This may explain why pain and tinnitus often are accompanied by affective symptoms such as depression and fear (for example phonophobia may occur in connection with severe tinnitus [132]). Expression of neural plasticity and establishment of new connections in the brain or spinal cord through expression of neural plasticity may therefore explain at least some of the affective attributes to pain.

Involvement of the sympathetic nervous system

The sympathetic nervous system can be involved in pain conditions in several ways. The sympathetic nervous system can influence the sensitivity of nociceptors (sensitize) and sympathetic activity can modulate pain transmission in the dorsal horn. Muscle activity (muscle tone) is affected by the degree of stress [177], and this is especially the case for the neck muscles. Increased sympathetic activity ("stress") is therefore a contributing factor to many pain disorders where increased muscle tension plays a role [177].

Pain conditions that are directly related to sympathetic activity are known as sympathetic maintained pain (SMP) [14, 77]. Partial nerve injury can cause injured and uninjured nerves to express α-adrenoreceptors causing such axons to discharge in response to circulating epinephrine and norepinephrine. Sympathetic afferent fibers enter the dorsal horn of the spinal cord and their activity can modulate neural transmission in pain circuits of the dorsal horn. Sprouting sympathetic nerve fibers that project to the dorsal root ganglia (DRG) may also be involved in causing SMP.

The term RSD has also been used as a general description of pain where the sympathetic nervous system is involved. More recently more differentiated groups of disorders have been identified and specific terminology has been adapted. RSD has been replaced by the term complex regional pain syndrome (CRPS Type I). CPRS Type I is similar to RSD and the symptoms follow noxious events and include spontaneous pain and possibly allodynia and hyperpathia, and skin edema and abnormal sudomotor (sweat glands activated by sympathetic nerves) activity, in larger anatomical regions of the body [166]. The term "causalgia" has been used earlier to describe pain where the sympathetic nervous system was involved. The term causalgia has been replaced by the term CRPS Type II, which relates to syndromes that have more anatomically localized symptoms than those of CRPS Type I, and which are often observed following peripheral nerve injury. CRPS II may include allodynia and hyperpathia, and skin edema, but in more localized body regions than that of CRPS Type I [124, 166].

Despite many attempts to divide these pain conditions into more homogenous groups, each diagnosis still includes conditions with great variations, and it is not known if the criteria that are used for the diagnosis relate consistently to the physiological and anatomical abnormalities that are important for generating the final outcome of interest, namely pain. Diagnostic tests are few and generally unspecific. However, changes in blood flow due to changes in vascular innervation may be demonstrated on bone scans.

The treatments used for these conditions are diverse, indicating that none is probably especially efficient. The effect of treatment with a beta-adrenergic blocker (such as propanolol) has not been extensively studied but such treatment has shown minimal effect in one study [165].

The sympathetic nervous system has two mainly opposite effects on pain. It can increase the sensitivity of nociceptors, and it can decrease (or block) pain transmission in the dorsal horn. Adrenergic substances (locally secreted or circulating catecholamines) can have the opposite effect on pain. The amplitude of C fiber compound action potentials increases after sympathetic stimulation [166, 170] supporting the hypothesis that sympathetic stimulation can increase the sensitivity of pain receptors. Circulating catecholamines can act on injured nerves which could explain some forms of pain that occur after trauma to nerves, such as after amputation where stump neuroma develops, and become sensitive to norepinephrine [25]. Sympathetic stimulation normally exerts inhibitory influence on dorsal horn pain cells (lamina I–II) as a part of the flight and fight reaction, but circulating catecholamines can also increase the sensitivity of central pain neurons, promoting plastic changes of WDR neurons. To further complicate matters, the effect of sympathetic activations (catecholamines) seems to change with time.

It is documented that sympathectomy can have a beneficial effect on pain such as phantom limb pain, stump pain and herpes virus induced pain [137]. While sympathectomy often produces good short term effects the long term effects are poor according to two studies [158, 186] and post–sympathectomy pain is an obstacle in that form of treatment. Sympathectomy, which is often beneficial in the early stage of SMP, thus loses its effect with time. Medical treatment aimed at reducing the effect of the sympathetic nervous system on pain has had little success. One reason is that it is mainly alpha-adrenergic receptors that are involved in these actions. Chemical sympathectomy using alpha-blocking agents such as phentolamine or phenoxybenzamine may be successful. Treatment with alpha-adrenergic blocking agents causes side effects such as orthostatic reactions observable when an individual attempts to rise from a prone position. Treatment with β adrenergic blockers such as those commonly used medications for heart ailments, is ineffective in treating pain [165]. Intravenous guanethidine that reduces norepinephrine in adrenergic neurons and blocks reuptake is effective in treatment of some patients with CRPS I, but some patients have experienced transient increase of pain following days or weeks of improvement.

The reduction in the beneficial response to manipulations of the sympathetic nervous system, with time, may be a form of expression of neural plasticity that is aimed at resetting the artificial changes induced by the therapy. The pain that sometimes occurs weeks after sympathectomy (interruption of the sympathetic chain) may also be caused by concomitant severing of other tracts that cause axon degeneration, and subsequently deprivation hypersensitivity. Sympathectomy at more peripheral locations does not seem to have that effect. In addition to catecholamines, prostaglandins seem to be involved in these very complex pain conditions. These substances may sensitize cells in the dorsal horn as a part of pain processes.

Again, the involvement of the sympathetic nervous system in pain is complex and incompletely understood. It has been questioned whether the sympathetic nervous system is always involved in pain conditions that are now known as CRPS [77]. It has been noted that similar symptoms may occur without the sympathetic

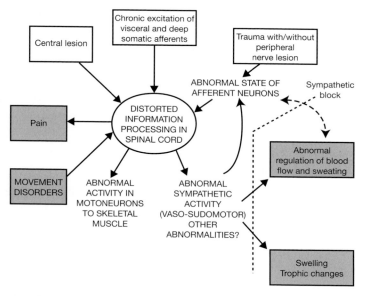

Fig. 4.36 Illustration of contemporary hypotheses of neural mechanisms involved in generating CRPS I and II following trauma. Adapted from Jänig, 1996 [76]

nervous system being involved. A recent hypothesis suggests involvement of many factors in generation of CPRS I and II syndromes (Fig. 4.36).

4.4.5   Visceral pain

The pathophysiology of pain from viscera is different from that of somatic pain [32]. Pain from the same parts of the viscera and the heart varies from individual to individual and the emotional components tend to be greater for visceral pain than pain caused by activation of nociceptors in the skin and muscles. Painful stimulation of the viscera and the heart are likely to produce referred pain and other sensations than pain, such as nausea and generally feeling unwell [149, 150]. The fact that ischemia of the heart can occur without noticeable symptoms in many individuals [85] or with non-pain symptoms (nausea and vomiting) [148, 149] is not generally recognized. The different symptoms of ischemia of the heart can only be partly explained by what is known about the neural pathways, and much regarding pain from the heart and viscera is unknown. In particular, it is unknown why there is such a great individual variation in the symptoms of insults to viscera and the heart [85]. Some investigators have ascribed anatomical and biochemical differences [138] in the heart to the differences in the symptoms and signs of ischemia, while others have suggested that differences in central processing of pain signals are the cause of the individual variations [149]. These matters are naturally of great importance

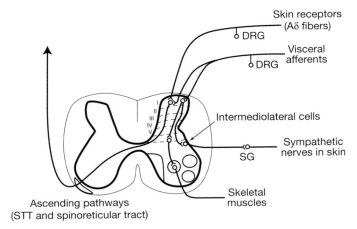

Fig. 4.37 Schematic diagram of the anatomical basis for one hypothesis for referred pain and sensitization of different nociceptors. Adapted from [34].

for diagnostics but are also of importance for individuals who need to know which signals should be interpreted as being indications of a serious condition that needs prompt medical attention.

Referred pain

Referred pain has been attributed to change (extension) of the receptive fields of neurons by activating dormant synapses, i.e. expression of neural plasticity. Pain from organs in the lower abdomen and reproductive organs is often referred to T_{12}-L_1, dermatomes, thus in accordance with the location where the afferent nerves enter the spinal cord [33]. However, as mentioned above, the receptors of some parts of pelvic organs are innervated by nerve fibers that follow the parasympathetic fibers entering the spinal cord as parts of dorsal roots of the sacral spine. This means that some pain from pelvic organs may be referred to the distribution (dermatomes) of sacral somatic nerves.

The anatomical basis for referred pain is not known in detail [32, 33]. Several hypotheses have been presented regarding the mechanisms. One hypothesis assumes that referred pain in connection with visceral pain is based on the assumption that the same cells in the dorsal horn receive input both from receptors in the viscera and from receptors in the skin (Fig. 4.34) [32] [34]. In fact the nerve cells in the dorsal horns that receive input from visceral organs also receive input from receptors in the skin and muscles.

Referred muscle pain may occur as a result of the diffusion of SP and calcitonin generated peptides in the dorsal horn of the spinal cord [123], which may explain the pathophysiology of trigger points[24] that is associated in muscle pain [71] (see p. 196). The sympathetic nervous system may be involved in referred pain (Fig. 4.37). (The sympathetic nervous system plays an important role by increasing the sensitivity of skin receptors, and activation of alpha motoneurons may occur causing contraction of skeletal muscles, which may cause pain, see p. 214). Referred pain may also be caused by convergence of pain impulses at more central locations such as the thalamus.

4.4.6   Itch

Itch can be caused by peripheral stimulation [83] as well as from central disturbances [47, 189]. The common forms of itch, such as for instance, from mosquito bites, is associated with release of histamine in the skin. Similar release of histamine can occur as an allergic reaction causing redness of the skin (associated with the effect of histamine), and the effect (skin changes and itch) can be lessened by antihistamines such as benadryl. Allergic reactions can cause itch by similar mechanisms.

Pruritus (itching) is related to pain, and assumed to use similar pathways as used by noxious stimulation, but different receptors, but itch rarely occurs together with pain and pain can inhibit itch [83]. The receptors for itch are similar to those that are activated by capsaicin but not identical and the targets for the information from these itch receptors are obviously different from that of the capsaicin receptor. Capsaicin causes a burning sensation and itch creates a desire to scratch. Stimulation of the receptors in the skin that mediate the sensation of itch are specialized unmyelinated chemoreceptors, and specialized circuitry in the spinal cord processes the information from these receptors [63, 168, 215]. Histamine and serotonin have been shown to activate superficial neurons in the dorsal horn [23]. These neurons may mediate the scratching behavior in response to itch [83].

Itch can be caused by injuries [199] and by functional changes in the CNS. Such forms of itch have similarities with central neuropathic pain and respond favorably to similar medications as are effective in treatment of central neuropathic pain (such as anticonvulsants and antidepressants). There is some clinical evidence that neuropathy (peripheral nerve disorders) can cause itch [31, 114, 220]. That itch can be elicited from the CNS is obvious from the observation that itch in the face often occurs when sleepy or just before sleep. Itch is also associated with depression and other affective disorders.

---

[24] Trigger points are locations on the skin (or in the mouth) where sensory stimulation (touch, cold or warmth) elicits an attack of pain. Many forms of pain have distinct trigger points from which pain can be elicited or from which attacks of pain can be initiated.

Another seemingly different type of itch is elicited as a side effect of, for example, opioids [91]. That form of itch is not caused by release of histamine, and it cannot be reduced by antihistamines, but antagonists to opioids (naloxone and naltrexone that inhibit μ and κ receptors) [99, 188] indicating that opioid receptors are involved in that kind of itch. While itch that is caused by local irritation responds to local treatment it would not be expected that itch that is caused by injury to the CNS would respond to such treatment. However, a recent study showed that itch that occurred as a result of a lesion to the spinal cord and occurred together with pain in a different region of the body, responded favorably to local application of a local anesthetic (Lidocain patch) [163].

It is believed that the information from "itch" receptors travels in similar ascending pathways as pain impulses [83, 168]. A specific class of cells of STT neurons in lamina I of the spinal horn have been found to respond selectively to histamine applied iontophoretically, simulating the cause of (peripheral) itch [38]. Since itch induces scratching, the central projection of the nerve fibers that mediate that must therefore be different from that of fibers that mediate the sensation of pain. The motor commands elicited by itch (scratching) may be initiated at subcortical levels as indicated by the fact that people scratch in their sleep, or it can be a highly coordinated motor activity that involves cerebral activity. There is a certain pleasure associated with scratching which indicates association with the old parts of the brain such as limbic structures and the cingulate gyrus. This shows that the generation of the neural activity that causes the sensation of itch is complicated, and the anatomical and physiological bases of itch are poorly understood.

4.5   Treatment of central neuropathic pain

Modern treatments of pain span a wide range of attempts to modify the function of the parts of the CNS that are involved in pain. We have already discussed some methods for treatment of central neuropathic pain. Other methods make use of making lesions in CNS structures.

> Some forms of chronic pain have been treated surgically by destruction of the dorsal root entry zones of the dorsal horn of the spinal cord through selectively destructing the layers that are dominated by C fiber entrances (Lissauer's tract) [174]. However, this dorsal root entry zone (DREZ) procedure is now largely abandoned except for brachialplexopathy.

Lesions have been made in almost all structures (including fiber tracts and nuclei) along the neuroaxis of pain pathways from the spinal cord (and the trigeminal nucleus) to the cerebral cortex, including thalamotomy [218] and cingulotomy [64, 143].

Administration of drugs for treatment of severe pain is still the most common means for controlling severe pain although the mechanisms of action are not completely understood. We will discuss some treatments that have been especially important in bringing new light to the understanding of the various forms of pain including central neuropathic pain.

4.5.1   Stimulation of peripheral nerves (TENS)

Electrical stimulation of peripheral nerves (TENS) [205] has been used for many years in treatment of pain. The underlying mechanisms for immediate pain reduction using TENS is most likely related to activation of large (Aβ) fibers that are inhibitory on dorsal horn pain neurons. Stimulation of peripheral nerves or dermatomes, such as occurs when using TENS, can probably activate several segments of the spinal cord if stimulating at a high rate because such stimulation can open dormant synapses [196]. This may in turn suppress neural activity in pain circuits at several segments up and down from the root that is stimulated because of the inhibitory effect of Aβ fiber stimulus. However, TENS may also promote expression of neural plasticity in the spinal cord and supraspinal structures (and the trigeminal nucleus), which may be the cause of the long-term effect of TENS on central neuropathic pain. The mechanisms for this action are poorly understood.

4.5.2   Stimulation of the dorsal column

The hypothesis behind dorsal column stimulation relates to the Melzak-Wall gating hypothesis [119], assuming that antidromic stimulation of dorsal column fibers influences neurons in the dorsal horn. The WDR neurons are most likely involved.

> Studies in rats have shown that ligation of the sciatic nerve produces signs of allodynia [212]. The spontaneous discharge of WDR neurons in such rats is higher than in controls. Spinal cord stimulation increased the spontaneous rate in 1/3 of such "allodynia" rats, but it had little effect on the spontaneous activity in controls. The effect lasted long after termination of the spinal cord stimulation in the rats with allodynia [212]. Depression of spontaneous activity from spinal cord stimulation was almost only seen in allodynia rats.

Orthodromic activation of dorsal column fibers is assumed to exert suppressive actions through descending pathways [126] but ascending activity may also have beneficial effect by inducing plastic changes in supraspinal structures.

4.5.3   Thalamic stimulation and lesioning

There is increasing evidence that the thalamus is involved in different forms of pain (p. 163), and this has intensified attempts to treat some forms of pain by making lesions or by electrical stimulation (DBS) of specific nuclei of the thalamus [56, 104, 216, 222]. DBS has now replaced many of the earlier used destructive procedures for treatment of severe pain. (DBS is also used for treatment of movement disorders, see Chapter 5.) The use of these techniques, besides providing a much-needed therapeutic tool, has brought new knowledge regarding the pathophysiology of some forms of neuropathic pain.

The way deep brain stimulation using implanted electrodes works is not entirely understood. Animal experiments have shown indications that high frequency electrical stimulation can block sodium and L- and T-type calcium current, and that should be the cause of the observed inhibition (inactivation of neurons) [159] [10] [133]. It has also been suggested that high frequency stimulation may re-synchronize abnormal impulse patterns that are associated with pathologic functions such as pain [159]. It has also been hypothesized that electrical stimulation work by inactivation of the tissue stimulated by constantly depolarizing nerve cells, achieves a similar effect to that of ablation but is reversible. The stimulation, however, may also activate structures beyond the location of the electrodes, possibly activating anatomically distant regions of the CNS in an abnormal and unanticipated way. While electrical stimulation may constantly hyperpolarize many nerve cells, the stimulation is also likely to activate many nerve fibers in adjacent fiber tracts. Such activation is abnormal and may cause temporally coherent high frequency firings of many fibers (rates of stimulation of 120–180 pps are commonly used).

4.5.4   Lesions of limbic structures

Lesions in the cingulate gyrus have been made to treat severe chronic pain with some success [64, 143]. Although lesions in other limbic structures are effective in treating psychiatric disorders, their efficacy in treating pain has not been established [59].

4.5.5   Stimulation of the prefrontal cortex and other CNS structures

The use of electrical stimulation of the motor cortex or the prefrontal cortex for control of neuropathic pain that is resistant to other treatments has recently been studied by many investigators [21, 86, 125, 140]. Stimulation of the motor cortex has also been found to reduce the pain elicited by stimulation of nociceptors [48].

The exact mechanisms for the beneficial effect of such stimulation are not known. Connections from the prefrontal motor cortex to the amygdala and other limbic structures could be responsible for the beneficial effect of electrical stimulation in pain but other connections to limbic structures could mediate the beneficial effect. Connections from the prefrontal motor cortex could activate the descending PAG pathways (Fig. 4.19). The fact that stimulation of the prefrontal cortex has a beneficial effect on some forms of pain has likewise increased our knowledge regarding the pathophysiology of neuropathic pain. The beneficial effect of motor cortex stimulation [21] decreases with time of use, as is the case for many other treatments of neuropathic pain.

Blockade or ablation and lesions in the sympathetic system has been used for treatment of some pain conditions [109]. Many or perhaps most of these methods were introduced without knowledge about their ways of action, but only later, if at all, has it become understood how these methods had their beneficial effect on the various forms of pain they were aimed at treating. The implementation of these methods and the experience with their action has brought much new understanding of the pathophysiology of many different pain conditions.

4.5.6   Stimulation of the vagus nerve

That electrical stimulation of the vagus nerve is beneficial in treatment of pain [90] was surprising when first introduced. It was discovered in connection with the use of electrical stimulation of the vagus nerve in controlling epileptic seizures. While the mechanisms for its effect on pain are still incompletely understood the use of vagus stimulation in pain control has provided evidence that the vagus nerve plays an important role in endogenous pain [54].

> Studies in cats and monkeys have shown that electrical stimulation of the vagus nerve attenuates the response from neurons in the dorsal horn to many different type types of noxious and innocuous stimuli [26]. Vagal activity elicited by endocrine stimulation from the adrenal medullae has a similar effect [78]. The effect seems to be related to anatomical connections between the vagus nerve and the dorsal horn neurons that mediate pain [54, 78].
>
> Other studies have shown that stimulation of the vagus nerve reduces the pain from controlled stimulation of nociceptors and it reduces the temporal integration of pain elicited by 5 consecutive impulses ("wind up") (see p. 205) and pain from tonic pressure [90]. However, the same study showed that pain associated with single impulses of heat was not affected [90]. This indicates that activity in the vagus nerve mainly affects the central processing of pain (central inhibition). Other studies have indicated that the effect of vagal activity on pain is mediated through the NA-serotonin descending system (Fig. 4.20) [185].

The vagus nerve seems to be involved in opioid-induced analgesia as studies in rats have shown that vagotomy decreases the analgesic effect of morphine administered intravenously in rats [54]. This means that intact function of the vagus nerve is necessary for the analgesic effect of morphine.

The involvement of the vagus nerve in sexual function especially in women has been the focus of a few studies that seem to show that the vagus nerve supplies sensory input to the brain that bypasses the spinal cord [96, 203, 204]. There are indications that the vagus nerve provides some sensory input to the brain from the lower abdomen (genitalia) and that such activation may decrease pain perception [39].

The use of electrical stimulation of CNS structures for pain and motor disorders may induce changes in the organization and function of parts of the nervous system. These changes may be responsible for some of the side effects of such treatment. Some form of neural plasticity may be responsible for the deterioration of the beneficial effect of making lesions in CNS structures or the use of DBS. The reduced efficacy of such intervention may thus be yet another example of expression of neural plasticity, which counteract the anticipated effects of treatment.

4.5.7   Psychoactive drugs

Antidepressants such as imipramine, amitriptylin, nortriptylin and some sodium channel blockers are effective in treating neuropathic pain [175]. However, the efficacy of the different kinds of these drugs varies as seen in Table 4.1. Sodium channel blockers such as carbamazepine and mexiletine were some of the least effective of these drugs. Selective serotonin reuptake inhibitors were less effective than imipramine. Studies of the effectiveness of antidepressants have indicated that the serotonin system is involved in central neuropathic pain but the fact that selective serotonin reuptake inhibitors are less effective than non-specific drugs such as imipramine and nortriptylin [175] may set that assumption in question and indicate a more complex relationship between central pain and the serotonin system.

4.5.8   Treatment of itch

Opioids are frequently used in the management of pain and itch. However, opioids, while having the ability to relieve both pain and itch, also have the possibility to cause itch. The mechanisms for that side-effect of opioids are not completely understood, but it has been hypothesized that the response of superficial neurons in the dorsal horn of the spinal cord to low concentrations of histamine is facilitated by morphine, and that may be involved in the development of itch [82].

Table 4.1 *Efficacy of different pharmacological treatments for neuropathic pain. (Adapted from [175]).*

Number of patients needed to be treated to obtain one patient with more than 50% pain relief. In case of more than one study on a drug in the pertinent pain type NNT is calculated for combined data. NA = Not active, ND = Not done, TCA = tricyclic antidepressants, SSRI = selective serotonin reuptake inhibitors

	Pain	Painful neuropathy Trigeminal neuralgia	Postherpetic neuralgia	Peripheral nerve injury	Central
Antidepressants					
all types (1.1±3.0)	ND	3.0 (2.4±4.0)	2.3 (1.7±3.3)	2.5 (1.4±10.6)	1.7
TCA all types (1.1±3.0)	ND	2.4 (2.0±3.0)	2.3 (1.7±3.3)	2.5 (1.4±10.6)	1.7
TCA serot./noradr. (1.1±3.0)	ND	2.0 (1.7±2.5)	2.4 (1.8±3.9)	2.5 (1.4±10.6)	1.7
TCA noradrenergic	ND	3.4 (2.3±6.6)	1.9 (1.3±3.7)	ND	ND
TCA serot./noradr. Optimal dose	ND	1.4 (1.1±1.9)	ND	ND	ND
SSRI	ND	6.7 (3.4±435)	ND	ND	NA
Ion channel blockers Mexiletine	ND	10.0 (3±1)	ND	ND	NA
Phenytoin	ND	2.1 (1.5±3.6)	ND	ND	ND
Carbamazepine (1.7±105)	2.6 (2.2±3.3)	3.3 (2±9.4)	ND	ND	3.4
Lamotrigin	2.1 (1.3±6.1)	ND	ND	ND	ND[a]
Gabapentin	ND	3.7 (2.4±8.3)	3.2 (2.4±5.0)	ND	ND
NMDA antagonists Dextromethorphan	ND	1.9 (1.1±3.7)	NA	ND[b]	NA
Memantine	ND	ND	NA	ND	ND
GABA_B agonist Baclofen	1.4 (1.0±2.6)	ND	ND	ND	ND[c]
Opioids Oxycodone	ND	ND[d]	2.5 (1.6±5.1)	ND	ND
Tramadol	ND	3.4 (2.3±6.4)	ND	ND	ND
Various Levodopa	ND	3.4 (1.5±1)	ND	ND	ND
Capsaicin	ND	5.9 (3.8±13)	5.3 (2.3±1)	3.5 (1.6±1)	ND

[a] Add on therapy to carbamazepine.

[b] Low dose of dextromethorphan.

[c] Add on therapy to carbamazepine or phenytoin in 4 of 10 patients.

[d] For 30% of patients add on therapy to tricyclic antidepressants.

Itch is often caused by chemical imbalances or by pathologies of the CNS. The mechanism for the efficacy of local treatment for itch that is assumed to be caused by pathologies of the CNS (spinal cord) is unknown. Some (normally benign) input from skin receptors may be necessary in order that the changes in central function can cause symptoms. This means that two factors that occur simultaneously could be necessary to cause symptoms, while each factor alone does not cause any noticeable symptoms. It is possible that the relief of itch through scratching has its effect by stimulating skin receptors that exert inhibitory influence on spinal (and trigeminal) pain (itch) neurons. Scratching in response to itch produces a sensation of pleasure but little is known about the central projections of activity that cause itch but it has been shown that the SMA and premotor areas are involved.

4.5.9   Paradoxical effects of opioids and benzodiazepines

Benzodiazepines (such as diazepam) are effective in management of pain that is caused by muscle contractions (spasm) because they are $GABA_A$ agonists and therefore increase inhibition in neurons that are involved in generating muscle activity (or which have facilitatory influence on motoneurons). However, GABAergic inhibition affects descending activity from the PAG that has inhibitory influence on pain-mediating neurons in the dorsal horn (the RVM pathway, see Fig. 4.18). This means that enhancement of GABAergic inhibition from administration of benzodiazepines may in fact decrease the (natural) inhibitory influence on transmission of pain signals in the spinal cord (and the trigeminal nucleus).

Administration of opioids can have beneficial effects on itch but itch can also be a side effect of opioids. Whichever one of these opposite effects is greatest will dominate, and there is no doubt that the analgesic and anti-pruritic effect of opioids normally is the dominating effect, as is the beneficial effect of muscle relaxation on muscle pain from administration of benzodiazepines. However, this balance between beneficial and non-beneficial effects may be shifted for unknown reasons and individual variations so that the paradoxical effects may become noticeable in some individuals under certain circumstances. If that occurs, effect of treatment of pain or itch may appear confusing both to the patient and the physician.

4.5.10   Placebo effect

It is well known that placebo treatment can have a positive effect on pain, and placebo treatment has been recognized as an effective form of treatment for pain [58, 106]. This means that patients who are given inactive medication (placebo), but told that they are treated for their pain, improve and experience a decrease in their pain symptoms. The placebo effect could be caused by endogenous opioids that were produced because of the expectation of pain relief from the assumed active medication (which was in fact inactive). One study of postoperative patients supported that hypothesis, and showed that those subjects, who responded positively to placebo, responded to subsequent administration of naloxone with increased pain. Those who did not respond to the first administration of placebo did not respond to naloxone either [106]. Considering the complexity of pain perception and the involvement of emotional factors in many forms of pain makes it understandable that additional mechanisms may be involved in the observed effect of placebo treatment for pain [58]. The limbic structures and descending pathways from the prefrontal cortex most likely play important roles in some forms of pain perception and the subsequent beneficial effect of treatment with placebos.

References

1. Abbadie, C., J. L. Brown, C. R. Mantyh, and A. I. Basbaum, Spinal Cord Substance P Receptor Immunoreactivity Increases in Both Inflammatory and Nerve Injury Models of Persistent Pain. *Neuroscience*, 1996. **70**: pp. 201–209.

2. Amaral, D. G., J. L. Price, A. Pitkanen, and S. T. Carmichael, Anatomical Organization of the Primate Amygdaloid Complex, in *The Amygdala*, J. P. Aggleton, Editor. 1992, Wiley-Liss: New York. pp. 1–66.

3. Arnettz, B. B. and B. Fjellner, Psychological Predictors of Neuroendocrine Responses to Mental Stress. *J. Psychosomatic Res.*, 1986. **30**: pp. 297–305.

4. Bach, S., M. F. Noreng, and N. U. Tjellden, Phantom Limb Pain in Amputees During the First 12 Months Following Limb Amputation, after Preoperative Lumbar Epidural Blockade. *Pain*, 1988. **33**: pp. 297–301.

5. Bandler, R. and M. T. Shipley, Columnar Organization in the Midbrain Periaqueductal Gray: Modules for Emotional Expression? *Trends Neurosci.*, 1994. **17**: pp. 379–389.

6. Basbaum, A. I., C. H. Clanton, and H. L. Fields, Three Bulbospinal Pathways from the Rostral Medulla of the Cat: An Autoradiographic Study of Pain Modulating Systems. *J. Comp. Neurol.*, 1978. **178**: pp. 209–224.

7. Basbaum, A. I. and H. L. Fields, Endogenous Pain Control Systems: Brainstem Spinal Pathways and Endorphin Circuitry. *Ann. Rev. Neurosci*, 1984. **7**(309–338).

8. Bennett, R. M., Fibromyalgia, in *Handbook of Pain*, P. D. Wall and R. Melzack, Editors. 1999, Churchill Livingstone: Edinburgh. pp. 579–601.

9. Berthoud, H. R. and W. L. Neuhuber, Functional and Chemical Anatomy of the Afferent Vagal System. *Autonomic Neurosci.*, 2000. **85**(1–3): pp. 1–17.

10. Beurrier, C., B. Bioulac, J. Audin, and Et Al., High-Frequency Stimulation Produces a Transient Blockade of Voltage-Gated Currents in Subthalamic Neurons. *J. Neurophys.*, 2001. **85**: pp. 1351–1356.

11. Blackburn-Munro, G. and R. E. Blackburn-Munro, Chronic Pain, Chronic Stress and Depression: Coincidence or Consequence? *J Neuroendocrinol*, 2001. **13**(12): pp. 1009–23.

12. Boivie, J. and B. A. Meyerson, A Correlative Anatomical and Clinical Study of Pain Suppression by Deep Brain Stimulation. *Pain*, 1982. **13**: pp. 113–126.

13. Boivie, J., Central Pain, in *Textbook of Pain*, P. D. Wall and R. Melzack, Editors. 1999, Churchill Livingstone: Edinburgh. pp. 879–914.

14. Bolay, H. and M. A. Moskowitz, Mechanisms of Pain Modulation in Chronic Syndromes. *Neurology*, 2002. **59**(5 Suppl. 2): pp. S2–7.

15. Bonomi, A. E., R. Shikiar, and M. W. Legro, Quality-of-Life Assessment in Acute, Chronic, and Cancer Pain: A Pharmacist's Guide. *J. Am. Pharmaceutical Association.*, 2000. **40**(3): pp. 402–16.

16. Borg-Stein, J. and S. A. Simon, Focused Review: Myofascial Pain. *Arch. Phys. Med. Rehab.*, 2002. **83**(3): pp. S40–7, S48–9.

17. Brodal, P., *The Central Nervous System*. 1998, Oxford University Press: New York.

18. Burstein, R., M. F. Cutrer, and D. Yarnitsky, The Development of Cutaneous Allodynia During a Migraine Attack Clinical Evidence for the Sequential Recruitment of Spinal and Supraspinal Nociceptive Neurons in Migraine. *Brain*, 2000. **123**(8): pp. 1703–9.

19. Cacace, A. T., J. P. Cousins, S. M. Parnes, D. J. McFarland, D. Semenoff, T. Holmes, C. Davenport, K. Stegbauer, and T. J. Lovely, Cutaneous-Evoked Tinnitus. Ii: Review of Neuroanatomical, Physiological and Functional Imaging Studies. *Audiol. Neurotol.*, 1999. **4**(5): pp. 258–268.

20. Campbell, J., S. Raja, and R. Meyer, Painful Sequelae of Nerve Injury, in *Proceedings of the Fifth World Congress on Pain*, R. Dubner, G. Gebhart, and M. Bond, Editors. 1988, Elsevier: Amsterdam. pp. 135–143.

21. Canavero, S., V. Bonicalzi, M. Dotta, S. Vighetti, and G. Asteggiano, Low-Rate Repetitive Tms Allays Central Pain. *Neurol. Res.*, 2003. 25: pp. 151–152.

22. Carli, G., Neuroplasticity and Clinical Pain. *Progr. Brain Res.*, 2000. **129**: pp. 325–330.

23. Carstens, E., Altered Spinal Processing in Animal Models of Radicular and Neuropathic Pain, in *Nervous System Plasticity and Chronic Pain*, J. Sandkühler, B. Bromm, and G. F. Gebhart, Editors. 2000, Elsevier: Amsterdam.

24. Cervero, F., Sensory Innervation of the Viscera: Peripheral Basis of Visceral Pain. *Physiol. Rev.*, 1994. **74**: pp. 95–138.

25. Chabal, C., L. Jacobson, L. C. Russell, and K. J. Burchiel, Pain Response to Perineuroneal Injection of Normal Saline, Epinephrine, and Lidocaine in Humans. *Pain*, 1992. **49**: pp. 9–12.

26. Chandler, M. J., S. F. Hobbs, D. C. Bolser, and R. D. Foreman, Effects of Vagal Afferent Stimulation on Cervical Spinothalamic Tract Neurons in Monkeys. *Pain*, 1991. **44**: pp. 81–87.

27. Cherny, N. I. and R. K. Portenoy, Practical Issues in the Management of Cancer Pain, in *Textbook of Pain*, P. D. Wall and R. Melzack, Editors. 1999, Churchill Livingstone: Edinburgh. pp. 1479–1522.

28. Cherny, N. I. and R. K. Portenoy, Cancer Pain: Principles of Assessment and Syndromes, in *Textbook of Pain*, P. D. Wall and R. Melzack, Editors. 1999, Churchill Livingstone: Edinburgh. pp. 1017–1064.

29. Coderre, T. J., J. Katz, A. L. Vaccarino, and R. Melzack, Contribution of Central Neuroplasticity to Pathological Pain: Review of Clinical and Experimental Evidence. *Pain*, 1993. **52**: pp. 259–285.

30. Coggeshall, R. E., P. M. Dougherty, C. M. Pover, and S. M. Carlton, Is Large Myelinated Fiber Loss Associated with Hyperalgesia in a Model of Experimental Peripheral Neuropathy in the Rat. *Pain*, 1993. **52**: pp. 233–242.

31. Cohen, A. D., R. Masalha, E. Medvedovsky, and D. A. Vardy, Brachioradial Pruritus: A Symptom of Neuropathy. *J. Am. Acad. Dermatol.*, 2003. **48**(6): pp. 825–8.

32. Cousins, M. and I. Power, Acute and Postoperative Pain, in *Textbook of Pain*, P. D. Wall and R. Melzack, Editors. 1999, Churchill Livingstone: Edinburgh. pp. 447–491.

33. Cousins, M. J. and G. D. Philips, *Acute Pain Management. Clinics in Critical Care Medicine.* 1986, Churchill Livingstone: Edinburgh.

34. Cousins, M. J. and P. O. Bridenbbaugh, *Neural Blockade in Clinical Anesthesia and Management of Pain.* 3rd ed. 1998, Lippincott-Raven: Philadelphia.

35. Crago, A., J. C. Houk, and W. Z. Rymer, Sampling of Total Muscle Force by Tendon Organs. *J. Neurophys.*, 1982. **47**: pp. 1069–1083.

36. Craig, A. D., M. C. Bushnell, E. T. Zang, and A. Blomquist, A Thalamic Nuclei Specific for Pain and Temperature. *Nature*, 1994. **372**(6508): pp. 770–3.

37. Craig, A. D. and J. O. Dostrovsky, Medulla to Thalamus, in *Textbook of Pain*, P. D. Wall and R. Melzack, Editors. 1999, Churchill-Livingstone: Edinburgh. pp. 183–214.

38. Craig, A. D., Spinothalamic Lamina I Neurons Sensitive to Histamine: A Central Pathway for Itch. *Nat. Neurosci.*, 2001. **4**(1): pp. 72–7.

39. Crowley, W. R., J. F. Rodriguez-Sierra, and B. R. Komisaruk, Analgesia Induced by Vagina Stimulation in Rats Is Apparently Independent of a Morphine-Sensitive Process. *Psychopharmacology*, 1977. **54**(3): pp. 223–5.

40. Dahlöf, C. G. H., Management of Primary Headaches: Current and Future Aspects, in *Pain 2002 – an Updated Review: Refresher Course Syllabus*, M. A. Giamberardino, Editor. 2002, IASP Press: Seattle.

41. Devor, M., The Pathophysiology of Damaged Peripheral Nerves, in *Textbook of Pain*, P. D. Wall and R. Melzack, Editors. 1994, Churchill Livingstone: Edinburgh. pp. 79–100.

42. Devor, M. and Z. Seltzer, Pathophysiology of Damaged Nerves in Relation to Chronic Pain, in *Textbook of Pain*, P. D. Wall and R. Melzack, Editors. 1999, Churchill Livingstone: Edinburgh. pp. 129–164.

43. Dickenson, A. H., NMDA Receptors Antagonists as an Analgesic. *Prog. in Pain Res. and Management*, 1994. **1**: pp. 173–187.

44. Dickenson, A. H., Balance between Excitatory and Inhibitory Events in the Spinal Cord and Chronic Pain. *Prog. Brain Res.*, 1996. **110**: pp. 225–231.

45. Doron, N. N. and J. E. Ledoux, Cells in the Posterior Thalamus Project to Both Amygdala and Temporal Cortex: A Quantitative Retrograde Double-Labeling Study in the Rat. *J. Comp. Neurol.*, 2000. **425**: pp. 257–274.

46. Doubell, T. P., R. J. Mannion, and C. J. Woolf, The Dorsal Horn: State-Dependent Sensory Processing, Plasticity and the Generation of Pain, in *Handbook of Pain*, P. D. Wall and R. Melzack, Editors. 1999, Churchill Livingstone: Edinburgh. pp. 165–181.

47. Drzezga, A., U. Darsow, R. D. Treede, H. Siebner, M. Frisch, F. Munz, F. Weilke, J. Ring, M. Schwaiger, and P. Bartenstein, Central Activation by Histamine-Induced Itch: Analogies to Pain Processing: A Correlational Analysis of O-15 H_2O Positron Emission Tomography Studies. *Pain*, 2001. **92**(1–2): pp. 295–305.

48. Farina, S., M. Tinazzi, D. Pera Le, and M. Valeriani, Pain-Related Modulation of the Human Motor Cortex. *Neurol. Res.*, 2003. **25**: pp. 130–142.

49. Fields, H. L. and A. I. Basbaum, Central Nervous System Mechanism of Pain Modulation, in *Textbook of Pain*, P. D. Wall and R. Melzack, Editors. 1999, Churchill Livingstone: Edinburgh. pp. 309–329.

50. Freund, B. J. and M. Schwartz, Relief of Tension-Type Headache Symptoms in Subjects with Temporomandibular Disorders Treated with Botulinum Toxin-A. *Headache*, 2002. **42**(10): pp. 1033–37.

51. Fu, Q. G., M. J. Chandler, D. L. McNeill, and R. D. Foreman, Vagal Afferent Fibers Excite Upper Cervical Neurons and Inhibit Activity of Lumbar Spinal Cord Neurons in the Rat. *Pain*, 1992. **51**: pp. 91–100.

52. Fusco, B. M., S. Marabini, C. A. Maggi, G. Fiore, and P. Geppetti, Preventive Effect of Repeated Nasal Applications of Capsaicin in Cluster Headache. *Pain*, **1994**(59): pp. 321–325.

53. Garonzik, I. M., S. E. Hua, S. Ohara, and F. A. Lenz, Intraoperative Microelectrode and Semi-Microelectrode Recording During the Physiological Localization of the Thalamic Nucleus Ventral Intermediate. *Movement Disorders*, 2002. **17**(3).

54. Gebhart, G. F. and A. Randich, Vagal Modulation of Nociception. *Am. Pain Soc. J.*, 1992. **1**: pp. 26–32.

55. Gerhart, K. D., R. P. Yezierski, and G. J. Giesler, Inhibitory Receptive Fields of Primate Spinothalamic Tract Cells. *J. Neurophys*, 1981. **46**: pp. 1309–25.

56. Gorecki, J., T. Hirayama, J. O. Dostrovsky, R. R. Tasker, and F. A. Lenz, Thalamic Stimulation and Recording in Patients with Deafferentation and Central Pain. *Stereotactic & Functional Neurosurgery*, 1989. **52**(2–4): pp. 219–26.

57. Graven-Nielsen, T. and S. Mense, The Peripheral Apparatus of Muscle Pain: Evidence from Animal and Human Studies. *Clin. J. Pain.*, 2001. **17**(1): pp. 2–10.

58. Grevert, P., L. H. Albert, and A. Goldstein, Partial Antagonism of Placebo Analgesia by Naloxone. *Pain*, 1983. **16**: pp. 129–143.

59. Gybels, J. M. and R. R. Tasker, Central Neurosurgery, in *Textbook of Pain*, P. D. Wall and R. Melzack, Editors. 1999, Churchill Livingstone: Edinburgh. pp. 1307–1339.

60. Hall, T. M. and R. L. Elvey, Nerve Trunk Pain: Physical Diagnosis and Treatment. *Manual Therapy*, 1999. **4**(2): pp. 63–73.

61. Hammond, D. L., G. M. Tyce, and T. L. Yaksh, Efflux of 5-Hydroxytryptamine and Noradrenaline into Spinal Cord Superfusates During Stimulation of the Rat Medulla. *J. Physiol.*, 1985. **359**: pp. 151–162.

62. Han, S. C. and P. Harrison, Myofascial Pain Syndrome and Trigger-Point Management. *Regional Anesthesia*, 1997. **95**(2): pp. 89–101.

63. Handwerker, H. O., W. Magerl, F. Klemm, and R. A. Westerman, Quantitative Evaluation of Itch Sensation, in *Fine Afferent Nerve Fibers and Pain*, R. F. Schmidt, H.-G. Schaible, and C. Vahle-Hinz, Editors. 1987, VCH Verlagsgesellschaft: Germany. pp. 462–473.

64. Hassenbusch, S. J., P. K. Pillay, and G. H. Barnett, Radiofrequency Cingulotomy for Intractable Cancer Pain Using Stereotaxis Guided by Magnetic Resonance Imaging. *Neurosurg.*, 1990. **27**(2): pp. 220–3.

65. Haws, C. M., A. M. Williamson, and H. L. Fields, Putative Nociceptive Modulatory Neurons in the Dorsolateral Pontomesencephalic Reticular Formation. *Brain Res.*, 1989. **483**: pp. 272–282.

66. Herbert, H. and C. B. Saper, Organization of Medullary Adrenergic and Noradrenergic Projections to Periaqueductal Gray Matter in the Rat. *J. Comp. Neurol.*, 1992. **315**: pp. 34–52.

67. Herndon, R. M., *Handbook of Neurologic Rating Scales*. 1997, Demos Vermande New York: New York.

68. Hirato, M., K. Watanabe, A. Takahashi, N. Hayase, S. Horikoshi, T. Shibaski, and C. Ohye, Pathophysiology of Central (Thalamic) Pain: Combined Change of Sensory Thalamus with Cerebral Cortex around Central Sulcus. *Stereotact. Funct. Neurosurg.*, 1994. **62**(1–4): pp. 300–3.

69. Hitzelberger, W. E. and R. M. Witten, Abnormal Myelograms in Asymptomatic Patients. *J. Neurosurg.*, 1968. **28**: pp. 204–6.

70. Hong, C. Z., Pathophysiology of Myofascial Trigger Point. *Journal of the Formosan Medical Association*, 1996. **95**(2): pp. 93–104.

71. Hong, C. Z. and D. G. Simons, Pathophysiologic and Electrophysiologic Mechanisms of Myofascial Trigger Points. *Arch Phys. Med. Rehab.*, 1998. **79**(7): pp. 863–72.

72. Hua, S. E., I. M. Garonzik, J. I. Lee, and F. A. Lenz, Microelectrode Studies of Normal Organization and Plasticity of Human Somatosensory Thalamus. *J. Clin. Neurophysiol.*, 2000. **17**(6): pp. 559–74.

73. Hubbard, D. R. and G. M. Berkoff, Myofascial Trigger Points Show Spontaneous Needle EMG Activity. *Spine*, 1993. **18**(13): pp. 1803–7.

74. Inui, K., D. T. Tran, M. Qiu, X. Wang, M. Hoshiyama, and R. Kakigi, Pain-Related Magnetic Fields Evoked by Intra-Epidermal Electrical Stimulation in Humans. *Clin. Neurophysiol.*, 2002. **113**: pp. 298–304.

75. Jaeger, B., Differential Diagnosis and Management of Craniofacial Pain, in *Endodontics*, J. I. Ingle and L. K. Bakland, Editors. 1994, Williams and Wilkins: Baltimore, MD. pp. 550–607.

76. Jänig, W., The Puzzle of "Reflex Sympathetic Dystrophy": Mechanisms, Hypotheses, Open Questions, in *Reflex Sympathetic Dystrophy: A Reappraisal*, W. Jänig and M. Stanton-Hicks, Editors. 1996, IASP Press: Seattle. pp. 1–24.

77. Jänig, W. and M. Stanton-Hicks, *Reflex Sympathetic Dystrophy – a Reapraisal*. 1996, ISAP: Seattle.

78. Jänig, W., S. G. Khasar, J. D. Levine, and F. J.-P. Miao, The Role of Vagal Visceral Afferents in the Control of Nociception. The Biological Basis for Mind Body Interaction. *Prog. Brain Res.*, 2000. **122**: pp. 271–285.

79. Jastreboff, P. J., Phantom Auditory Perception (Tinnitus): Mechanisms of Generation and Perception. *Neurosci. Res.*, 1990. **8**: pp. 221–254.

80. Jastreboff, P. J., Tinnitus as a Phantom Perception: Theories and Clinical Implications, in *Mechanisms of Tinnitus*, J. A. Vernon and A. R. Møller, Editors. 1995, Allyn & Bacon: Boston. pp. 73–93.

81. Jensen, R., Peripheral and Central Mechanisms in Tension-Type Headache: An Update. *Cephalalgia*, 2003. **23**(Suppl. 1): pp. 49–52.

82. Jinks, S. L. and E. Carstens, Superficial Dorsal Horn Neurons Identified by Intracutaneous Histamine: Chemonociceptive Responses and Modulation by Morphine. *J. Neurophys.*, 2000. **84**: pp. 616–627.

83. Jinks, S. L. and E. Carstens, Responses of Superficial Dorsal Horn Neurons to Intradermal Serotonin and Other Irritants: Comparison with Scratching Behavior. *J. Neurophys.*, 2002. **87**(3): pp. 1280–9.

84. Kakigi, R., T. Diep, Y. Qiu, X. Wang, T. B. Nguyen, K. Inui, S. Watanabe, and M. Hoshiyama, Cerebral Responses Following Stimulation of Unmyelinated C-Fibers in Humans: Eletro- and Magneto-Encephalographic Study. *Neurosci. Res.*, 2003.

85. Kannel, W. B. and R. D. Abbott, Incidence and Prognosis of Unrecognized Myocardial Infarction. *N. Eng. J. Med.*, 1984. **311**: pp. 1144–1147.

86. Katayama, Y., T. Tsubokawa, and T. Yamamoto, Chronic Motor Cortex Stimulation for Central Deafferentation Pain: Experience with Bulbar Pain Secondary to Wallenberg Syndrome. *Stereotact. Funct. Neurosurg.*, 1995. **34**: pp. 42–48.

87. Keay, K. A., and R. Bandler, Parallel Circuits Mediating Distinct Emotional Coping Reactions to Different Types of Stress. *Neurosci Biobehav Rev*, 2001. **25**(7–8): pp. 669–78.

88. Keay, K. A., C. I. Clement, A. Depaulis, and R. Bandler, Different Representations of Inescapable Noxious Stimuli in the Periaqueductal Gray and Upper Cervical Spinal Cord of Freely Moving Rats. *Neurosci Lett*, 2001. **313**(1–2): pp. 17–20.

89. Kilgard, M. P. and M. M. Merzenich, Cortical Map Reorganization Enabled by Nucleus Basalis Activity. *Science*, 1998. **279**: pp. 1714–1718.

90. Kirchner, A., F. Birklein, H. Stefan, and H. O. Handwerker, Left Vagus Nerve Stimulation Suppresses Experimentally Induced Pain. *Neurology*, 2000. **55**(8): pp. 1167–71.

91. Kjellberg, F. and M. R. Tramer, Pharmacological Control of Opioid-Induced Pruritus: A Quantitative Systematic Review of Randomized Trials. *Europ. J. Anaesthesiol.*, 2001. **18**(6): pp. 346–57.

92. Knighton, R. S. and P. R. Dumke, *Pain*. 1966, Little Brown: Boston.

93. Koch, B. D., G. F. Faurot, J. R. McGuirk, D. E. Clarke, and J. C. Hunter, Modulation of Mechano-Hyperalgesia by Clinically Effective Analgesics in Rats with Peripheral Mononeuropathy. *Analgesia*, 1996. **2**: pp. 157–164.

94. Koerber, H. R., K. Mirnics, A. M. Kavookjian, and A. R. Light, Ultrastructural Analysis of Ectopic Synaptic Boutons Arising from Peripherally Regenerated Primary Afferent Fibers. *J. Neurophysiol*, 1999. **81**: pp. 1636.

95. Kohama, I., K. Ishikawa, and J. D. Kocsis, Synaptic Reorganization in the Substantia Gelatinosa after Peripheral Nerve Neuroma Formation: Aberrant Innervation of Lamina II Neurons by Beta Afferents. *J. Neurosci.*, 2000. **20**: pp. 1538–1549.

96. Komisaruk, B. R., C. A. Gerdes, and B. Whipple, 'Complete' Spinal Cord Injury Does Not Block Perceptual Responses to Genital Self-Stimulation in Women. *Arch. Neurol.*, 1997. **54**(12): pp. 1513–20.

97. Kruit, M. C., M. A. Buchem Van, P. A. Hofman, J. T. Bakkers, G. M. Terwindt, M. D. Ferrari, and L. J. Launer, Migraine as a Risk Factor for Subclinical Brain Lesions. *JAMA*, 2004. **291**(4): pp. 427–34.

98. Kugelberg, E., Activation of Human Nerves by Ischemia. *Arch. Neurol. Psychiat.*, 1948. **60**: pp. 140–152.

99. Kuraishi, Y., T. Yamaguchi, and T. Miyamoto, Itch-Scratch Responses Induced by Opioids through Central Mu Opioid Receptors in Mice. 2000. 7(3): pp. 248–52.

100. Kwiat, G. C. and A. I. Basbaum, The Origin of Brainstem Noradrenergic and Serotonergic Projections to the Spinal Cord Dorsal Horn in the Rat. *Somatosensory and Motor Res.*, 1992. **9**: pp. 157–173.

101. Layzer, R. B., Muscle Pain, Cramps, and Fatigue, in *Myology, 2nd Ed*, A. G. Engel and C. Franzini-Armstrong, Editors. 1994, McGraw-Hill: New York. pp. 1754–1768.

102. LeDoux, J. E., Brain Mechanisms of Emotion and Emotional Learning. *Curr. Opin. Neurobiol.*, 1992. **2**: pp. 191–197.

103. Lenz, F. A., R. H. Gracely, A. J. Romanoski, E. J. Hope, L. H. Rowland, and P. M. Dougherty, Stimulation in the Human Somatosensory Thalamus Can Reproduce Both the Affective and Sensory Dimensions of Previously Experienced Pain. *Nature Medicine*, 1995. **1**(9): pp. 910–3.

104. Lenz, F. A., R. H. Gracely, F. H. Baker, R. T. Richardson, and P. M. Dougherty, Reorganization of Sensory Modalities Evoked by Microstimulation in Region of the Thalamic Principal Sensory Nucleus in Patients with Pain Due to Nervous System Injury. *J. Comp. Neurol.*, 1998. **399**(1): pp. 125–38.

105. Lenz, F. A., M. Rios, A. Zirh, D. Chau, G. Krauss, and R. P. Lesser, Painful Stimuli Evoke Potentials Recorded over the Human Anterior Cingulate Gyrus. *J. Neurophys.*, 1998. **79**(4): pp. 2231–4.

106. Levine, J. D., N. C. Gordon, and H. L. Fields, The Mechanism of Placebo Analgesia. *Lancet*, 1978: pp. 654–657.

107. Liu, H., C. R. Mantyh, and A. I. Basbaum, NMDA-Receptor Regulation of Substance-P Release from Primary Nociceptors. *Nature*, 1997. **386**: pp. 721–724.

108. Loder, E. and D. Biondi, Use of Botulinum Toxins for Chronic Headaches: A Focused Review. *Clin. J. Pain*, 2002. **18**(6): pp. 169–176.

109. Loh, L. and P. W. Nathan, Painful Peripheral States and Sympathetic Blocks. *J. Neurol. Neurosurg. Psychiat.*, 1978. **41**: pp. 664–671.

110. Long, D. M., Chronic Back Pain, in *Handbook of Pain*, P. D. Wall and R. Melzack, Editors. 1999, Churchill Livingstone: Edinburgh. pp. 539–538.

111. Lumb, B. M., Inescapable and Escapable Pain Is Represented in Distinct Hypothalamic-Midbrain Circuits: Specific Roles of Ad- and C-Nociceptors. *Exp. Physiol.*, 2002. **87**: pp. 281–86.

112. Malmberg, A. B., Central Changes, in *Pain in Peripheral Nerve Diseases. Pain Headache*, C. Sommer, Editor. 2001, Karger: Basel. pp. 149–167.

113. Mason, P., S. A. Back, and H. L. Fields, A Confocal Laser Microscopic Study of Enkephalin-Immunoreactive Appositions onto Physiologically Identified Neurons in the Rostral Ventromedial Medulla. *J. Neuro. Sci.*, 1992. 12: pp. 4023–4036.

114. Massey, E. W. and J. M. Massey, Forearm Neuropathy and Pruritus. *Southern Medical J.*, 1986. **79**(10): pp. 1259–1260.

115. Mathews, E. S. and S. J. Scrivani, Percutaneous Stereotactic Radiofrequency Thermal Rhizotomy for the Treatment of Trigeminal Neuralgia. *Mount Sinai J. Med.*, 2000. **67**(4): pp. 288–99.

116. Mäurer, M. and K. Reiners, Mononeuropathies, in *Pain in Peripheral Nerve Diseases. Pain Headache*, C. Sommer, Editor. 2001, Karger: Basel. pp. 37–52.

117. McDonald, A. J., Cortical Pathways to the Mammalian Amygdala. *Progr. Neurobiol.*, 1998. **55**(3): pp. 257–332.

118. McQuay, H., Do Preemptive Treatments Provide Better Pain Control?, in *Progr. Pain Res. Management*, G. F. Gebhart, D. L. Hammond, and T. Jensen, Editors. 1994, IASP Press: Seattle, WA. pp. 709–723.

119. Melzack, R. and P. D. Wall, Pain Mechanisms: A New Theory. *Science*, 1965. **150**: pp. 971–979.

120. Melzack, R., Phantom Limbs. *Sci. Am.*, 1992. **266**: pp. 120–126.

121. Mendell, L. M., Modifiability of Spinal Synapses. *Physiol Rev*, 1984. **64**: pp. 260–324.

122. Mense, S. and M. H., Bradykinin-Induced Modulation of the Response Behaviour of Different Types of Feline Group Iii and Iv Muscle Receptors. *J. Physiol.*, 1988. **398**: pp. 49–63.

123. Mense, S., Referral of Muscle Pain: New Aspects. *Am. Pain Soc. J.*, 1994. **3**: pp. 1–9.

124. Merskey, H. and N. Bogduk, Classification of Chronic Pain. 1994, IASP Press: Seattle. pp. 1–222.

125. Meyerson, B. A., U. Lindblom, B. Linderoth, and G. Lind, Motor Cortex Stimulation as Treatment of Trigeminal Neuropathic Pain. *Acta Neurochir. – Suppl.*, 1993. **58**: pp. 105–3.

126. Meyerson, B. A. and B. Linderoth, Mechanism of Spinal Cord Stimulation in Neuropathic Pain. *Neurol. Res.*, 2000. **22**: pp. 285–292.

127. Møller, A. R., M. B. Møller, and M. Yokota, Some Forms of Tinnitus May Involve the Extralemniscal Auditory Pathway. *Laryngoscope*, 1992. **102**: pp. 1165–1171.

128. Møller, A. R., Cranial Nerve Dysfunction Syndromes: Pathophysiology of Microvascular Compression, in *Neurosurgical Topics Book 13, 'Surgery of Cranial Nerves of the Posterior Fossa,' Chapter 2*, D. L. Barrow, Editor. 1993, American Association of Neurological Surgeons: Park Ridge. IL. pp. 105–129.

129. Møller, A. R., Similarities between Chronic Pain and Tinnitus. *Am. J. Otol.*, 1997. **18**: pp. 577–585.

130. Møller, A. R. and T. Pinkerton, Temporal Integration of Pain from Electrical Stimulation of the Skin. *Neurol. Res*, 1997. **19**: pp. 481–488.

131. Møller, A. R., *Sensory Systems: Anatomy and Physiology*. 2003, Academic Press: Amsterdam.

132. Møller, A. R., Pathophysiology of Tinnitus, in *Otolaryngologic Clinics of North America*, A. Sismanis, Editor. 2003, W. B. Saunders: Amsterdam. pp. 249–266.

133. Montgomery, E. B. J. and K. B. Baker, Mechanisms of Deep Brain Stimulation and Future Technical Developments. *Neurol Res*, 2000. **22**: pp. 259–66.

134. Morgan, M. M. and P. Carrive, Activation of Periaqueductal Gray Reduces Locomotion but Not Mean Arterial Blood Pressure in Awake, Freely Moving Rats. *Neuroscience*, 2001. **102**: pp. 905–10.

135. Narins, C. R., W. Zareba, A. J. Moss, R. E. Goldstein, and W. J. Hall, Clinical Implications of Silent Versus Symptomatic Exercise-Induced Myocardial Ischemia in Patients with Stable Coronary Disease. *J. Am. Col. Cardiol.*, 1997. **29**(4): pp. 756–63.

136. Nasreddine, Z. S. and J. L. Saver, Pain after Thalamic Stroke: Right Diencephalic Predominance and Clinical Features in 180 Patients. *Neurology*, 1997. **48**(5): pp. 1196–9.

137. Nathan, P. W., On the Pathogenesis of Causalgia in Peripheral Nerve Injuries. *Brain*, 1947. **70**: pp. 145–70.

138. Neri Serneri, G. G., M. Boddi, L. Arata, C. Rostagno, P. Dabizzi, M. Coppo, M. Bini, S. Lazzerini, A. Dagianti, and G. F. Gensini, Silent Ischemia in Unstable Angina Is Related to an Altered Cardiac Norepinephrine Handling. *Circulation*, 1993. **87**(6): pp. 1928–37.

139. Newham, D. J. and K. R. Mills, Muscles, Tendons and Ligaments, in *Handbook of Pain*, P. D. Wall and R. Melzack, Editors. 1999, Churchill Livingstone: Edinburgh. pp. 517–538.

140. Nguyen, J. P., Y. Keravel, A. Feve, T. Uchiyama, P. Cesaro, C. Le Guerinel, and B. Pollin, Treatment of Deafferentation Pain by Chronic Stimulation of the Motor Cortex. Report of a Series of 20 Cases. *Acta Neurochiur. Suppl. (Wien)*, 1997. **8**(54–60).

141. Oppenheimer, S. M., N. Kulshreshtha, F. A. Lenz, Z. Zhang, L. H. Rowland, and P. M. Dougherty, Distribution of Cardiovascular Related Cells within the Human Thalamus. *Clinical Autonomic Research.*, 1998. **8**(3): pp. 173–9.

142. Pagni, C. A., M. Lanotte, and S. Canavero, How Frequent Is Anesthesia Dolorosa Following Spinal Posterior Rhizotomy? A Retrospective Analysis of Fifteen Patients. *Pain*, 1993. **54**(3): pp. 323–7.

143. Pillay, P. K. and S. J. Hassenbusch, Bilateral Mri-Guided Stereotactic Cingulotomy for Intractable Pain. *Stereotac. & Funct. Neurosurg.*, 1992. **59**(1–4): pp. 33–8.

144. Podivinsky, F., Torticollis, in *Handbook of Clinical Neurology, Diseases of the Basal Ganglia*, P. J. Vinken and G. W. Bruyn, Editors. 1968, North Holland Publishing Co: New York. pp. 567–603.

145. Porta, M., A Comparative Trial of Botulinum Toxin Type A and Methylprednisolone for the Treatment of Myofascial Pain Syndrome and Pain from Chronic Muscle Spasm. *Pain*, 2000. **85**(1): pp. 101–105.

146. Price, D. D., *Psychological and Neural Mechanisms of Pain*. 1988, Raven: New York.

147. Price, D. D., S. Long, and C. Huitt, Sensory Testing of Pathophysiological Mechanisms of Pain in Patients with Reflex Sympathetic Dystrophy. *Pain*, 1992. **49**: pp. 163–173.

148. Procacci, P., M. Zoppi, L. Padeletti, and M. Maresca, Myocardial Infarction without Pain. A Study of the Sensory Function of the Upper Limbs. *Pain*, 1976. **2**: pp. 309–313.

149. Procaccio, P. and M. Zoppi, Pathophysiology and Clinical Aspects of Visceral and Referred Pain, in *Proceedings of the Third World Congress on Pain*, J. J. Bonica, U. Lindblom, and A. Iggo, Editors. 1983, Raven Press: New York. pp. 643–658.

150. Procacci, P., M. Zoppi, and M. Maresca, Heart, Vascular and Haemopathic Pain, in *Textbook of Pain*, P. D. Wall and R. Melzack, Editors. 1999, Churchill Livingstone: Edinburgh. pp. 621–639.

151. Quasthoff, S. and C. Sommer, Peripheral Mechanisms, in *Pain in Peripheral Nerve Diseases. Pain Headache*, C. Sommer, Editor. 2001, Karger: Basel. pp. 110–148.

152. Quinn, C., C. Chandler, and A. Moraska, Massage Therapy and Frequency of Chronic Tension Headaches. *Am. J. Public Health*, 2002. **92**(10): pp. 1657–61.

153. Raja, S. N., J. N. Campbell, and R. A. Meyer, Evidence for Different Mechanisms of Primary and Secondary Hyperalgesia Following Heat Injury to the Glabrous Skin. *Brain*, 1984. **107**: pp. 1791–1188.

154. Randich, A. and G. F. Gebhart, Vagal Afferent Modulation of Nociception. *Brain Res. Rev.*, 1992. **17**: pp. 77–99.

155. Rapkin, A. J., Chronic Pelvic Pain, in *Textbook of Pain*, P. D. Wall and R. Melzack, Editors. 1999, Churchill Livingstone: Edinburgh. pp. 641–659.

156. Reichling, D. B. and A. I. Basbaum, Contribution of Brainstem GABAergic Circuitry to Descending Antinociceptive Controls: I. GABA-Immunoreactive Projection Neurons in the Periaquaductal Gray and Nucleus Raphe Magnus. *J. Comp. Neurol.*, 1990. **302**: pp. 303–377.

157. Rexed, B. A., Cytoarchitectonic Atlas of the Spinal Cord. *J. Comp. Neurol.*, 1954. **100**: pp. 297–379.

158. Rocco, A. G., Radiofrequency Lumbar Sympatholysis. *Regional Anesthesia*, 1995. **20**: pp. 3–12.

159. Rosenow, J. M., A. Y. Mogilner, A. Ahmed, and A. R. Rezai, Deep Brain Stimulation for Movement Disorders. *Neurol. Res.*, 2004. **26**: pp. 9–20.

160. Roychowdhury, S. M. and H. L. Fields, Endogenous Opioids Acting at a
     Medullary Mμ-Opioid Receptors Contribute to the Behavioral Antinociception
     Produced by GABA Antagonism in the Midbrain Periaqueductal Gray.
     Neuroscience, 1996. **74**: pp. 863–72.

161. Ruch, T. C., Pathophysiology of Pain, in *The Brain and Neural Function*, T. C. Ruch
     and H. D. Patton, Editors. 1979, W. B. Saunders: Philadelphia. pp. 272–324.

162. Sandkühler, J., J. Benrath, C. Brechtel, R. Ryuscheweyh, and B. Heinke, Synaptic
     Mechanisms of Hyperalgesia, in *Nervous System Plasticity and Chronic Pain*, J.
     Sandkühler, B. Bromm, and G. F. Gebhart, Editors. 2000, Elsevier: Amsterdam.
     pp. 81–100.

163. Sandroni, P., Central Neuropathic Itch: A New Treatment Option? *Neurology*,
     2002. **59**: pp. 778–780.

164. Sastry, B. R., Substance P Effects on Spinal Nociceptive Neurons. *Life Sci.*, 1979.
     24: pp. 2178.

165. Scadding, J. W., P. D. Wall, C. B. Parry, and D. M. Brooks, Clinical Trial of
     Propranolol in Post-Traumatic Neuralgia. *Pain*, 1982: pp. 283–92.

166. Scadding, J. W., Complex Regional Pain Syndrome, in *Textbook of Pain*, P. D. Wall
     and R. Melzack, Editors. 1999, Churchill Livingstone: Edinburgh. pp. 835–849.

167. Schäfers, M. and C. Sommer, Polyneuropathies, in *Pain in Peripheral Nerve
     Diseases. Pain Headache*, C. Sommer, Editor. 2001, Karger: Basel. pp. 53–108.

168. Schmelz, M., Itch – Mediators and Mechanisms. *J. Dermatol. Sci.*, 2002. **28**:
     pp. 91–96.

169. Sessle, B. J., Recent Development in Pain Research: Central Mechanism of
     Orofacial Pain and Its Control. *J. Endodon.*, 1986. **12**: pp. 435–444.

170. Shyu, B. C., N. Danielsen, S. A. Andersson, and L. B. Dahlin, Effects of
     Sympathetic Stimulation on C-Fiber Response after Peripheral Nerve
     Compression: An Experimental Study in the Rabbit Common Peroneal Nerve.
     Acta Physiol. Scand, 1990. **140**: pp. 237–243.

171. Siegfried, J., Sensory Thalamic Neurostimulation for Chronic Pain. *Pacing &
     Clin. Electrophysiol.*, 1987. **10**(2): pp. 209–210.

172. Simone, D. A., L. S. Sorkin, U. Oh, J. M. Chung, C. Owens, R. H. Lamotte, and
     W. D. Willis, Neurogenic Hyperalgesia: Central Neural Correlates in Responses
     of Spinothalamic Tract Neurons. *J. Neurophys.*, 1991. **66**: pp. 228–246.

173. Simons, D. G. and S. Mense, Understanding and Measurement of Muscle Tone
     as Related to Clinical Muscle Pain. *Pain*, 1998. **75**(1)(1): pp. 1–17.

174. Sindou, M. and D. Jeanmonod, Microsurgical-Drez-Otomy for Treatment of
     Spasticity and Pain in the Lower Limbs. *Neurosurgery*, 1989. **24**: pp. 655–670.

175. Sindrup, S. H. and T. S. Jensen, Efficacy of Pharmacological Treatments of
     Neuropathic Pain: An Update and Effect Related to Mechanism of Drug Action.
     Pain, 1999. **83**: pp. 389–400.

176. Sola, A. E., M. L. Rodenberg, and B. B. Getty, Incidence of Hypersensitive Areas
     in the Neck and Shoulder Muscles. *Am. J. Phys. Med.*, 1955. **34**: pp. 585–90.

177. Sola, A. E., Upper Extremity Pain, in *Handbook of Pain*, P. D. Wall and R.
     Melzack, Editors. 1999, Churchill Livingstone: Edinburgh. pp. 559–578.

178. Sommer, C., Why Do Some Patients Develop Neuropathic Pain and Others Not?, in *Pain in Peripheral Nerve Diseases*, C. Sommer, Editor. 2001, Karger: Basel. pp. 168–170.

179. Sorensen, J., A. Bengtsson, E. Backman, K. G. Henrikson, and M. Bengtsson, Pain Analysis in Patients with Fibromyalgia: Effects of Intravenous Morphine, Lidocaine and Ketamine. *J. Rheumatology*, 1995. **24**: pp. 360–365.

180. Sorensen, J., A. Bengtsson, J. Ahlner, and E. Al, Fibromyalgia – Are There Different Mechanisms in the Processing of Pain? A Double Blind Crossover Comparison of Analgesic Drugs. *J. Rheumatology*, 1997. **24**: pp. 1615–1621.

181. Stubhaug, A., H. Breivik, P. K. Eide, M. Kreunen, and A. Foss, Mapping of Punctuate Hyperalgesia around a Surgical Incision Demonstrates That Ketamine Is a Powerful Suppressor of Central Sensitization to Pain Following Surgery. *Acta Anaesthesiologica Scand.*, 1997. **41**(9): pp. 1124–1132.

182. Sugar, O., Victor Horsley, John Marshall, Nerve Stretching, and the Nervi Nervorum. *Surg. Neurol.*, 1990. **34**(3): pp. 184–7.

183. Sugimoto, T., G. J. Bennett, and K. C. Kajander, Transsynaptic Degeneration in the Superficial Dorsal Horn after Sciatic Nerve Injury: Effects of Chronic Constriction Injury, Transection, and Strychnine. *42*, 1990: pp. 205–213.

184. Sweet, W. H., Deafferentation Pain after Posterior Rhizotomy, Trauma to a Limb, and Herpes Zoster. *Neurosurgery*, 1984. **15**(6): pp. 928–32.

185. Tanimoto, T., M. Takeda, and S. S. Matsumoto, Suppressive Effect of Vagal Afferents on Cervical Dorsal Horn Neurons Responding to Tooth Pulp Electrical Stimulation in the Rat. *Experimental Brain Research*, 2002. **145**(4): pp. 468–79.

186. Tasker, R. R., Reflex Sympathetic Dystrophy – Neurosurgical Approaches, in *Reflex Sympathetic Dystrophy*, M. Stanton-Hicks, W. Jänig, and R. A. Roas, Editors. 1990, Kluwer Academic: MA. pp. 125–34.

187. Thompson, S. W. N., A. E. King, and C. J. Woolf, Activity-Dependent Changes in Rat Ventral Horn Neurons in Vitro: Summation of Prolonged Afferent Evoked Post-Synaptic Depolarization Produce a D-Apv Sensitive Wind-Up. *Eur. J. Neurosci.*, 1990. **2**: pp. 638–649.

188. Tohda, C., T. Yamaguchi, and Y. Kuraishi, Intracisternal Injection of Opioids Induces Itch – Associated Response through Mμ-Opioid Receptors in Mice. *Jap. J.Pharmacol.*, 1997.

189. Torebjoerk, H. E. and J. L. Ochoa, Pain and Itch from C-Fiber Stimulation. *Society for Neuroscience Abstracts*, 1981. **7**: pp. 228.

190. Tran, T. D., K. Inui, M. Hoshiyama, K. Lam, and R. Kakigi, Conduction Velocity of the Spinothalamic Tract Following Co2 Laser Stimulation of C-Fibers in Humans. *Pain*, 2002. **95**: pp. 125–131.

191. Travell, J., S. Rinzler, and M. Herman, Pain and Disability of the Shoulder and Arm, Treatment with Infiltration with Procaine Hydrochloride. *JAMA*, 1942. **120**(6): pp. 417–22.

192. Travell, J. and D. G. Simons, *Myofascial Pain and Dysfunction, the Trigger Point Manual*. 1983, Williams and Wilkins: New York.

193. Urban, M. O. and G. F. Gebhart, Supraspinal Contribution to Hyperalgesia. *Proc. Nat. Acad. Sci*, 1999. **96**: pp. 7687–7692.

194. Valbo, A. B., K. E. Hagbarth, H. E. Torebjoerk, and B. G. Wallin, Somatosensory Proprioceptive, and Sympathetic Activity in Human Peripheral Nerves. *Physiol. Rev.*, 1979. **59**: pp. 919–957.

195. Vandenheede, M. and J. Schoenen, Central Mechanisms in Tension-Type Headaches. *Curr. Pain Headache Rep.*, 2002. **6**(5): pp. 392 400.

196. Wall, P. D., The Presence of Ineffective Synapses and Circumstances Which Unmask Them. *Phil. Trans. Royal Soc. (Lond.)*, 1977. **278**: pp. 361–372.

197. Wall, P. D. and M. Devor, Sensory Afferent Impulses Originate from Dorsal Root Ganglia as Well as from Periphery in Normal and Nerve Injured Rats. *Pain*, 1983. **17**: pp. 321–339.

198. Wall, P. D. and R. Melzack, *Textbook of Pain, Fourth Ed.* 4th ed. 1999, Churchill-Livingstone: Edinburgh.

199. Wallengren, J., E. Tegner, and F. Sundler, Cutaneous Sensory Fibers Are Decreased in Number in Peripheral and Central Nerve Damage. *J. Am. Acad. Dermatol.*, 2002. **46**(2): pp. 215–7.

200. Walsh, E. G., *Muscles, Masses and Motion: The Physiology of Normality, Hypotonicity, Spasticity and Rigidity*. 1992, Blackwell: Oxford.

201. Weber, H., The Natural History of Disc Herniation and the Influence of Intervention. *Spine*, 1994. **19**: pp. 2234–2238.

202. Weltz, C. R., S. M. Klein, J. E. Arbo, and R. A. Greengrass, Paravertebral Block Anesthesia for Inguinal Hernia Repair. *World Journal of Surgery*, 2003. **27**(4): pp. 425–9.

203. Whipple, B., C. A. Gerdes, and B. R. Komisaruk, Sexual Response to Self-Stimulation in Women with Complete Spinal Cord Injury. *J. Sex. Res.*, 1996. **33**: pp. 231–240.

204. Whipple, B. and B. R. Komisaruk, Brain (Pet) Responses to Vaginal-Cervical Self-Stimulation in Women with Complete Spinal Cord Injury: Preliminary Findings. *J. Sex & Marital Therapy*, 2002. **28**(1): pp. 79–86.

205. Willer, J. C., Relieving Effect of Tens on Painful Muscle Contraction Produced by an Impairment of Reciprocal Innervation: An Electrophysiological Analysis. *Pain*, 1988. **32**: pp. 271–274.

206. Willis, W. D., From Nociceptor to Cortical Activity, in *Pain and the Brain*, B. Bromm and J. E. Desmedt Editors. 1995, Raven Press: New York. pp. 1–19.

207. Woolf, C. J., Evidence of a Central Component of Postinjury Pain Hypersensitivity. *Nature*, 1983. **308**: pp. 686–688.

208. Woolf, C. J. and S. W. N. Thompson, The Induction and Maintenance of Central Sensitization Is Dependent on N-Methyl-D-Aspartic Acid Receptor Activation: Implications for the Treatment of Post-Injury Pain Hypersensitivity States. *Pain*, 1991. **44**: pp. 293–299.

209. Woolf, C. J., P. Shortland, and R. E. Cogershall, Peripheral Nerve Injury Triggers Central Sprouting of Myelinated Afferents. *Nature*, 1992. **355**: pp. 75–78.

210. Woolf, C. J. and R. J. Mannion, Neuropathic Pain: Aetiology, Symptoms, Mechanisms, and Managements. *The Lancet*, 1999. **353**: pp. 1959–1964.

211. Woolf, C. J. and M. W. Salter, Neural Plasticity: Increasing the Gain in Pain. *Science*, 2000. **288**: pp. 1765–1768.

212. Yakhnitsa, V., B. Linderoth, and B. A. Meyerson, Spinal Cord Stimulation Attenuates Dorsal Horn Hyperexcitability in a Rat Model of Mononeuropathy. *Pain*, 1999. **79**: pp. 223–233.

213. Yaksh, T. L., Preclinical Models of Nociception, in *Anesthesia: Biological Functions*, T. L. Yaksh, *et al.*, Editors. 1997, Lippincott-Raven Publishers: Philadelphia.

214. Yaksh, T. L., Central Pharmacology of Nociceptive Transmission, in *Textbook of Pain*, P. D. Wall and R. Melzack, Editors. 1999, Churchill Livingstone: Edinburgh. pp. 253–308.

215. Yosipovitch, G., C. Szolar, X. Y. Hui, and H. Maibach, Effect of Topically Applied Menthol on Thermal, Pain and Itch Sensations and Biophysical Properties of the Skin. *Arch. Arch. Dermatol. Res.*, 1996. **288**: pp. 245–8.

216. Young, R. F., R. Kroening, W. Fulton, R. A. Feldman, and I. Chambi, Electrical Stimulation of the Brain in Treatment of Chronic Pain. Experience over 5 Years. *J. Neurosurg.*, 1985. **62**: pp. 389–396.

217. Young, R. F., V. Tronnier, and P. C. Rinaldi, Chronic Stimulation of the Kolliker-Fuse Nucleus Region for Relief of Intractable Pain in Humans. *J. Neurosurg*, 1992. **76**: pp. 979–985.

218. Young, R. F., D. S. Jacques, R. W. Rand, B. C. Copcutt, S. S. Vermeulen, and A. E. Posewitz, Technique of Stereotactic Medical Thalamotomy with the Leksell Gamma Knife for Treatment of Chronic Pain. *Neurol. Res.*, 1995. **17**(1): pp. 59–65.

219. Young, R. F., Deep Brain Stimulation for Failed Back Surgery Syndrome, in *Textbook of Stereotactic Surgery*, P. L. Gildenberg and R. R. Tasker, Editors. 1998, McGraw Hill: New York. pp. 1621.

220. Zakrzewska-Pniewska, B. and M. Jedras, Is Pruritus in Chronic Uremic Patients Related to Peripheral Somatic and Autonomic Neuropathy? Study by R-R Interval Variation Test (RRIV) and by Sympathetic Skin Response (SSR). *Neurophysiol Clinique*, 2001. **311**(3): pp. 181–93.

221. Zimmermann, M., Physiological Mechanisms of Pain in Muscloskeletal System, in *Muscle Spasms and Pain*, M. Emre and H. Mathies, Editors. 1988, Parthenon Publishing: Carnforth. pp. 7–17.

222. Zirh, A., S. G. Reich, P. M. Dougherty, and F. A. Lenz, Stereotactic Thalamotomy in the Treatment of Essential Tremor of the Upper Extremity: Reassessment Including a Blinded Measure of Outcome. *J. Neurol. Neurosurg. Psych.*, 1999. **66**(6): pp. 772–5.

223. Zochodne, D. W., Epineurial Peptides: A Role in Neuropathic Pain? *Canadian. J. Neurol. Sci.*, 1993. **20**(1): pp. 69–72.

5

Movement disorders

Introduction

The somatic[1] motor system controls voluntary movement, locomotion and posture. The motor system is the output organ for all conscious communications. The motor system is complex and it includes sophisticated control systems with many loops, most of which are integrated with one another. The motor system includes a large degree of redundancy, and it has a high degree of plasticity. Therefore, motor systems can be reorganized through expression of neural plasticity, and such reorganization can be activated by new or differing use (exercise), changing demands or injury. Expression of neural plasticity can also cause symptoms and signs of disease.

Disorders of the motor system may cause negative phenomena such as loss of voluntary movement and strength of fine motor control, muscle spasm, tremor, twitches and synkinesis,[2] involuntary movements (chorea, athetosis) and deficits in coordination (ataxia), or positive phenomena such as increased reflexes and increased tone. Reorganization and change in function that are primarily aimed at compensating for deficits may cause symptoms and signs that are not directly related to the primary injury.

---

[1] Somatic motor system; distinguished from the motor system that consists of smooth muscles and glands.

[2] Synkinesis means that voluntary contraction of muscles is accompanied by involuntary contractions of other muscles. Synkinesis is a form of altered neural processing of motor information that may occur as a sequel of regenerating injured peripheral nerves. Synkinesis may be regarded as a form of lateral spread of motor activity, thus similar to the reorganization of sensory systems that occur after deficits or changes in demand (see Chapter 3).

Understanding the function of motor systems is a challenge. It is an even greater challenge to understand the causes of various symptoms and signs of injury and diseases that affect the motor systems of the spinal cord and brain. We will therefore devote a part of this chapter to describing the basic organization and function of the motor system.

Studies of the function of the spinal cord motor system were pioneered by Sherrington and Eccles, and later by Lundberg, Jankowska and Burke, as well as other investigators. These individuals contributed to our basis of understanding the motor system derived from animal experiments. There are considerable differences, however, between the motor system of humans and that of animals. We owe much of our understanding of motor system functioning in humans to a few individuals who used the neurosurgical operating room as their laboratory to study the function of the normal, as well as the diseased, human motor system. Currently, some contributions to our understanding of motor system functioning and plasticity come from studies using recent technological developments such as functional imaging, like fMRI, as well as other sophisticated imaging methods.

In this section, we will first describe some important disorders of the motor system and then discuss the general organization and basic functions of the motor system. After that, we turn to discussing the causes and the pathophysiology of some common disorders of the motor system. Lastly, we will discuss movement disorders where expression of neural plasticity plays an important role in generating the symptoms and signs of these diseases.

5.1   Disorders of motor systems

Spinal cord injuries (SCI), disorders of the basal ganglia and the motor cortex are the most common causes of movement disorders. Pathologies of the CNS such as multiple sclerosis (MS), and degenerative disorders such as Parkinson's disease (PD) and Huntington's disease (HD), cause various forms of movement disorders. Traumatic injuries and ischemic insults to the CNS such as strokes, birth injuries, surgically-induced trauma, etc., are other common causes of movement disorders. Traumatic injuries to the spinal cord (SCI) cause severe movement disorders including paresis or paralysis and spasticity, changed reflexes, etc., and present with clinical signs such as hypotonia, hypertonia and paresthesia. These deficits and abnormal functions are associated with morphological changes, but changes in function that have no detectable morphological correlates may also cause movement disorders. It is only recently that neural plasticity has been recognized as a cause of symptoms and signs of movement disorders. Some movement disorders are accompanied by different forms of pain conditions (see Chapter 4).

Movement disorders were earlier divided into disorders of pyramidal and extrapyramidal origin. Extrapyramidal signs were earlier assumed to be associated with disorders of the basal ganglia, while pyramidal disorders were assumed to have their origin in the pyramidal tract (the corticospinal tract). The distinction between disorders with pyramidal and extrapyramidal signs lost its anatomical relevance when it became known that information from the basal ganglia could reach the primary motor cortex (MI) and thereby reach the spinal cord through the corticospinal tract. The term *extrapyramidal signs* is still in clinical use for describing symptoms that are related to the basal ganglia.

Changes in peripheral nerves that resemble those that occur in neuropathies, specific diseases such as diabetes, MS (and earlier poliomyelitis) or alcohol-induced changes, may cause difficulties with movement although these are not clinically referred to under the classification of "movement disorders."

Traumatic SCI may alter processing of information in specific segments of the spinal cord, impair or disrupt input from supraspinal structures, and interrupt or impair communication between neighboring spinal segments. These changes have immediate effects on motor function, and most likely result in delayed effects through the expression of neural plasticity.

Injury to motor nerves and irritation of motor nerves may cause motor abnormalities (deficits or abnormal function) such as spasm and synkinesis by altering the processing in cranial motor nuclei such as the facial nucleus [93] (see Chapter 6), and in the ventral horn of the spinal cord. Some forms of spasm and synkinesis are, however, often caused by more complex mechanisms, including abnormal proprioceptive or other somatosensory input. The involvement of proprioception in causing signs of movement disorders is important and will be discussed below.

Aging is an important factor in causing changes in motor functioning. Age-related changes include deficits in neural transmitters and subsequent degeneration of neural tissue such as occurs in PD and HD. Decrease in the production of gamma amino butyric acid (GABA) that occurs in the CNS with age [28] is important as is the subsequent sensitizing of GABA receptors [29], which shifts the relation between excitation and inhibition in the CNS. The changes that occur as a function of age occur at different rates in different individuals. Many disorders have an increasing incidence with age, which indicate that age-related changes play a role in many movement disorders. The question then is: is aging in itself pathological? If it is regarded as pathological, what constitutes normal age-related changes must be defined.

Table 5.1 *Summary of some differences between pyramidal and extrapyramidal signs.*

Lesion Type	Tone	Adventitious Movements	Muscle Groups	Distal/Proximal	Reflexes	Weakness
Pyramidal	Clasp-knife	No	Flexors more than extensors in upper extremities Extensors more than flexors in lower extremities	Distal>Proximal	Increased	Yes
Extrapyramidal	Lead-pipe	Yes	Both	Both	Normal	No

Treatments of patients with SCI and cerebral palsy have been aimed at reducing the abnormal muscle activity and treatment of the deficits. So far, little improvements in function have been achieved, but some of the abnormal muscle activities – such as those associated with spasticity – can be controlled by medication or various kinds of surgical intervention, although often not completely alleviated. A better understanding of such disorders is needed to develop better treatments. The symptoms that are caused by plastic changes in the nervous system that often accompany morphological changes may be reversed by appropriate rehabilitative training, which already is an important part of the treatment of many motor disorders. Better understanding of the role of neural plasticity in movement disorders could lead to development of better training methods for reversing these changes, and thereby alleviate many symptoms.

Studies of the diseased motor system can also aid in understanding how the motor system normally functions. Studies of patients with SCI, where supraspinal input to the spinal cord is reduced or changed, have provided important information regarding the mechanisms of other spinal cord disorders, as well as improved understanding of normal motor system functioning.

5.1.1   Paresis and paralysis

Paresis or paralysis may occur because of damage to any parts of the motor system; however, when it occurs at levels above the α motoneuron, paresis is usually accompanied by abnormal muscle activity in one form or another. The symptoms and signs of injuries to motor nerves (see Chapter 2) are primarily decreased functions, which cause paralysis (loss of power of muscles) or paresis (partial paralysis).

The function of the α motoneurons (the "final common pathway") is impaired in amyotrophic lateral sclerosis (ALS), which is a progressive degenerative disorder that affects not only α motoneurons but also fiber tracts and cortical neurons. Disorders that influence the function of interneurons in the spinal cord and the input from proprioceptors and cutaneous afferents can also cause paresis and paralysis, which may be accompanied by movement disorders such as spasm, clonus and deficits in coordination. SCI are often accompanied by complex movement disorders (spasticity) in addition to paresis and paralysis.

Upper motoneuron disorders may also cause paresis, but this is usually accompanied by other symptoms and signs such as hyperactivity (spasm, tremor, etc.) of different muscle groups. Cerebral palsy is a common name for a group of non-progressive motor disorders that occur parenterally, or which is acquired at birth or early in life. Strokes, bleeding and inflammation may affect CNS structures involved in motor control and are common causes of paresis or paralysis.

Demyelinating disorders such as MS that affect fiber tracts in the spinal cord or brain may cause paresis, in addition to symptoms from sensory systems and higher order CNS functions (mood, etc.).

Paresis and paralysis may be caused by inadequate facilitation of alpha motoneurons, even when descending motor pathways are intact. The facilitatory and inhibitory input to the alpha motoneurons from spinal and supraspinal sources may be altered because of injuries such as SCI or strokes. This is often overlooked, but better understanding of how such facilitation occurs may aid in the development of treatments for paresis and paralysis.

5.1.2   Dyskinesia (hypokinesis and hyperkinesis)

Hypokinesia refer to movement disorders characterized by decreased amplitude of movement. The term is also used to describe conditions of abnormal ability to move, such as bradykinesia (reduced speed of movement). The term Parkinsonism is used synonymously with hypokinesis. The most common forms of hypokinesia occur in PD.

Hyperkinesia means excessive movements and the term is used for a wide variety of abnormal involuntary muscle activity, including spasm, tremor etc., but the term is typically not used for involuntary movements in connection with attention deficit disorders or psychiatric disorders. Terms such as chorea, myoclonus, tremor, tics, spasms, athetosis and ballism are used to describe hyperkinetic disorders. In general, the degree of pathological signs in these very different disorders varies from individual to individual, and the symptoms of many of these disorders are slowly progressive.

There are distinct differences between upper motoneuron disorders and lower motoneuron disorders. Lower spinal motoneuron deficits often cause flaccid paresis or paralysis on the same side as the lesion occurs, while upper motoneuron disorders are likely to include more complex symptoms that often include spasms and spasticity which mostly affect the side opposite to the lesion although occasionally can be bilateral.

Other movement disorders that are related to supraspinal structures are congenital movement disorders like hyperkinesia syndromes, which include tremor, spasm and various forms of chorea. Tremor is an oscillating movement that may consist of alternating contractions of antagonist muscles. It can be inherited or caused by systemic diseases such as thyroid disorders, drugs, or age-related changes. Certain forms of tremor may be associated with ataxia.

The many different types of chorea are often congenital and involve both cortical and subcortical structures with diffuse morphological abnormalities. Chorea often occurs together with mental disorders. Involuntary sound production ranging from nonverbal sounds to obscenities (coprolalia) also occurs.

Common for all these disorders is that their cause is poorly understood, and even the anatomical location of the physiological abnormality is often incompletely known. Some of these disorders have been associated with abnormalities of specific neurotransmitters.

Spinal cord disorders

SCI may cause a total or partial lack of motor function, and it may involve inadequate function such as weakness, spasticity, clonus and spasm. Injuries, tumors, and inflammatory processes that affect the spinal cord can cause a host of complex symptoms. The symptoms and signs depend on the level where the spinal cord is affected and of its nature and extension.

Many forms of reduced function of motor systems may be related to the alpha motoneurons (the "final common pathway", see p. 123). An example is poliomyelitis and ALS causing death or impairment of function of alpha motoneuron. That may be caused by a combination of many factors such as increased oxidative stress, glutamate excitotoxicity, disruption of calcium homeostasis and subsequent apoptosis.

> Several processes are initiated when motoneurons are lost to aging or disease processes [56]. In the beginning of loss of motoneurons, sprouting from intact motoneurons to replace lost motoneurons occurs. This occurs in aging, and early stages of ALS and poliomyelitis. This means that motor units[3] of the surviving motoneurons expand. Axonal sprouting is thus a normal compensatory mechanism in motoneuron diseases and in normal aging. Muscle paralysis induces sprouting in normal muscles (cf discussion on the effect of botulinum toxin); direct stimulation of muscles inhibits such sprouting, as does exercise. Increased oxidative stress with increasing age is assumed to be responsible for the progressive decline in the number of motoneurons. Enlarged motor units from disorders such as poliomyelitis become progressively vulnerable with age and nerve terminals degenerate [56]. The higher level of activity of a fewer motor units further compromises the function of the surviving motoneurons and their ability to sprout. Similar accelerated deficits are seen in ALS. Increased levels of neuromuscular activity in a reduced number of motor units inhibit the outgrowth of sprouts. These factors may explain the progression of motor deficits with age in diseases such as ALS and late poliomyelitis.

However, many disorders are caused by inadequate input to alpha motoneurons from supraspinal sources, or from local circuitry in the spinal horns at the

---

[3] Motor units: Motoneuron and its innervated muscle fibers. The size of motor units in normal muscles varies from ten to thousands of muscle fibers.

same segment or at higher or lower segments of the spinal cord (ALS, strokes, upper SCI).

Traumatic spinal cord injuries

Traumatic SCI that occur from automobile accidents, falls, gunshots, etc., rarely involve total anatomical transection (approximately 33%), yet many patients with such incomplete anatomical transection have neurologically total transection (approximately 50%). Surgical operations can cause SCI in conjunction with removal of tumors, arterial-venous malformations, etc., or as a complication to operations on the spine. Operations for scoliosis was earlier a not uncommon cause of SCI, but the introduction of intraoperative neurophysiologic monitoring and improved surgical techniques have reduced the risk to very small numbers [25, 39, 77, 101, 134].

The symptoms and signs of patients with SCI likely go through several phases after the occurrence of the injury, each one being characterized by different signs and different forms of abnormal spinal reflexes. Initially, the symptoms are characterized by spinal shock, which are often followed by spasticity,[4] and weakness or flaccid paresis from spinal shock may subsequently be replaced by the characteristic hyperkinetic signs of spasticity [62].

Spasticity usually occurs several months after the injuries have occurred. During the first 4–6 month period after the injury, flexor and extensor spasms may alternate, and after 6–12 months a final phase may be reached, where the spasms are predominantly affecting extensor muscles. The extensor reflexes may be abnormally affected by input from cutaneous receptors while innocuous (non-nociceptive) stimulation of specific skin areas may also provoke extensor reflexes. Stimulation of skin receptors may also cause autonomic responses such as changes in blood pressure.

The flexor spasm that is typical for spasticity may be regarded as an exaggerated withdrawal reflex that is uncontrolled because of the lack of supraspinal input to the reflex circuit (cf movements of newborns). Delwaide and Oliver showed indications that the tendon reflex (Ib inhibition) is reduced or not active in spasticity [41].

Spasticity often (but not always) occurs in conjunction with damage to descending corticospinal (pyramidal) motor tracts at any point of their course: the cortex, the internal capsule or the spinal cord [27]. However, selective section of the pyramidal tract alone may not produce spasticity in animals nor in

---

[4] Spasticity is characterized by increased muscle tone and abnormal spinal reflexes, mainly due to increased resistance to passive stretch that is velocity dependent, and is greater for flexor muscles than extensor muscles. Typically, deep tendon reflexes are exaggerated.

humans. The only deficits of selective section of the corticospinal tract in non-human primates are small; only the ability to perform precise tasks is reduced, and is most pronounced for hands and fingers. Strokes that are associated with spasticity rarely involve the pyramidal tracts in the brainstem.

Basal ganglia and upper motor neuron diseases

The anatomical location of the physiological abnormality that causes the symptoms of many movement disorders is the basal ganglia and the motor cortex. Strokes are common causes of movement disorders affecting supraspinal structures. Some movement disorders that are related to supraspinal disorders are congenital and others are acquired; some are progressive and some are non-progressive. Abnormal movements (hypokinesia and hyperkinesia) often occur together with paresis and paralysis, such as can be seen in cerebral palsy. Acquired disorders of the basal ganglia and motor cortex are from injuries (accident or iatrogenic), and from strokes and intracranial bleeding. The term cerebral palsy is used for a group of non-progressive disorders that are caused by intrauterine events or during birth.

Parkinsonism

The term Parkinsonism is synonymous with the hypokinetic syndrome. Neurologists use the term Parkinsonism for a group of disorders that are characterized by slowness of movement, but other symptoms often accompany these disorders, including tremor, bradykinesia or hypokinesia, flexed posture, loss of postural reflexes, gait dysfunction and freezing. PD is the most common type of parkinsonism, and it is the best-known neurodegenerative motor disorder (for details, see [55]). Similar symptoms may occur as a side effect of various medications including the designer drug methylphenyltetrahydropyridine (MPTP), in hepatic failure, or in the class of degenerative disorders known as multi-symptom atrophies (MSA).

Parkinson's disease

PD is a disorder of older individuals [19] although some few individuals acquire PD or Parkinson-like disorders at a young age. PD is a progressive disease that is dominated by slowness of movement and it is categorized as a hypokinetic disorder, but other signs such as muscular rigidity and tremor at rest are normally present in patients with PD. Sometimes "freezing" occurs.

> The occurrence of PD increases with age and it is estimated that 1% of the population above 50 years of age has PD, and 2% above the age of 70. These values of prevalence have been questioned, and some investigators

[17] have estimated the occurrence of parkinsonism (including patients with PD) to as much as 14.9% between the age of 65 and 74, 29.5% between the age of 75 and 84, and 52.4% for individuals of 85 and older.

PD has attracted more attention than many other movement disorders and several treatments have been developed during the past 100 years. These treatments have focused almost exclusively on the motor deficits. Before the introduction of levodopa approximately 40 years ago, surgical treatment using localized lesions in the basal ganglia was the only effective treatment. After introduction of medical treatment with levodopa, surgical treatment became almost totally abandoned, but surgical treatment has re-appeared as an effective alternative when medical treatment fails, or when it has serious side effects. Modern surgical treatment of PD makes use of better knowledge about pathologies and the function of the basal ganglia, and it uses better methods for localizing the targets than older methods. Surgical lesions have now largely been replaced by electrical stimulation (deep brain stimulation, DBS) using electrophysiological guidance in the placement of electrodes. The use of inactivation of central structures such as the thalamus and basal ganglia, through electrical stimulation (DBS) is perhaps the most important therapeutical means for many movement disorders. Optimal use of such treatment requires thorough understanding of both the normal function of motor systems and of the pathophysiology of PD.

Multi-symptom atrophies

Many of the disorders that are associated with a Parkinson-like syndrome are known as multi-symptom atrophies (MSA). Some, like striato-nigral degeneration, produce Parkinson-like symptoms, but do not respond to levodopa since the pathology is in the striatum and not the substantia nigra. Progressive supranuclear palsy also produces PD-like symptoms, but is associated with prominent eye motion abnormalities and increased axial tone, and also does not respond to levodopa. Some of these syndromes are referred to as Parkinson Plus syndromes. These include the Shy-Drager syndrome in which autonomic dysfunction is prominent in addition to Parkinson symptoms. Many related syndromes now classified as SCA (spinocerebellar atrophies – older names included olivopontocerebellar atrophy, dentatepalidoluysian atrophy, Machado Joseph disease, etc.) most prominently are characterized by abnormalities in the cerebellar systems, but are also associated with parkinsonian symptoms. It is common to see some parkinsonian symptoms even in unrelated degenerative diseases such as Alzheimer's disease.

Tardive dyskinesia[5] is a category to itself and is not really a PD-like syndrome. Tardive dyskinesia occurs as a side effect to some antipsychotic and neuroleptic drugs used in treating primarily schizophrenia; these antipsychotic and neuroleptic drugs are increasingly used in the treatment of other disorders, including disorders in children.

Huntington's disease

HD is a hereditary, progressive neurodegenerative disorder characterized by abnormal, involuntary movements and cognitive and behavioral impairments. HD is caused by a known genetic error and affects 1 in 10,000. The onset of HD occurs earlier than PD (often in the fourth decade of life) and the symptoms of HD progress over 10–25 years to death. The symptoms of HD are different from PD in that the abnormal movements are quick and random (chorea) with time sustained movements (dystonia). In later states of the disease, Parkinson's-like signs appear such as rigidity, bradykinesia and dystonia. The motor signs in HD are accompanied by dementia, and behavioral disturbances and depression are common. These additional signs are often more debilitating to the individuals with HD than the motor disorders.

5.1.3   Strokes

Any clinical event that relates to impaired cerebral circulation and lasts more than 24 hours is generally known as a (ischemic) stroke. Such strokes cause focal destruction of cerebral tissue with symptoms related to the structures affected. Bleeding, such as from hemorrhagic strokes, causes less localized damage to brain tissue. Strokes are different from diffuse deficits in perfusion such as from low blood pressure, which causes general symptoms of ischemia typically with loss of consciousness. Transient ischemic attacks (TIA) are short lasting strokes with full recovery from neurologic deficits (generally less than a few hours).

5.2   General organization of motor systems

Voluntary contraction of skeletal muscles that are innervated by spinal nerves can be initiated from the motor cortex, but many muscles can also contract involuntarily in response to signals that are generated in the spinal cord from sensory input, or in subcortical cerebral structures like the brain stem.

---

[5] Tardive dyskinesia: Affect mainly the facial muscles and the tongue, with involuntary movements (also known as oral buccal dyskinesia).

Voluntary motor commands are transformed in various ways by processing in the basal ganglia (including the thalamus) and the cerebellum before they reach the spinal cord, where further and extensive processing occurs.

Motor systems have usually been divided into two sub-systems: upper and lower motor neurons. We will start at the top, first describing the cortical control of motion, and then discuss the descending pathways and the processing that occurs at the spinal segmental level. We will consider the processing that occurs at the spinal segmental level and in supraspinal structures including the cerebral motor cortex as separate entities. We will discuss the control of descending information occurring in the brainstem, and explore the processing that occurs in the basal ganglia and the cerebellum.

5.2.1   Upper motoneuron

Voluntary motor control is initiated by the cerebral motor cortex. Cortical neurons in the MI (Brodmann's area 4 together with neurons in the adjacent Brodmann's area 6) supply much of the descending activity that controls voluntary muscle activity. The neurons in the MI receive input from many other cortical areas and other parts of the CNS such as the basal ganglia and the thalamus. Premotor areas (PMA) and somatosensory cortical areas such as the primary somatosensory cortex (SI) have extensive connections with neurons in the motor areas. The anatomy and function of these structures are outside the scope of this book (see Brodal [22]).

The organization of the MI is complex with many internal connections. In general, the MI is organized somatotopically similar to that of the SI (see Chapter 3, p. 85). The corticospinal system activates flexor and extensor muscles of the limbs and activation of flexor muscles causes inhibition of extensor muscles [109]. Extensor and flexor muscles are activated from individual pyramidal cells in layer V of the motor cortex (MI). Those cells that excite flexor muscles inhibit motoneurons of extensor muscles. There are extensive cortico-cortical connections in the motor cortex, with connections to other motor areas such as the supplementary motor area (SMA); and to somatosensory cortical areas (SI).

The neurons of the MI have overlapping projections to muscles (Fig. 5.1) [13], but these cortical maps are not static, and the representation of different muscles can be altered through the expression of neural plasticity. Studies of limb amputations have demonstrated that considerable reorganization of the corticospinal system can occur, and the territories of the motor cortex that belonged to an amputated limb may be given to other muscles [59]. It has also been shown that the output map of the motor cortex can be altered by application of a GABA antagonist (bicuculine), which unmasks latent connections [66].

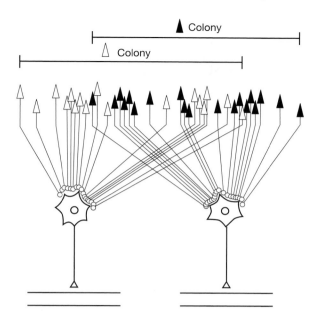

Fig. 5.1 Monosynaptic connections from cells in the motor cortex to the muscles, as revealed by microstimulation of the motor cortex. The diagram shows the cortical cells that connect to two motoneurons of a single muscle of the hand of a baboon [13].

Proprioception relays information about the movements and the position of the body through the activation of proprioceptors. Proprioceptors are mechano-receptors that are located in muscles, tendons and joints. Their afferent fibers travel together with other sensory fibers in mixed peripheral nerves and enter the spinal cord as dorsal roots. Proprioception has many similarities with the somatosensory system, but activation of proprioceptors normally does not cause any conscious perception. Therefore, proprioception is often excluded when sensory systems are discussed [94]. Proprioceptive information reaches the cortex mostly via the cerebellum, through the spinocerebellar tract.

The spinothalamic tract (STT) (see Chapter 4, p. 168) is important in mediating proprioceptive feedback. The STT consists of a dorsal and a ventral part. The dorsal part provides feedback information to the cerebellum about the resulting movement, while the ventral spinocerebellar tract provides feed-forward information about the activity of the motor neuron. Both parts originate in neurons in the middle part of the spinal horn and contain large diameter myelinated fibers, which are among the fastest conducting fibers in the spinal cord and provide information to the ipsilateral cerebellum.

The output of cortical neurons is the result of considerable intracortical processing [51]. The connections from the cortex to other structures such as the basal ganglia, the thalamus and the cerebellum (see pp. 264, 290, 293) build feed-back and feed-forward loops that provide considerable processing of motor commands that descend to the spinal cord and the nuclei of cranial motor nerves.

The internal organization of motor cortices is dynamic [109]. Many studies have demonstrated that connections in the motor cortex are not "hard-wired." Rather, its organization and function are subjected to changes through the expression of neural plasticity in response to changing demands or from injuries to CNS structures such as may result from strokes or trauma. (Early mention of neural plasticity in the motor system by Eccles [47] seems to have been directed to ontogenetic development rather than to what we now understand to be neural plasticity.) There is considerable evidence that ineffective synapses can be unmasked through the expression of neural plasticity (see Chapter 1). Ineffective synapses that have become effective (unmasked) can establish new functional connections between adjacent cortical areas [66, 109] and between neurons in MI and other regions of the CNS. Re-organization of the MI may occur in response to extensive use of certain muscles such as certain fingers of string players [49], or as a result of amputations [59, 109]. The changes in the organization of the MI that occur after amputations seem to occur in response to altered sensory and proprioceptive input to the motor cortex (via SI).

> In this connection, it is interesting to note that the transection of the facial nerve causes the cortical area of the forelimb to expand [45, 109, 117]. Donoghue *et al.* 1990 [45] showed that within 1–4 hours after facial nerve transection, electrical stimulation of the vibrissa area of the motor cortex elicited contractions of the biceps and wrist extensor muscles. It is also interesting to note that this reorganization occurs with a short delay, which means that it cannot be due to new morphological changes. That expansion of the cortical territorium of the forelimb muscles is more likely the result of changes in synaptic efficacy (unmasking of dormant synapses), or changes in protein synthesis in the cells [123]. The information about the severance of the motor nerve may reach the motor cortex through the sensory nervous system. The facial nerve, however, does not carry somatosensory or proprioceptive fibers (but taste fibers [94]), and the trigeminal nerve is regarded to provide proprioceptive feedback for face movements.
>
> Jacobs and Donoghue [45, 66] showed that changes in the cortical representation occurring after section of the facial motor nerve can be mimicked by injection of bicuculine (a GABA$_A$ antagonist) in the cortex, which indicates that changes in GABAergic inhibition is involved in the creation of the observed cortical re-organization.
>
> Animal experiments have shown evidence that changes in the function of neurons in the dorsal horn of the spinal cord occur after interruption of motor nerves [63]. Severing of the motor nerve fibers caused

a decrease in the response to stimulation of large myelinated fibers (A fibers) from the cut nerve 2–5 hours after axotomy. The efficacy of C fiber input to the lateral dorsal horn increased after axotomy, thus, a similar reaction as occurs in acute myositis [63]. This indicates that neural plasticity can be an important factor in establishing muscle tone. Cortical motor maps can also reorganize after SCI. It has been shown that the motoneuron pool recruited by magnetic stimulation of a particular location within the cerebral cortex, which activates muscles that are innervated by spinal segments immediately rostral to the injury, is larger in individuals after SCI than it is in control subjects [137]. This was taken to indicate that a (limited) flexible relationship exists between parts of the motor cortex and the muscles they innervate. Motor-evoked potentials were also different in patients with SCI than in normal individuals. The potentials recorded from individuals with SCI had a shorter latency than those recorded from normal individuals, indicating enhanced excitability and a reorganization of the motor pathways after SCI, with a possible expansion of the cortical territorium occupied by muscles that are innervated from spinal segments immediately rostral to the injury. These results are convincing evidence of the role of neural plasticity in generating some of the symptoms and signs that are present in patients with SCI. (Neural plasticity is discussed in more detail in Chapter 1).

5.2.2   Descending spinal pathways

Central (supraspinal) control of movements is mediated through several descending pathways (Figs. 5.2 and 5.3), of which the corticospinal tract, reticulospinal, vestibulospinal, rubrospinal and tectospinal tracts are the most important ones conveying information to the individual segments of the spinal cord. These descending spinal pathways provide commands for voluntary and involuntary movements and they modulate spinal reflexes and spinal (segmental) processing of motor and sensory information.

Kuypers (1981) [78] distinguished between two different groups of descending pathways: the medial system and the lateral system. The (dorso) lateral pathways (Fig. 5.2) comprise the corticospinal and rubrospinal tracts, and the (ventro) medial system (Fig. 5.3) consists of the vestibulospinal, reticulospinal and tectospinal tracts. The lateral system provides voluntary, sophisticated motor control for fine movements, mainly of distal muscles of the upper limbs. Flexors are activated more than extensors by the lateral system. The lateral system superimposes on the medial system, which mainly provides control of posture, breathing, ambulation and orientation of the head. The medial system activates extensors more than flexors.

The two most direct pathways from the MI are the corticospinal tract (also known as the pyramidal tract) and the rubrospinal tract (Fig. 5.2). The

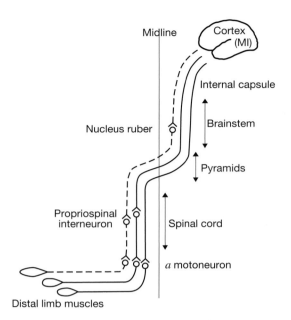

Fig. 5.2 Simplified schematic diagram of the lateral descending motor pathways from the MI, showing the corticospinal and rubrospinal pathways.

rubrospinal tract originates in the red nucleus (nucleus ruber), which receives input from the MI. The tracts of the medial system are less direct pathways (Fig. 5.3). The tectospinal tract originates in the tectum (mainly the superior colliculus, SC) and the reticulospinal tract originates in the pontine and medullary reticular formation; the vestibulospinal tract originates in the vestibular nuclei (Fig. 5.3). The nuclei from which these tracts originate and from which they have their names all receive input from the MI through more or less direct pathways.

It is important to point out that the fibers of all descending pathways have many collateral fibers. These collateral fibers not only connect to neurons in the spinal cord directly related to motor control, but they also supply input to neurons that control spinal reflexes. In fact, much control of movement is mediated by supraspinal control of spinal reflexes (see p. 269). Some types of stereotyped movements such as walking and breathing can be performed without supraspinal input and can thus be controlled by neural circuits in the spinal cord. Some collaterals of descending motor fibers (possibly corticospinal tract fibers that originate from the sensory cortex) can control sensory functions, particularly the sensitivity of neurons in the dorsal horn of the spinal cord that are involved in transmission of pain signals to the CNS. Collaterals also terminate on neurons in the different parts of the basal ganglia and cerebellum.

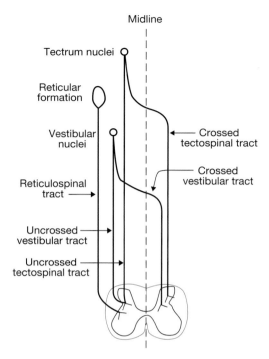

Fig. 5.3 Simplified schematic diagram of medial descending motor pathways showing the vestibular, tectospinal and reticulospinal tracts.

The involvement of the basal ganglia and the cerebellum in motor control is complex, and shall be discussed last in this chapter (pp. 290, 293).

Lateral spinal pathways

The dorsolateral pathways are mostly crossed tracts that terminate mainly on propriospinal interneurons that are located anatomically in the inter-mediate zone of the spinal horn. These propriospinal interneurons connect by short axons to alpha motoneurons that supply muscle on distal extremities. Some (few) fibers connect uninterrupted to α motoneurons. (Alpha motoneu-rons are located in lamina of the ventral spinal cord, see Fig. 5.4.)

Corticospinal (pyramidal) tract

The corticospinal tract originates in cells of the MI (Brodmann's area 4), and also cells in Brodmann's area 6 and in the SI. The fibers of this tract descend through the internal capsule and cross to the opposite side at the pyramids in the lower medulla. From there, most fibers travel in the lateral part of the spinal cord. Most of the fibers of the corticospinal tract cross the midline at

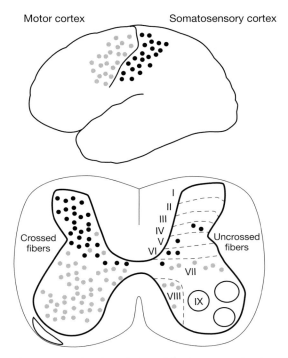

Motor cortex   Somatosensory cortex

Crossed
fibers

Uncrossed
fibers

I
II
III
IV
V
VI
VII
VIII
IX

Fig. 5.4 Termination of the corticospinal tract in the spinal cord. (Adapted from Brodal [22].)

the lower medulla (medullary pyramid), but some fibers travel to targets in the ipsilateral spinal cord. Some, mostly uncrossed fibers, travel ventrolaterally near the midline as the ventral corticospinal tract. Some fibers of cells in the MI innervate cranial motor nerve nuclei (see Chapter 6) and other brainstem cell groups, the so-called corticobulbar pathways.

The descending spinal fibers terminate in the ventral horn within the different segments of the spinal cord (Fig. 5.4). It has been stated that 15% of the fibers do not cross the midline (Fig. 5.4), but large individual variations exist [22]. For example, the fraction of crossed to uncrossed corticospinal fibers in humans varies from one individual to another, and the corticospinal tract is asymmetric in about 75% of the population [22], with both the lateral and the ventral portions being larger on one side (most often on the right side) [22]. This is of importance for assessing the effect of SCI, and may be responsible for some of the observed individual variations.

The corticospinal tract mainly controls fine motor movements, particularly the upper limbs and hands. Some of these fibers terminate directly (monosynaptically) on alpha motoneurons (Fig. 5.5). This is particularly the case for motoneurons that control the small muscles in the hand. Most corticospinal fibers,

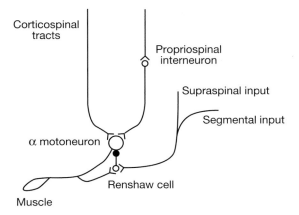

Fig. 5.5 Input from corticospinal tract to α motoneurons.

however, terminate on interneurons (propriospinal neurons), which in turn connect to alpha motoneurons through short axons [22, 110] (Fig. 5.5). The axons of
these propriospinal interneurons terminate on alpha motoneurons, which are
located in the different parts of layer IX of the ventral horn of the spinal cord.

> The corticospinal tract is most developed in primates, and probably more
> developed in humans than in the monkey, where the corticospinal fibers
> terminate on interneurons located in several layers of the ventral horn
> (especially layers VII and VIII) [22, 110]. Some authors claim that only 10%
> of corticospinal fibers terminate directly on alpha motoneurons [122] in
> humans. There is a slight overlap with sensory neurons in layer VI [22]
> Fig. 5.4).

Most of the fibers of the corticospinal tract originate in neurons in the MI,
but some fibers originate in the somatosensory area 3a of the SI (cells in area 3a
are known for receiving input from proprioceptive fibers). These terminate predominantly in the dorsal horn, where they can modulate sensory processing.

> The corticospinal tract is phylogenetically young (and it may therefore
> bear similarities with the classical sensory pathways that also evolved
> late, see p. 77). Evolution seems to have shifted from the red nucleus and
> rubrospinal system to the cortex and corticospinal system. The function
> of the corticospinal tract is different in primates and animals like cats,
> and the size of the corticospinal tract in the spinal cord varies among
> animal species [109]. Furthermore, the corticospinal tract differs among
> different primate species, and there is evidence that the corticospinal
> tract in humans is also different from that of any other primates. In
> great apes and humans, the corticospinal tract extends throughout the
> spinal cord and terminates in large parts of the spinal gray including
> the dorsal horn, but the projections are mostly segregated in the ventral

horn area. The ventral shift of the projections of corticospinal tracts has occurred in higher animals, and these fibers connect either directly to alpha motoneurons or via propriospinal neurons with short axons (see Figs. 5.2, 5.5) [109].

The corticospinal tract is small and only slightly developed in animals such as the rat. In the cat, only a few corticospinal fibers in the neck terminate monosynaptically on alpha motoneurons (lamina IX Fig. 5.4). In primates, the number of fibers that connect monosynaptically to alpha motoneurons has increased, and includes motoneurons that innervate lower extremities. In the monkey, severance of the corticospinal tract mainly influences the ability to use hands for precision grips. However, the effect of lesions to the corticospinal tract in humans is wider, and includes an effect on spinal reflexes. This contributes to the signs of spasticity. Anthropoid monkeys such as the chimpanzee have the largest number of monosynaptic connections [22]. It is likely that there are even more monosynaptic connections in humans. The monosynaptic innervation mostly regards α motoneurons that innervate muscles in the distant limbs (hands, fingers).

The activity in the corticospinal tract can also control processing in the spinal cord through propriospinal interneurons in laminas VII and VIII of the spinal horn. These interneurons make direct (monosynaptic) contacts with motoneurons as well as with other interneurons to form complex circuitries.

Corticospinal fibers have collaterals that make connections with neurons in subcortical centers [65, 78]. The collateralization of the fibers of the corticospinal tract is extensive and very complex [109]; some of these corticospinal fibers have collaterals that innervate neurons in different areas of the spinal cord. Perhaps the most surprising findings are that micro-stimulation of a specific site on the cortex can evoke contraction of many different muscles, and it can cause descending activity in many different tracts due to connections from the MI to the basal ganglia and the red nucleus [109]. Morphological studies show connections to the striatum, specific and non-specific thalamic nuclei, the red nucleus, pontine nuclei, the mesencephalic, pontine and medullary parts of the reticular formation, dorsal column and trigeminal sensory nuclei, and the lateral reticular nucleus [145]. Again, it must be pointed out that the connections commonly shown in diagrams are based on morphological studies, and it is not known how many of these connections are active at any given time. The pool of non-conducting synapses represents redundancy that may be activated through expression of neural plasticity that can be initiated by injuries or changes in demand.

It has been estimated that a motonucleus that consists of 300 motoneurons receives inputs from 4,500 to 6,000 last-order interneurons, some being excitatory and some inhibitory [109]. Again, as discussed earlier, these data are based on histological studies and, as Jankowska and her co-workers have pointed out, we know little about the synaptic efficacy in these pathways. There may be great differences in these different pathways [68].

Rubrospinal tract

The rubrospinal tract (Fig. 5.2) is a major projection pathway from the red nucleus, which is located in the midbrain and receives input from the MI [22] as well as other motor centers like the cerebellum. The rubrospinal tract terminates in the same parts of the spinal gray matter as the corticospinal tract, and it supplements the cerebrospinal tract in mediating voluntary movements. The rubrospinal fibers are few, estimated to be only 1% of the number of the corticospinal tract in monkey and man, and its importance in humans has been questioned [22]. However, the red nucleus has a strong influence on the spinal cord via the cerebellum (see p. 294) [22].

Medial pathways

The medial descending pathways consist of the medial and lateral vestibulospinal pathways, the medial and lateral reticulospinal and the tectospinal pathways, which are phylogenetically the oldest motor pathways. These tracts all have their nuclei in the brainstem, while some, but not all of these nuclei, have input from the motor cortex (MI).

The tracts of the medial system are crossed and uncrossed (Fig. 5.3) and terminate on neurons in the ventromedial zone of the spinal gray, where they control propriospinal interneurons and the motoneurons that control muscle on the trunk and girdle, mostly extensor postural or "anti-gravity" muscles. The tectospinal and vestibulospinal fibers are crossed pathways [109] (Fig. 5.3) that terminate predominantly on propriospinal neurons and other interneurons.

While the lateral pathways (corticospinal and rubrospinal tracts) control finer movements of extremities, the medial group of descending tracts controls locomotion, posture and reaching. The medial tracts supply both voluntary and involuntary control of muscle activity. Since the activity in these tracts can modulate spinal reflexes, they are important for automatic functions such as posture, and many other functions that do not require conscious attention.

Reticulospinal pathways

The reticulospinal pathway has its cell bodies in the reticular formation of the pons and medulla. These cells receive input from the cerebral cortex through corticoreticular fibers from motor areas 4 and 6 [22]. The reticulospinal pathway also receives input from other nuclei such as vestibular nuclei, the colliculi and the cerebellum. The fibers from the pontine reticular formation travel in the ventral funiculus, while those from the medullary portion travel in the ventral part of the lateral funiculus [22]. The fibers of this tract have many collaterals that terminate in the spinal cord on both sides. Electrical stimulation of the reticular formation can have both inhibitory and excitatory influence on spinal motoneurons [22], and these tracts influence both alpha and gamma motoneurons. The reticulospinal tract is important for maintaining posture, and serves to orient the body in fairly crude stereotyped movements [22].

Tectospinal pathways

Many of the fibers of the tectospinal tract originate in cells in the SC, which receives input from the visual system and the auditory system, as well as the SI and MI cortices. The SC also receives abundant input from the vestibular system. This tract is especially involved in and coordinates movements of the head and eyes. The fibers from the SC also innervate neurons of the motor nuclei of the cranial nerves (CN), and that control the external eye muscles (see Chapter 6). The fibers of the tectospinal tract terminate mainly in the rostral spinal cord innervating muscles of the neck and upper body.

Vestibular spinal pathways

The vestibulospinal tract consists of the lateral vestibulospinal and medial vestibulospinal tracts (Fig. 5.6). The lateral vestibulospinal tract originates in the lateral vestibular nucleus and reaches all parts of the spinal cord, where the fibers provide excitatory input to both alpha and gamma motoneurons [22]. Its main influence, like the reticulospinal fibers, is on the motoneurons in the medial part of the ventral horn that control muscles on the trunk and the proximal muscles of the extremities. These muscles are important for antigravity control of posture, so the main function of this tract is to control antigravity muscles (muscles that oppose the force of gravity). The medial vestibulospinal tract reaches only the cervical spinal cord, and it is therefore mostly involved in head movements in response to vestibular input. Since the vestibular nuclei have little, if any, input from the cerebral cortex, the vestibulospinal tract mediates mostly automatic reflex movements that have to do with adjustment of muscle tone. The vestibular nuclei have input from the reticular formation, which forms an indirect route to the vestibular nuclei from the cerebral cortex. A major input to the vestibular nuclei is the midline cerebellum.

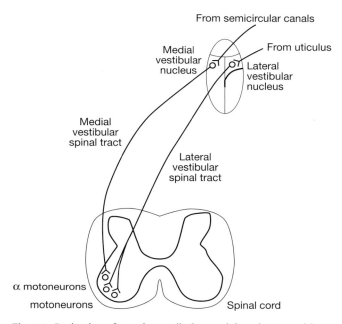

Fig. 5.6 Projections from the vestibular nuclei to the ventral horn of the spinal cord.

While the vestibular system is important for posture, it is possible to maintain normal posture and locomotion without any input from the vestibular system. Individuals without a functioning vestibular organ can have a normal life with little noticeable signs or symptoms, provided that the loss of vestibular function occurs early in life. Since loss of input to the vestibular system has little noticeable symptoms and signs, the function of the vestibulospinal tract may be regarded as redundant – at least partly – and its function can be replaced by that of other systems.

Other descending pathways (norepinephrine-serotonin)

In addition to these specific motor tracts described above, there are descending connections that have neuromodulatory functions on the motor system. The raphe nuclei [22] are the source of serotonin, and project to the spinal cord through noradrenalin (NA)-serotonin pathways. The locus coeruleus is the source of norepinephrine, and projects to the spinal cord (both the raphe nuclei and the locus coeruleus also send connections to many regions of the brain) [22].

The cells in the raphe nuclei receive their input from many sources, including the cerebral cortex and the hypothalamus. The cells in the locus coeruleus receive most of their input from two groups of cells in the reticular formation.

One such group of cells is located in the ventrolateral part of the reticular formation, and these cells provide excitatory input to the locus coeruleus cells. The input from the other group located in the dorsomedial part of the reticular formation is inhibitory [22].

The fibers of the NA-serotonin pathways are slow conducting and terminate throughout the gray matter in the spinal cord, where they modulate segmental neural activity including the excitability of alpha motoneurons. Both serotonin and norepinephrine increase the excitability of alpha motoneurons [144] (for an overview see [37]) and these descending pathways are involved in adjusting muscle tone. Both of these tracts excite the interneurons of the locomotor central pattern generator (CPG). During REM sleep, these descending monoaminergic neurons have their lowest activity, which may explain the suppression of movements of muscles that are controlled by the spinal cord [22]. (These descending tracts have sometimes been included in the description of the reticulospinal tract, see p. 261.)

The fibers of the descending monoaminergic tracts have many collaterals, some of which reach the dorsal horn, where they can suppress pain impulses from reaching higher CNS structures by reducing the excitability of dorsal horn cells that respond to noxious stimulation [22] (see pp. 178, 208, 263). These descending systems are activated during stressful situations when muscle tone is increased and pain sensitivity is reduced.

5.2.3   Basal ganglia

The corticospinal tract alone passes through the pyramids, while the other descending motor tracts pass through other parts of the medulla. This is why a distinction was made earlier between the pyramidal and the extrapyramidal systems. This division of the motor systems was regarded to reflect phylogenetic development, with the pyramidal system being the newer of the two systems. This distinction was commonly used in conjunction with movement disorders, where disorders related to the basal ganglia were known as "extrapyramidal" disorders. The division into pyramidal and extrapyramidal motor systems was abandoned when it was found that the basal ganglia connect backwards to the cerebral cortex (MI), enabling the basal ganglia to provide input to what was earlier known as the pyramidal system (Fig. 5.7). This division is therefore misleading because the basal ganglia provide input to the MI via the thalamus, and input from the basal ganglia can reach the spinal cord not only through pathways that do not pass through the pyramids but also through the corticospinal tract. The fact that the MI receives input from the basal ganglia means that disorders of the basal ganglia may affect transmission of information in the corticospinal tract.

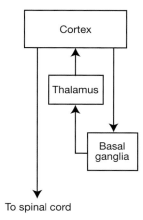

Fig. 5.7 Connections between the basal ganglia and the motor cortex (MI).

Section of the pyramids[6] fails to give spasticity, just weakness and lost fine motor skills. This is evidence that the pyramidal system functions also through the extrapyramidal system. This means that a stroke in the motor cortex will cause spasticity due to its influence on both pyramidal and extrapyramidal systems.

5.2.4   *Activation of the primary motor cortex*

Descending pathways can be activated by electrical stimulation of the MI, and motor activity can be initiated in muscles in different parts of the body. Stimulation of the motor cortex in humans can be done by electrical stimulation from electrodes placed on the scalp [91] (transcranial electrical stimulation). Recordings from the exposed spinal cord in animals have confirmed that such stimulation activates cortical neurons because of its ability to activate the corticospinal tract [48, 76]. Stimulation of the somatosensory cortex (SI) can also elicit muscle contractions, but it requires a higher intensity than stimulation of the MI.

Transcranial electrical stimulation is associated with considerable pain and therefore cannot be used in awake individuals. Impulses of a magnetic field generated by a coil placed outside the scalp (transcranial magnetic stimulation[7]) induces electrical current in intracranial

---

[6] Pyramids: an anatomically distinct structure of the lower medulla. The two-motor system hypothesis regards the extrapyramidal system to be a system that includes the basal ganglia, while the pyramidal system was the corticospinal system.

[7] Magnetic stimulation consists of a strong magnetic impulse delivered by passing an impulse of electrical current through a coil that is placed over the region that is to be activated [114]. The resulting magnetic impulse induces an electrical current in the brain tissue that can activate neural structures [10]. The magnetic field is not attenuated by the skull bone (only by the distance), and this is why such stimulation can be applied non-invasively and without eliciting pain.

tissue and can thereby activate cells in the motor cortex in humans [10, 16]. (For an overview of the techniques of magnetic stimulation, see Rösler, 2001 [114].) Such stimulation is painless and can be applied to awake individuals without noticeable discomfort. Studies using transcranial magnetic stimulation have shown that magnetic stimulation is useful for intraoperative neurophysiologic monitoring in operations where the spinal cord may be at risk of being injured (iatrogenic injuries) [11, 39, 129].

Transcranial magnetic and electrical stimulation of the motor cortex elicit responses in descending motor tracts that can be recorded from the exposed spinal cord. Recordings of such responses from the exposed spinal cord in cats, monkeys and humans to electrical stimulation of the MI have contributed to our knowledge about the function of the corticospinal tract. The responses to stimulation of the MI consist of a series of distinct (negative) waves [11, 39, 76] that are often labeled D and I waves. Responses evoked by transcranial magnetic and electrical stimulation in awake human individuals who had epidural electrodes placed at the C1-C2 spinal levels have been studied [79]. The D waves that are elicited by stimulation of axons of pyramidal cells of the motor cortex seem to be generated by descending volleys in the corticospinal tract. The I waves are generated by activity in the same tracts that are elicited by stimulation of other cells in the motor cortex. The direction (and thus the position of the stimulating coil) affects the waveform of the recorded potentials [73].

When recorded at the T_{11} level in a monkey, at least six waves can be identified in response to electrical or magnetic stimulation of the MI. The earliest wave occurs with a latency of approximately 3 msec (Fig. 5.8) [76]. This wave (the D wave) represents the direct response from the corticospinal tract caused by activation of pyramidal cells in MI that sends their axons descending in the corticospinal tract. The D wave is followed by a series of 5–6 negative waves (I waves or indirect waves). The I waves occur with an interval of 1.5–2 msec in cats, monkeys [76] (Fig. 5.8) and humans (Fig. 5.9) [39]. These I waves are assumed to be caused by subsequent activation of interneurons within the different layers of MI [9]. The later (longer latency) I waves are probably generated in neurons that are located closer to the surface of the cortex [12, 76] (see Fig. 5.8). The direction of the applied electrical current is important for the generation of the D and I waves, and if the electrode placement on the scalp is altered, the recorded wave pattern changes [39].

It appears that the activity that is represented by both the D wave and the I wave is necessary for activating alpha motoneurons. Transcranial electrical stimulation acts slightly differently on the motor cortex from electrical stimulation [76], and elicits I waves to a greater extent than magnetic stimulation [76].

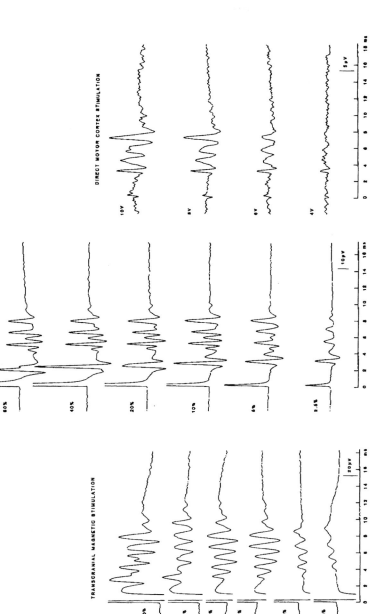

Fig. 5.8 Effect of stimulus intensity on the response from the surface of the exposed spinal cord in a monkey to different forms of cortical stimulation. Left column: transcranial magnetic stimulation. Middle column: transcranial electrical stimulation. Right hand column: direct electrical stimulation of the exposed cortex. The responses were recorded from the spinal epidural space by a monopolar electrode placed on the dorsal surface of the dura at the T_{11} level. Negativity is shown as an upward deflection. The initial negative wave (D wave) is followed by a series of negative waves (I waves). (From Kitagawa and Møller, 1993 [76]. *Clin. Neurophys.* vol. 93, 57–67; 1994, reprinted with permission from Elsevier.)

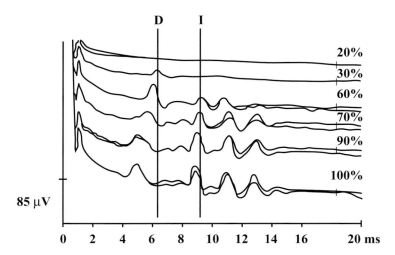

Fig. 5.9 Similar recordings as in Fig. 5.8, done in a patient undergoing a scoliosis operation. D and I waves are shown from a 14-year-old child with idiopathic scoliosis. The stimuli were applied through electrodes placed at Cz and 6 cm anterior. 100% = 750 volts (Adapted from Deletis, 2002 [39].)

Studies in monkeys and humans have shown that the D wave elicited in response to electrical activation of the cells in the MI cortex reflects the neural activity that descends in the dorsolateral funiculus without any synaptic interruption. The potentials with the latency of that of the first I wave have their maximum in the ventromedial funiculus, in agreement with anatomical data [78]. The ventral corticospinal tract may contribute to the I waves, but the I waves are most likely a result of intracortical processing. This pathway has bilateral projections, some of which may be mediated through the reticulospinal tract [8].

5.2.5   *Lower motoneuron (α and γ motoneuron)*

Alpha and gamma motoneurons are the targets of the descending motor tracts. These motoneurons are located together in the different parts of layer IX of the ventral horn of the spinal cord. Their axons form the ventral spinal roots that innervate skeletal (extrafusal) muscles and the (intrafusal) muscles of muscle spindles. Alpha motoneurons are also found in the cranial nerve motonuclei. Alpha motoneurons are among the largest nerve cells in the body, and each cell has many synapses that connect input from different sources (estimated to be approximately 10,000–50,000). The alpha motoneurons are known as the "final common pathway" (Sherrington) of the motor system.

Alpha motoneurons receive convergent input from propriospinal neurons and other local segmental interneurons (excitatory and inhibitory). These interneurons receive their input from supraspinal sources through long descending pathways (corticospinal, rubrospinal, vestibulospinal, and reticulospinal tracts), and from local spinal sources. As mentioned above, some of the fibers of the corticospinal tracts (pyramidal tracts) provide monosynaptic input to alpha motoneurons directly from cells in the MI [13, 109] (Fig. 5.2.), but most corticospinal fibers activate alpha motoneurons through propriospinal interneurons. These interneurons provide a means of modifying input from supraspinal sources before it reaches the alpha motoneurons and integrating afferent input. The lateral system of descending pathways provides disynaptic and polysynaptic input from different parts of the cerebral motor areas and from other supraspinal sources.

5.2.6   Segmental control of motion

The neural circuits in the spinal cord can generate commands for many forms of motion. Spinal reflexes play an important role in that respect. The CPG is an example of spinal cord circuits that can generate commands for complex motion without supraspinal input. The CPG plays an important role in locomotion together with spinal reflexes that are under control from the brainstem [43].

The spinal control of motion is modulated by supraspinal input, and by proprioceptive input. Processing of information in the spinal cord can be modified or modulated through expression of neural plasticity. This means that abnormal motor function may not only be caused by abnormal input from the descending motor pathways, but also by plastic changes in spinal cord and changes in proprioceptive feedback. We will discuss these matters in the sections that follow.

Spinal reflexes

Spinal reflexes are important for posture and for conscious and unconscious movements. Voluntary control of motion depends to a great extent on modulation of spinal reflexes, from intra- or intersegmental spinal cord neurons and from supraspinal sources. Motor systems of cranial nerves have similar reflexes, but their organization is more diverse than those of the spinal cord (see Chapter 6). A typical spinal reflex arc consists of a receptor, an afferent pathway (sensory nerve), a reflex center (in gray matter of the spinal cord), and an efferent pathway that passes the output to the effector organ (striated or smooth muscle or gland).

Some reflexes are simple and involve only one synapse in the spinal cord (monosynaptic stretch reflexes), whereas the reflex center of other (disynaptic and polysynaptic) reflexes involves several synapses. The two most basic spinal

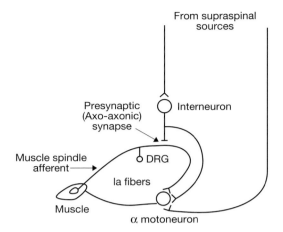

Fig. 5.10 Simplified diagram of the monosynaptic stretch reflex, showing the modulatory input from supraspinal and spinal sources via an interneuron.

reflexes are the stretch reflex, which is a monosynaptic reflex that opposes stretch of a muscle, and the tendon reflex, which is a disynaptic reflex. Other spinal reflexes are more complex and involve supraspinal structures in the brainstem and the cerebral cortex. Spinal reflexes form different "layers" that interact with each other in various ways.

Spinal reflexes are subjected to modulation through proprioceptive input, from circuits in the spinal cord and from supraspinal circuits. That far-away segments can influence excitability is evident from the Jendrassik maneuver[8] that can alter the excitability of lower-extremity stretch reflexes by activating upper limb segments. The gain in spinal reflexes can be changed by expression of neural plasticity [27, 69, 146], thus subject to the effect of training and adaptation to injuries and altered demands.

Monosynaptic stretch reflex

The monosynaptic stretch reflex is the simplest of the spinal reflexes (Fig. 5.10). The reflex arc consists of a muscle spindle, the afferent fibers of which travel in peripheral nerves, and enters the dorsal horn of the spinal cord in dorsal roots as Ia fibers. In the spinal cord, these fibers travel to the ventral horn, where collaterals connect to the alpha motoneurons of several agonist muscles. (Collaterals of Ia fibers also connect to Ia interneurons and to other internal spinal cord neurons, see p. 274.)

---

[8] The Jendrassik maneuver that is used clinically is a way to increase the excitability of lower extremity stretch reflexes. It is performed by having the subject hook the hands together by the flexed fingers and pulling against them with all possible strength.

The muscle spindles measure the absolute length and rate of length change of muscles. The firing of Ia and group fibers innervating muscle spindles increases when a muscle is stretched and decreases when it is shortened, such as occurs during normal contraction. In this way, the muscle spindles provide feedback to the spinal cord regarding the length of muscles. When a muscle contracts (shortens), the input from its muscle spindles decreases, which decreases the excitatory input to its alpha motoneurons. This is known as negative feedback because it tends to decrease the contraction. Negative feedback stabilizes control systems.

There are two ways that the stretch reflex can be modulated. One way is through presynaptic modulation of the afferent input to the alpha motoneuron mediated by an axo-axonic synapse (Fig. 5.10). The other way is through the gamma motor system that controls the resting length of the muscle spindles (see below). Presynaptic inhibition through the axo-axonic synapses is induced by input from fibers of descending tracts via an interneuron, the output of which then can control the flow of impulses in Ia fibers and thus the input to the stretch reflex (Fig. 5.10). This is a means to adjust the efficiency of the stretch reflex [109]. The dorsal reticulospinal tract also provides inhibitory effect on stretch reflexes through its input to the interneuron that mediates the presynaptic inhibition on the Ia fibers [27] (Fig. 5.10). The medial reticulospinal tract and, to some extent, the vestibulospinal tract mediate facilitatory effects on extensor tone [24], and intersegmental spinal sources provide input to the interneuron as can be demonstrated by the Jendrassik's maneuver (see pp. 278, 286) and the H-reflex can be up- and downregulated with training.

Examining the response of the stretch reflex by applying a brief force to the patellar tendon below the knee is a test included in most neurologic examinations. Observing the subsequent stretch of the leg assesses the excitability of alpha motoneurons. The effect of activation of Ia fibers and group II afferents on alpha motoneurons can be assessed quantitatively by electrically stimulating a peripheral nerve (containing fibers from muscle spindles) and recording the electromyographic (EMG) responses from the muscle. This response is known as the Hoffman (H) reflex. (Recordings of the H-reflex are used clinically to assess alpha motoneuron excitability.) The stimulation used to elicit the H-reflex activates the stretch reflex and thereby provides excitatory input to alpha motoneurons (Fig. 5.11). For example, stimulating the tibialis nerve behind the knee electrically and recording EMG potentials from the soleus muscle show two separate responses. One component (the M-wave) originates from direct activation of the muscle from the stimulation of motor fibers in the nerve. The other component of the response (the H-wave) is from activation of proprioceptive sensory fibers in the nerve eliciting a

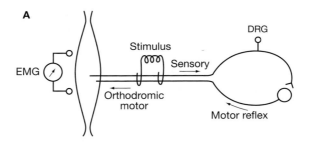

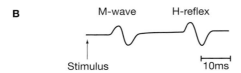

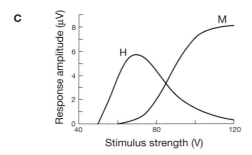

Fig. 5.11 Illustration of the Hoffmann reflex.

A: A mixed peripheral nerve containing both motor and proprioceptive fibers from muscle spindles is stimulated electrically, eliciting activity that progresses both distally, eliciting a direct muscle contraction (M-wave), and proximally, activating the monosynaptic stretch reflex that causes another and later muscle response (the H-reflex).

B: Recording of the direct muscle (M-wave) and the H-reflex from electrodes placed on the muscle.

C: Amplitude of the M-wave and H-reflex as a function of the stimulus intensity.

The H-response is separated in time, and the amplitude of these two responses has different relationships to the stimulus intensity.

response from the stretch reflex. When the nerve is stimulated at a location that is close to the muscle it innervates, the direct muscle response will occur with a much shorter latency than the H-response, which makes the two kinds of responses occur separately (Fig. 5.11) [120].

The amplitude of the Hoffmann reflex response first increases when the stimulus intensity is increased from threshold values; when the stimulus is further increased, the response decreases while the amplitude of the direct muscle response continues to increase (Fig. 5.11) [72, 120]. The reason that the H-reflex response decreases when the stimulus strength is increased above a certain value is that the strong stimulation elicits activity in motor fibers, which prevents the reflex response from the motoneuron to propagate towards the muscle from which the recordings are made (Fig. 5.11) [120].

When stimulating a mixed nerve electrically, a third kind of response from the target muscle, the F-response, may be observed. This response is a result of firing α motoneurons antidromically.

Gamma motor systems

The spinal neurons that receive their input from corticospinal fibers not only make monosynaptic contact with α motoneurons but also innervate γ motoneurons, which control the length and thereby sensitivity of the muscle spindles. Input to the γ motoneuron thereby adjusts proprioceptive feedback provided by the stretch reflex [22, 27, 99, 107] and thus modulates the stretch reflex. In this way, the corticospinal tract not only activates alpha motoneurons directly by input from the corticospinal tract, but also affects motor functions indirectly through Ia afferents from muscle spindles that activate the monosynaptic stretch reflex.

There is evidence that central commands that reach the individual segments of the spinal cords through the corticospinal and rubrospinal tracts exert much of their motor control through their activation of gamma motoneurons and thereby activate muscle spindle afferents [52]. There is also evidence for alpha and gamma co-activation.

Reciprocal inhibition

The reciprocal reflex causes the antagonist muscle to relax when the agonist muscle contracts (Fig. 5.12). Collateral fibers from Ia afferents contact Ia inhibitory interneurons, which in turn make synaptic contact with alpha motoneurons of the antagonist muscles. The reciprocal reflex is closely related to the monosynaptic stretch reflex because it gets its main input from the Ia afferents from muscle spindles via an interneuron (Fig. 5.12). Through this reflex, a decrease in the output of muscle spindles causes a decrease in the inhibition of the alpha motoneurons that innervate antagonist muscles (through the Ia inhibitory interneuron).

Lundberg 1979 [89] demonstrated the importance of Ia inhibitory interneurons (Fig. 5.12) in experiments in cats. He and his group showed that the main output of the Ia interneurons is directed to the antagonist muscle's alpha motoneuron, and that many supraspinal, close and distant segmental sources serve as input to the Ia interneurons. Fibers

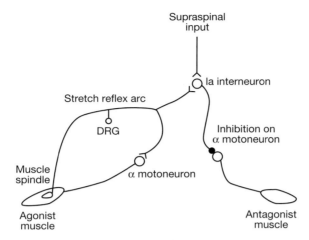

Fig. 5.12 Schematic diagram of the reflex arc of the reciprocal spinal reflex. Input from muscle spindles inhibits the antagonist muscle's motoneuron through the Ia interneuron.

of the corticospinal and vestibulospinal tracts terminate either directly or through their propriospinal interneurons on the Ia interneurons. This input can modulate the inhibition of the antagonist muscle when the stretch reflex is activated [87]. The Ia interneuron has numerous other inputs from the same and other segments of the spinal cord [89, 109] and the inhibition it provides on alpha motoneurons is therefore complex and can affect motor output across multiple motoneuron pools at multiple spinal levels.

Tendon reflex

The tendon reflex is a disynaptic reflex that receives its afferent input from the Golgi tendon organs via (Ib) interneurons (Fig. 5.13). The tendon reflex provides inhibitory input to α motoneurons that innervate agonist muscles. Golgi tendon organs that provide the main inputs to Ib interneurons measure the force of muscle contraction.

Since Golgi tendon organs measure the tension of muscle contractions and are inhibitory on alpha motoneurons, the tendon reflex provides some protection for overloading muscles. This was earlier regarded to be the main function of the tendon reflex, but more recently it has become apparent that Golgi tendon organs do not have a high threshold. Rather, they respond over a larger range of muscle tensions [32]. This means that the tendon reflex provides important and continuous feedback to motor systems similar to that of the stretch reflex, which is controlled by the length of a muscle.

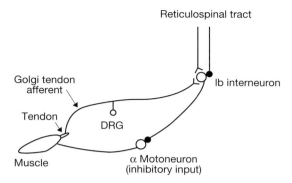

Fig. 5.13 Tendon reflex. The output of tendon receptors (Golgi organs) inhibits alpha motoneurons on the same muscle through the Ib interneuron. The reflex can be modulated by supraspinal input mainly from the reticulospinal tract. Some descending fibers have an inhibitory influence while some are excitatory.

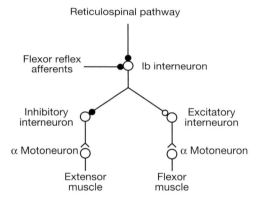

Fig. 5.14 Flexor reflex. Flexor reflex afferents (FRA) provide inhibitory input to Ib (inhibitory) interneurons that have excitatory influence on the motoneurons of flexor muscles and inhibitory influence on extensor muscles.

Afferent (Ib) fibers from joint receptors and some cutaneous receptors also converge on to cells in the dorsal horn of the spinal cord and serve as input to Ib interneurons, which supply inhibitory input to alpha motoneurons of the agonist muscle (Fig. 5.13). The Ib inhibitory interneurons receive input from corticospinal and rubrospinal tracts, and from interneurons that receive input from flexor reflex afferents (FRA) (Fig. 5.14).

The flexor reflex

The flexor reflexes can be elicited by stimulation of several different afferents, known as the FRA. The flexor reflex is mediated through inhibitory

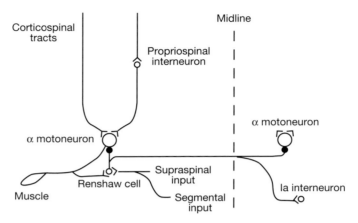

Fig. 5.15 Schematic diagram of Renshaw inhibition.

Ib interneurons (Fig. 5.14), which are inhibited by the input from Aδ fibers that innervate nociceptors in the skin. The Ib interneurons connect to alpha motoneurons that innervate extensor muscles through at least two synapses, and they send many collaterals up and down the spinal cord to activate muscles that are innervated from several segments [22]. Collaterals that reach other spinal segments make synaptic contact with cells that provide inhibitory input to alpha motoneurons of extensor muscles. The flexor reflex is also known as the withdrawal reflex.

The activity in the pathway of the FRA is subjected to supraspinal modulation by the dorsal reticulospinal system (Fig. 5.14) [27], which descends bilaterally from the pontomedullary reticular formation through the dorsolateral funiculus. These fibers inhibit first-order interneurons of the FRA reflex pathways. The corticospinal and the rubrospinal pathways facilitate transmission in the FRA reflex [88].

Crossed extensor reflex

The crossed extensor reflex is a flexor reflex that is elicited from the opposite side. For example, stepping on a sharp object with one foot causes the other leg to extend to prevent falling.

Renshaw inhibition

Another important circuit in the spinal cord is the recurrent (Renshaw) inhibition circuit that plays an important role in normal spinal reflexes [27] (Fig. 5.15).

The Renshaw feedback system consists of a cell that acts as an interneuron with input from collaterals of motor nerves. The output of Renshaw cells

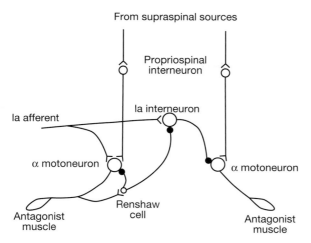

Fig. 5.16 Compound schematic diagram of Renshaw inhibition and the reciprocal reflex illustrating how inhibitory input from Ia interneurons on the antagonist muscle can be modulated by Renshaw cells. This allows switching from agonist to antagonist, such as from flexor to extensor, and back again as occurs in cyclic movements like stepping.

provides inhibitory input to the same alpha motoneuron and to other agonist motoneurons as well (Fig. 5.16). Renshaw neurons receive supraspinal input (such as from the corticospinal tract) that can modulate the recurrent inhibition. Renshaw feedback is an important source of negative feedback in motor systems. Renshaw cells also connect to Ia interneurons and can thereby modulate the stretch reflex.

Although Renshaw inhibition is not a reflex in the strictest meaning of the word, it has similarities with both the monosynaptic stretch reflex and the tendon reflex in that it provides negative feedback to motor control. Negative feedback stabilizes muscle control, similar to the negative feedback that is used in man-made control systems.

Long reflex arcs

Proprioceptive signals travel in the dorsal column and the spinocerebellar tract to form the afferent path of long reflex arcs. The MI cortex also receives input from proprioceptors. The efferent paths are the descending (corticospinal and other) tracts. The fibers in the dorsal column mainly project to the ventral posterior lateral (VPL) nucleus of the thalamus and these fibers also send collaterals that connect to neurons in the corticospinal motor system via thalamo-cortical and cortico-cortical connections. The medial lemniscus and corticospinal system are the ascending and descending limbs of long loop (spinal) reflexes. Such reflexes have much longer latency than the spinal reflexes, and they are affected by many factors such as the degree of wakefulness.

Inter- and intraspinal segmental processing

Most input to cells in the gray matter of the spinal cord originates in other cells in the gray matter of the spinal cord. This complex network of connections between neurons in the spinal cord provides extensive intra- and intersegmental processing, which is important for the normal function of the motor system.

Local spinal cord connections provide powerful processing of information at the segmental level of the spinal cord, and extensive connections between the segments adds to the complexity of the internal processing of information occurring in the spinal cord. The integration of somatosensory and proprioceptive information with supraspinal motor commands makes the spinal cord a complex system, with wide ranges of computational capabilities regarding voluntary and automatic motor control. Spinal cord processing involves multiple feedback loops (including reflexes), the gain of which is affected by several sources of supraspinal input as well as proprioceptor input. There are extensive connections between segments of the spinal cord, extending many segments. The existence of connections between lumbar and cervical segments of the spinal cord is evident, for instance, in the locomotion of quadrupedal animals. Humans have a vestige of this manifestation in the tendency of swinging the arms opposite to leg movements while crawling as infants and walking as adults.

Another example elucidating the extensive intersegmental connections is the Jendrassik's maneuver (see p. 270) that enhances the stretch reflex of the lower limb (such as the patellar reflex) by upper limb motor action. This is a clear indication of the interaction between spinal segments, which are far apart.

Interneurons are the most common type of cells in the spinal cord. Interneurons are not only an important path to motoneurons from supraspinal motor centers, but these neurons have a much more complex role in motor control; most commands from supraspinal sources pass through interneurons. Interneurons receive input not only from descending motor tracts, but also from several types of proprioceptive receptors such as muscle spindles, tendon organs and joint receptors. Skin receptors also provide input to interneurons. This provides a means to modulate motor commands that are issued at supraspinal structures. Interneurons send collaterals to many laminas in the dorsal and ventral horns of the spinal cord, and extend their connections to several segments. This means that interneurons are not just relays, but they perform extensive processing of information in their function as links to supraspinal structures and modify motor activity.

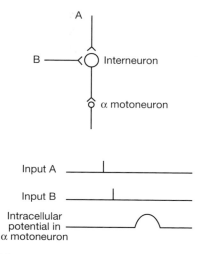

Fig. 5.17 Convergence of two excitatory inputs onto an interneuron (facilitation).

This complex role of interneurons was investigated by Lundberg and his co-workers who provided much experimental evidence for the complex role of interneurons in the spinal cord [69]. These investigators also showed that each input alone may not be able to activate interneurons. Some neurons may require input from more than one source to become activated (Fig. 5.17).

The processing that occurs at segmental levels can be modulated by supraspinal input, and by proprioceptive and sensory input from receptors in muscles, tendons and joints, and in the skin. For example, the spinal proprioceptive interneurons that receive their input from corticospinal neurons also receive excitatory and inhibitory input from many segmental sources. This input can modulate the descending input to alpha motoneurons as well as modulate spinal reflexes [22, 27, 99, 107]. The reciprocal inhibition of the antagonist muscle that occurs during stretch reflexes can be modulated by supraspinal input through the corticospinal tract (Fig. 5.12) [22].

The organization and function of the inter- and intrasegmental spinal connections have received less attention than the processing that occurs in supraspinal structures. The processing that normally occurs in the spinal cord and the extensive intra- and intersegmental communication are factors that are often underestimated. The diagrams of spinal circuitry, such as that for reflexes, and those which appear in textbooks (including this one), are highly simplified and usually omit intersegmental processing.

This complex system is normally a stable control system, but pathologic factors can introduce instability that can cause such symptoms as weakness,

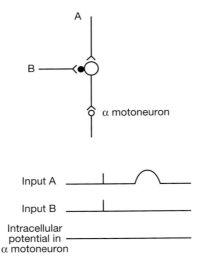

Fig. 5.18 Convergence of an excitatory and an inhibitory input onto an interneuron (counteraction).

incoordination and spasm from, for example, SCI (see p. 299). Paresis, paralysis and abnormal muscle activity such as spasm and tremor can be related to changes in the processing that occurs at segmental levels of the spinal cord, in addition to changed supraspinal input.

Sensory input entering through dorsal spinal roots contributes to motor control via the Ia and Ib system and propriospinal neurons, which receive input from peripheral receptors [15, 69, 109] (Figs. 5.14, 5.15, 5.16) including muscle afferents.

> Propriospinal interneurons were identified in the cat at the C_3-C_4 level of the spinal cord as reported in a series of papers by Alstermark *et al.* [8] (summarized by Porter and Lemon [109]) (see p. 259). Indications that similar propriospinal interneurons are present in humans were presented by Pierrot-Deseilligny (1989) [106].

The balance of active circuitry in the spinal cord is task specific. For example, when the spinal cord CPGs are turned on during locomotion, Ib neurons are turned off and there is now synaptic excitation to extensor motoneurons [90].

The interneurons that relay descending motor information to alpha motoneurons and interneurons that receive input from peripheral receptors may be involved in modification of motor control at a pre-motor neuron level [69].

These complex connections make it possible to modulate spinal reflexes from spinal and supraspinal sources. Presynaptic inhibition induced by corticospinal

Descending motor tracts

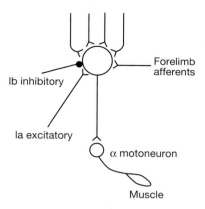

Fig. 5.19 Input to propriospinal neurons of the forelimb of the cat [15].

fibers through axo-axonic synapses can control spinal reflexes, including those that involve Ia spindle afferents and large afferents from the skin (Fig. 5.19) [15, 115]. Control of spinal reflexes and control of muscle spindles through activation of gamma motoneurons are other examples of ways in which the motor cortex can control movement, in addition to their direct activation of alpha motoneurons, either monosynaptic or via propriospinal interneurons.

Even simple reflexes such as the withdrawal reflex can be modulated by willful actions. For example, it is possible to abort or modify the withdrawal reflex normally elicited by input from skin receptors. The proprioceptive input from the vestibulospinal (descending) tract to the spinal cord can be modified by training and affected by its use, as is evident from being on a boat. Such changes in function may be described as a form of neural plasticity (see p. 357), and it can be used in therapy for vestibular disorders.

5.2.7   Brainstem control of motor activity

The brainstem, together with the basal ganglia, cerebellum and the spinal cord, coordinates basic voluntary motor programs that are issued by the motor cortex. The brainstem also generates commands for basic motor functions such as swallowing, chewing and breathing without input from the cerebral cortex. Some of the control circuitry for eye movements is also located in the brainstem.

Brainstem structures exert several important influences on descending spinal motor pathways as they pass through the brainstem. All the descending motor tracts (except the corticospinal and the rubrospinal tracts) are interrupted in the brainstem. Synaptic contact with neurons in the brainstem provides the substrate for modulation of descending motor commands in the brainstem. Brainstem structures can thereby control the flow of impulse activity in descending motor tracts, as well as generate motor control activity in tracts such as the reticulospinal tract. Brainstem structures cannot affect the corticospinal and rubrospinal tracts directly because they pass brainstem structures uninterrupted. The motor control by the corticospinal tract can be affected indirectly by ascending activity from brainstem structures that terminate on neurons of the MI cortex and by descending activity that controls the excitability of propriospinal interneurons and alpha motoneurons.

Blocking of descending activity

It is generally known that activity of skeletal muscles of the body and head (except the eye muscles and those involved in respiration) are blocked during rapid eye movement (REM) sleep (also known as paradoxical sleep), and probably also during other sleep stages. Blockage of skeletal muscle movement is apparent during REM stage of sleep because the eye muscles are active during that sleep stage but other muscles are not, at least not normally.

The ability to activate skeletal muscles through transcranial magnetic stimulation of the motor cortex area is reduced during normal surgical anesthesia, which is another sign that the degree of wakefulness affects the ability to activate skeletal muscles. The effect of anesthesia may be caused by its effect on cortical neurons, but most of the depressive effect is likely to be caused by reduction of descending facilitatory input to spinal motoneurons.

Startle and freezing reactions

The startle response and the freezing[9] reactions are the result of opposite kinds of commands that originate in the brainstem. The startle response activates most skeletal muscles, while freezing involves arrest of all body movements.

The "freezing" reaction occurs in many animals, and it is present in humans. The freezing reaction is caused by blockage of skeletal muscle contractions similar to what occurs normally during rapid eye movement (REM) (or paradoxical) sleep. The freezing reaction that causes all body motion to arrest is elicited by extreme fear or fright. The "freezing reaction" is an example of an unconscious influence on motor activity.

While the startle and freezing reactions seem to be opposite in nature, both are influenced by input from the central nucleus of the amygdala [37].

---

[9] Freezing reactions occur in response to fear and in some pathological conditions such as Parkinson's disease (PD).

The amygdala is involved in fear reactions, and the cells in its nuclei connect to many structures of the CNS. The freezing reaction is an example of the amygdala's influence on descending motor pathways (via brainstem nuclei). The central nucleus of the amygdala exerts its control on the motor systems through its connections to the PAG [37]. Cessation of behavior in freezing occurs by blockage of descending motor activity at the brainstem level [37].

The acoustic startle response is a reflex response that is also related to fear. It occurs most often in response to a strong transient sensory stimulation, but the cause of the response is similar to freezing, namely fear or fright. Startle responses are mediated by circuitry in the brainstem, the main input to which originates in the auditory system. It is mainly elicited by a sharp and loud sound [37]. The acoustic startle response is a short 3-synapse reflex in the brainstem, consisting of the ventral cochlear nucleus (VCN), the paralemniscal zone of the ventral nucleus of the lateral lemniscus (VLL), and the nucleus reticularis pontis caudalis (RPC) [36]. This reflex can be modulated by activity in other structures, in particular the amygdala (rostral part of the medial subdivision) [112]. The input from the amygdala is mediated through the nucleus RPC [37, 112]. The startle response can be modified by behavioral interventions, indicating that expression of neural plasticity can change the function of the reflex. The same is the case for the freezing reaction.

Shivering

Shivering or trembling may occur as a result of cold or because of fear. This reaction is yet another example of a non-conscious form of muscle activity. Shivering that occurs because of cooling of the skin is mediated without conscious control, and can occur even though the temperature in the hypothalamus is normal. The increased heat production that is the purpose of shivering occurs in anticipation of a decrease in core temperature [97]. While this is an advantage to the organism because it can restore body temperature by generating heat, the value of shivering that occurs because of fear is questionable.

Muscle tone

Muscle tone[10] (or resting tone) is the background contraction of muscles that occurs without any voluntary commands or by changes in the viscoelastic properties of muscle, tendon and connective tissue.

---

[10] Words like muscle tone and muscle tension are sometimes used synonymously, but some authors [124] define muscle tone only to mean viscoelastic changes in a muscle that occur in absence of contractile activity. Increased muscle tone may also give pain and is discussed in Chapter 4.

Abnormally increased muscle tone can be caused either by contractile activity mediated by the motor nerve and the motoneurons or by changes in the viscoelastic properties of muscles [124]. Abnormally low muscle tone is known as hypotonus, while abnormally high muscle tone is hypertonia, as may occur in spasticity. Our understanding of normal muscle tone is, however, incomplete, which hampers our understanding of many pathologic conditions of the motor system.

There are three different forms of contractile activation of muscles: (1) electrogenic stiffness caused by activation of motoneurons and neuromuscular endplates (having observable EMG activity); (2) electrogenic spasm (pathological and involuntary electrogenic contraction), and (3) contracture (occurring within the muscle fibers independent of EMG activity [124] and more a function of tissue properties than activity).

The resting muscle tone is often assumed to be caused by a low rate of firings of motor nerves but this assumption seems to rest on a misconception according to Simons and Mense [124]. These investigators described methods to measure muscle tone mechanically, and they credited Walsh [142] for clarifying the misconception that muscle tone was caused by electrical activation of the contractile apparatus of muscles. Some forms of increased muscle tone are thus not caused by activity of alpha motoneurons; instead, the resistance to stretching a muscle is caused by mechanical properties (compliance) of the muscle itself.

Altered muscle tone is an important sign in disorders such as spasticity, which may include an abnormal high degree of muscle tone. The non-neural muscle tone (compliance) is an important contributor to the signs of spasticity, one cause being an increase in connective tissue within muscles as muscle contraction tissue decreases. Loss of muscle sarcomeres that occurs when muscles are immobilized in a shortened position also contributes to the change in muscle tone. (Another contributor to signs of spasticity arises from hyperreflexia [27], see pp. 301, 303.)

Here we will discuss the muscle tone that is induced by neural activity (thus alpha motoneuron activity), and not the passive resistance that a muscle always has against being extended and which depends on a muscle's passive mechanical properties [124].

Muscle tone varies among healthy individuals, and it is affected by many factors such as autonomic activation. The form of muscle tone caused by neural plasticity is affected by the degree of wakefulness and increased sympathetic activity. High levels of stress may cause spontaneous contraction (tremble) while the lowest level of sympathetic activation can cause complete relaxation. Since involuntary shaking causes a feeling of stress, a vicious circle may be the result. Many drugs such as benzodiazepines and alcohol are effective in reducing muscle tonus. These drugs reduce sympathetic activity and thereby lower blood pressure and heart rates. Central muscle relaxants such as benzodiazepines that reduce muscle activity may also make the person feel less stressed, and this may be an effect of the GABA$_A$ receptor agonist on other CNS systems or a result of reduced muscle contractions.

Activation of gamma motoneurons by input from supraspinal sources can influence the tone of skeletal musculature through the stretch reflex. Brain-stem structures are known to exert strong modulatory influence on gamma motoneuron (fusimotor) activity [64]. The reticulospinal tract, and especially the serotonin-norepinephrine tract, exerts considerable influence on the excitability of neurons within the spinal cord, and they modulate the excitability of spinal reflexes and innervate some gamma motoneurons. The tegmental area of the upper brainstem is important in regulating muscle tone in general, which may occur by activation of the serotonin-norepinephrine descending pathways (see pp. 177, 263). It has also been shown that some of the antidepressive drugs of the selective serotonin re-uptake inhibitor (SSRI) class can cause excessive eye movements [118], thus signs of activating neurons of the tectum. These drugs can also increase spasticity in SCI.

> In one study [74], electrical stimulation of the common peroneal nerve was found to increase the excitability of the motor system, as demon-strated by magnetic stimulation of the motor cortex. When elicited by magnetic stimulation, the amplitude of the motor evoked potentials (MEP) that can be recorded from the tibialis anterior increased an aver-age of 104% by stimulation of the common peroneal nerve and the effect lasted up to 110 minutes after the cessation of the stimulation. The excitability to transcranial electrical stimulation was also increased, but to a lesser extent (approximately only half of that of magnetic stimula-tion). The monosynaptic stretch reflex was not increased, indicating that the effect of peroneal stimulation was not caused by increased excitabil-ity of the motoneuron pool. It was speculated that the anatomical site of increased excitability was the motor cortex.

Much effort has been spent on reducing muscle tone. Such simple measures as taking a deep breath can reduce the tonus in most skeletal muscle. The reduced muscle tension occurs immediately and lasts for some time, and it can easily be repeated.

5.2.8   Other descending control of excitability

In the awake individual, many factors can affect the excitability of alpha motoneurons. Descending influence from high cerebral centers, from spinal seg-mental circuitry receiving input from proprioceptors in muscles innervated by their respective motoneurons, and from other muscle groups, all contribute to the excitability of alpha motoneurons and thereby also to their resting activity. Chemical factors can also facilitate alpha motoneuron excitability.

Descending norepinephrine and serotonin pathways (see p. 265) contribute to regulating the excitability of the α motoneurons and thereby muscle tone. The reticulospinal tract and the rubrospinal tract also play important roles in regulating the excitability of α motoneurons. (Some investigators have included the norepinephrine-serotonin pathway in their description of the reticulospinal pathway.)

The role of the reticular formation on muscle tone was mentioned above (pp. 255, 261), thus, the reticulospinal tract plays an important role in control of α motoneuron excitability. Too much activity causes increased excitability. Too little activation results in difficulty eliciting the stretch reflex, yet input from other segments of the spinal cord can increase excitability (cf. the Jendrassik's maneuver). The reticular system has a similar effect on the motor system as it has on sensory systems [94]. The excitability of both the sensory and motor systems depends on the degree of wakefulness controlled by the reticular formation and other centers in the CNS like the amygdala [94]. This means that voluntary movements require both a voluntary command and adequate excitability of α motoneurons.

> An example of the effect of descending excitatory input to α motoneurons is demonstrated by the observation that anesthesia reduces the ability to elicit muscle contractions by transcranial electrical or magnetic stimulation of the cerebral cortex [129, 130]. Transcranial stimulation is effective in eliciting contractions of skeletal muscles in awake individuals, but the effectiveness of such stimulation was much diminished in patients under general (surgical) anesthesia [16]. This reduction in excitability of the motor system that is seen when the motor cortex (MI) is stimulated electrically or by transcranial magnetic stimulation during anesthesia is assumed to be caused by reduced facilitatory input to the spinal cord from supraspinal sources. While one impulse is sufficient to elicit a muscle contraction in the awake individual, trains of impulses are necessary in anesthetized individuals. This means that the EPSPs that are evoked in alpha motoneurons by a single impulse stimulating the MI are not sufficient to reach threshold and, consequently, temporal summation of EPSPs of several descending impulses are necessary to exceed the threshold of alpha motoneurons in anesthetized individuals. The advantage of electrical transcranial stimulation over magnetic stimulation is that trains of electrical impulses are technically easier to generate than trains of magnetic stimulation (see pp. 177, 263).
>
> It is probably the decrease in the descending activity in tracts originating in the reticular formation that causes the lower excitability that

recording from
left abductor digiti minimi

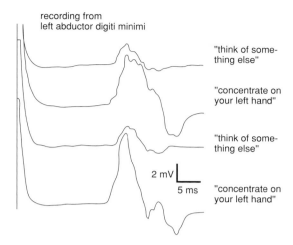

"think of some-
thing else"

"concentrate on
your left hand"

"think of some-
thing else"

2 mV

5 ms

"concentrate on
your left hand"

Fig. 5.20 Illustration of facilitatory and inhibitory influence from high CNS levels on the response of a muscle in the hand of an awake human subject in response to transcranial magnetic stimulation of the motor cortex. (From Rösler, 2001 [114].) Reprinted from *News Physiol. Sci.* vol. 16, 297–302; 2001, with permission from the American Physiological Society.

is observed in anesthetized individuals. In the awake individual, input from supraspinal sources facilitate excitation of α motoneurons and the EPSP that is generated by a single impulse is sufficient to reach the firing threshold of motoneurons.

Activation of skeletal muscles through (magnetic) stimulation of the motor cortex is also affected by attention (Fig. 5.20). This means that descending activity from high CNS structures is capable of modulating the excitability of α motoneurons. The effect of supraspinal activity on the excitability of muscles in the hand of an awake human subject is illustrated by the response to transcranial magnetic stimulation of the motor cortex (Fig. 5.20). The amplitude of the recorded EMG response increases when the subject "thinks of the hand," while the amplitude decreases when "thinking of something else" [114]. The response from magnetic stimulation of the cortex is also facilitated by a weak voluntary contraction of the muscles in question, which illustrates the multitude of factors that influences the excitability of alpha motoneurons.

Experience from intraoperative neurophysiologic monitoring in which the motor cortical areas are stimulated transcranially (electrically or magnetically) [12], shows that the response recorded from the corticospinal tract of the spinal cord is relatively insensitive to anesthesia, while EMG responses are suppressed by general anesthesia. This indicates that the MI excited by transcranial electrical stimulation is relatively insensitive to anesthesia. (In fact, it is believed that the major location of neural activation from transcranial electrical stimulation is in

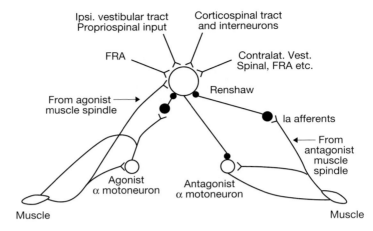

Fig. 5.21   Input to an Ia inhibitory interneuron [89].

the deep white matter and not at the level of the cortex.) The reason that the excitability of α motoneurons is affected by anesthesia may be that anesthesia causes the facilitatory input to the alpha motoneurons to decrease. The reduced supraspinal facilitatory input to motoneurons may make it difficult to excite α motoneurons. EMG response naturally also depends on the function of the muscle endplates, but these are less sensitive to anesthesia, as is evident from the possibility to elicit muscle contractions by electrical stimulation of motor nerves in surgically anesthetized (but not paralyzed) patients.

The fact that muscle contractions are difficult to evoke from stimulation of the motor cortex during surgical anesthesia [130] shows that the cortico-spinal tract alone cannot elicit muscle contractions, and that facilitation is also required to elicit muscle contractions. (This is again a similarity with sensory systems, where input from sensory receptors is not sufficient to elicit a sensory response, but facilitation of cortical neurons from the reticular system is also needed [94].)

The Ia inhibitory interneurons are important for controlling muscle tone. These neurons receive excitatory input from muscle spindles in the agonist mus-cle, and inhibitory influence from the antagonist muscle spindles in addition to input from many sources that converge on these Ia inhibitory interneurons (Fig. 5.21). These Ia neurons have excitatory input from supraspinal sources (cor-ticospinal and rubrospinal tracts, ipsilateral and contralateral vestibulospinal tracts), and from many interneurons in the spinal cord that receive supraspinal input. Some interneurons that have excitatory influence on inhibitory Ia interneurons receive input from cutaneous receptors (FRA) from both sides [89, 109] (Fig. 5.21). Since the Ia interneurons exert inhibitory influence on alpha

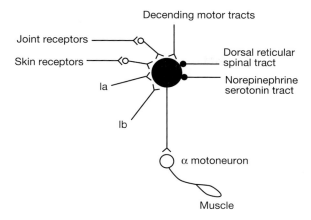

Fig. 5.22 Input to an Ib (inhibitory) interneuron (based on Jankowska and Lundberg, 1981) [69].

motoneurons of the agonist muscle, reduced input to these neurons from any of these multiple sources will increase the excitability of alpha motoneurons, and subsequently facilitate spinal reflexes and increase the tone of the muscles involved.

The Ib inhibitory interneurons (Fig. 5.22) receive excitatory input from Golgi tendon organs in the agonist muscle and are inhibitory on agonist alpha motoneurons [89] (p. 274). The Ib interneurons also receive input from supraspinal sources (excitatory input via the corticospinal tract and inhibitory from the reticulospinal tract), and they receive excitatory input from interneurons that receive cutaneous input (FRA). Again, elimination or reduction of such input may increase the excitability of alpha motoneurons and thereby increase muscle tone [14, 89, 109]. The functions of these circuits are plastic and subject to modifications in their response to demands and in response to injuries.

Control of locomotion and posture depends on subthalamic, mesencephalic and medullary (locomotor strips) – structures of the brainstem that communicate through the reticulospinal pathway. These structures exert control over the spinal cord CPG that controls motion (initiation and speed). The same structures control postural tone and modulate the force that is generated by muscles activated by CPGs. The cerebellum that refines these commands is involved in coordination of movements. It was earlier believed that the cerebellum was the anatomical site for learning motor skills, but it has later been found that motor skills can be learned without the cerebellum, thus involving other structures, sometimes just the spinal cord.

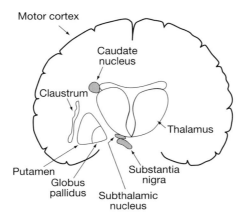

Fig. 5.23 Anatomical organization of the basal ganglia and the motor thalamus.

5.2.9 Basal ganglia

The term basal ganglia is defined differently by different investigators, but the term commonly includes the caudate nucleus, the putamen and the globus pallidus (Fig. 5.23). Some authors also include the substantia nigra and the subthalamic nucleus (STN) because they are functionally related to the other components of the basal ganglia [22]. The putamen and the globus pallidus are commonly known as the lentiform nucleus. The caudate nucleus and the putamen have similarities, and these two nuclei are often referred to as the striatum or neostriatum.

The basal ganglia do not issue motor commands, but process information that they receive from the cerebral cortex and send it back to the cerebral cortex via the motor thalamus (Figs. 5.7, 5.23). The basal ganglia are involved in many movement disorders, most characteristically in common disorders such as PD and HD. The role that the basal ganglia play in PD has caused rapid increase in the interest in these nuclei. It has been demonstrated that various forms of specific manipulations (surgical lesions, electrical stimulation) can have beneficial effects and can alleviate symptoms and signs of movement disorders. This increased interest has also resulted in a more differentiated view of these ganglia, and several subdivisions of these nuclei are now recognized. Thus, the globus pallidus is commonly divided into an external segment (globus pallidus external part, GPe) and an internal segment (globus pallidus internal part, GPi). A part of the substantia nigra pars reticulata (SNr), and the substantia nigra pars compacta (SNc), are of particular interest in connection with movement disorders (Fig. 5.24).

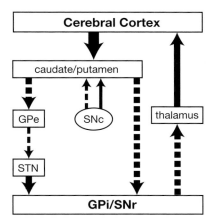

Fig. 5.24 Simplified scheme of the connections between the cerebral cortex and some of the nuclei of the basal ganglia and the thalamus. Black arrows show excitation and interrupted arrows show inhibition.

The functional organization of the basal ganglia is complex, and is not completely understood. The function of the basal ganglia must be seen with regard to the interrelationship between components of multiple segregated circuits, including many other structures of the CNS [7]. The circuitry of the basal ganglia can be viewed as starting in the primary motor and somatosensory cortices that connect to portions of the putamen, GPe and GPi, the SNr, and the STN (Fig. 5.24). The pathway through these nuclei returns the information they receive from the motor cortex (and somatosensory cortex) to the same (precentral) motor area (MI) through the motor thalamus (ventralis lateralis, pars oralis, VLo, and ventralis anterior, VA) [7].

The basal ganglia communicate closely with each other, and with specific parts of the thalamus that connects to the motor cortex (Fig. 5.24) [22]. The striatum is the main receiving part of the basal ganglia. Input from the cortex (MI) converges on the striatum (caudate nucleus and putamen), the centromedian nucleus (CM) of the thalamus and the substantia nigra (Fig. 5.24). The putamen receives input from both motor cortex (MI) and somatosensory cortex (SI), but the cortical input to the caudate nucleus mostly originates from association cortices [22] (Fig. 5.25). The nuclei of the striatum provide "direct" inhibitory input to the GPi and SNr. An "indirect" route projects to the GPi/SNr via the GPe and the STN. GPi and SNr nuclei thus receive input from the striatum with and without interruption in the GPe and STN [7].

All intrinsic connections of the basal ganglia are inhibitory, except the connections between the STN and the Gpi/SNr, which are excitatory. There is

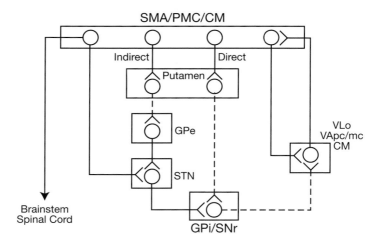

Fig. 5.25 Schematic diagram of direct and indirect pathways of the basal ganglia [6]. SMA: Supplementary motor area; PMC: Premotor cortex.

evidence that the output of GPi and SNr provides tonic inhibition on thalamo-cortical neurons [147], whereas the direct dopaminergic nigrostriatal pathway from SNc may modulate the activity in the two striato-pallidal pathways in two different ways by using two different dopamine receptors. One of these two ways facilitates transmission in the "direct" pathway, while the other inhibits transmission in the "indirect" pathway [4].

The STN connects to the globus pallidus and the substantia nigra, in a reciprocal way, and the STN receives input from the motor cortex (Fig. 5.26). The output from the basal ganglia mainly originates from the globus pallidus and the substantia nigra.

The fact that the basal ganglia receive input from the MI and deliver output to the MI makes descending pathways from the MI (corticospinal tract) contain information from the basal ganglia (Figs. 5.7 and 5.25). This is why the distinction between pyramidal and extrapyramidal tracts has become invalid from an anatomical and physiological point of view, but that old distinction may have some relevance regarding the collection of symptoms in disorders of the motor system.

Several hypotheses have been presented regarding the role of the basal ganglia in control of motor activity. One hypothesis claims that the basal ganglia are involved in the planning of movements [6]. This hypothesis is supported by the existence of connections to PMA, SMA and prefrontal cortex (PF) (Fig. 5.26).

Much of our understanding of the role of the basal ganglia in motor control has been gained from studies done in patients with PD and other motor disorders

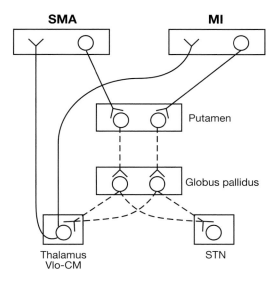

Fig. 5.26 Connections between the basal ganglia and MI and SMA cortical motor areas.

who are treated using either lesions in the basal ganglia or by implantation of electrodes for DBS.

> The fact that recordings of electrical activity from cells of the target nuclei are essential for making precise lesions or implantation of electrodes for DBS has provided opportunities for studies not previously possible. The methods that are used involve recordings from single nerve cells or small groups of nerve cells using microelectrodes. This method of recording from deep brain structures in humans with microelectrodes was introduced by Albe-Fessard and her co-workers [3]. The methods these investigators developed were later used routinely in intraoperative guidance and for basic studies of normal and pathological functions of the motor system [80–86, 138, 139]. These studies have produced a wealth of information about the pathophysiology of movement disorders, and much information on the normal function of the basal ganglia and various parts of the thalamus has been gained through such studies.

5.2.10   Cerebellum

The cerebellum is involved in the control of movements, but like the basal ganglia, it does not initiate movements. Rather, the cerebellum modifies and processes information from other CNS structures. The cerebellum consists of many different parts that have different functions. Earlier, it was assumed that the cerebellum was only involved in the control of movements, but more

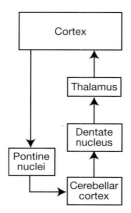

Fig. 5.27 Schematic diagram showing some important connections from the cortex to the cerebellum (cerebro-cerebellum) [22].

recently, it has become evident that the cerebellum also plays a role in many other functions, including cognitive functions. It has been hypothesized that the cerebellum is involved in the shifting of attention, and since attention deficits are marked in individuals with developmental disorders such as autism, the dysfunction of the cerebellum has been implicated in the symptoms of such disorders [31].

Aside from connecting to the basal ganglia and the spinal cord, neurons in the MI also connect to the cerebellum and to brainstem nuclei (Fig. 5.27). The cerebellum plays an important role in shaping motor commands issued by the MI, but as is the case for the basal ganglia, the cerebellum is not believed to issue commands on its own.

The cerebellum receives input from different areas of the cerebral cortex that are involved in control of movements via the pontine nuclei. The cerebellum sends information to motor cortical areas, red nucleus, and to the reticular formation of the brainstem (Fig. 5.28). There are extensive connections between the basal ganglia and the cerebellum. The cerebellum also receives extensive input from sensory and proprioceptive sources such as the skin, joints and muscle spindles through the spinocerebellar tract, and from the vestibular system.

The pontine nuclei are important relays between the motor and sensory cortices (MI and SI) and the cerebellar cortex. The cerebellar cortex in turn provides input to the cerebral cortex via the dentate nucleus of the cerebellum. The dentate nucleus also provides input to the red nucleus, which is the origin of the rubrospinal tract. The thalamus receives input from the dentate nucleus and conveys that input to the cerebral motor cortex. The cerebellar hemispheres receive input from the inferior olive in the medulla, which in turn receives input from many nuclei including the SC, pretectal nuclei and the red nucleus [22].

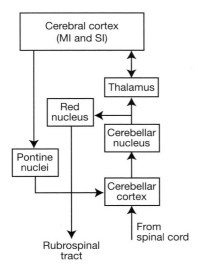

Fig. 5.28 Schematic diagram of the connections of the intermediate zone of the cerebellum [22].

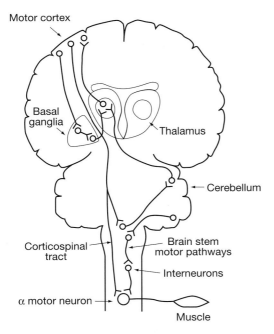

Fig. 5.29 Anatomical location of major motor pathways.

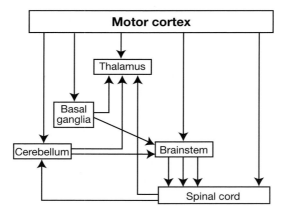

Fig. 5.30 Simplified diagram of the motor systems including the cerebellum.

The cerebellum connects to the red nucleus, to pontine nuclei (inferior olive) via the central tegmental tract, and back to the cerebellum via the unique inputs of the climbing fibers. This is called the Mollaret's triangle, and lesions along this pathway cause different deficits from rubral (postural) tremor (mixture of rest, postural and kinetic tremor) to myoclonus.

The dorsal and ventral spinocerebellar tracts carry proprioceptive information about the function of the motor neuron pools to the cerebellum and this information can modify muscle control, but does not normally reach consciousness; it acts to smooth muscle activity, and faults in that system cause signs of ataxia.

Below T_1 level of the spinal cord, the dorsal spinocerebellar tract originates in the dorsal nucleus of Clarke's column, the neurons of which receive input from muscle spindles and low threshold cutaneous fibers. Above T_1, proprioceptive fibers do not travel in Clarke's column or the dorsal spinocerebellar tract. Instead, such information ascends in the fasciculus cuneatus of the dorsal column, the fibers of which make synaptic contact with cells in the accessory nucleus cuneatus in the lower medulla. The axons of these cells form the cuneocerebellar tract that joins the dorsal spinocerebellar tract (from the lower body) to reach the restiform body (the larger part of the cerebellar peduncle). The restiform body is an input path to the cerebrum.

The ventral spinocerebellar tract has a complex path. The fibers originate in cells in the lateral border of the ventral horn of the lumbar spinal cord. These cells receive input from proprioceptive afferent fibers and from descending supraspinal pathways that innervate motor neurons (propriospinal interneurons and alpha motoneurons). The axons of the spinal border cells cross the midline and ascend as the ventral spinocerebellar tract, through the medulla and pons and enter the cerebellum through the superior cerebellar peduncle. The fibers cross the midline in the posterior fossa, which implies that this tract innervates predominantly the ipsilateral cerebellum. Afferent fibers from the upper spinal cord also reach cells predominantly in the ipsilateral cerebellum, via the rostral part of the spinocerebellar tract.

The spinocerebellar tract thus provides information to the cerebellum about motor activity. One part of this tract conveys information from muscle spindles, tendon organs and cutaneous mechanoreceptors to the cerebellum. The other part of the spinocerebellar tract provides information to the cerebellum from spinal cord interneurons.

The reticulospinal and vestibulospinal tracts receive input from the cerebellum and vestibular nuclei, and the cells in the reticular formation provide input to the cerebellum. The number of fibers that connect to the cerebellum is much larger than the number of fibers that provide output from the cerebellum (40:1 in humans [22]).

5.2.11   Control of sexual functions

Neural control of sexual functions is complex and little studied. Consequently, our understanding of the normal physiology of sexual functions such as the mechanisms for erection, lubrication and orgasm is limited. Studies of individuals with SCI have brought some light to some of these mechanisms [128]. These studies have shown that sexual arousal that can be caused by central processes (psychogenically evoked) and those caused by stimulation of genitalia use separate routes and different circuits in the spinal cord. Thus, studies of women with SCI by Sipski and her colleagues [128] seem to show that intact T_{12}-L_2 segments, as revealed by response to pin pricks in the distribution areas of the skin (T_{12}-L_2 dermatomes), are necessary for psychogenetically mediated genitalia vasoconstriction, whereas sexual arousal from stimulation of genitalia depended on sacral segments in the spinal cord. Genital vasoconstriction is mediated by the parasympathetic activity (the only vessels that are controlled by the parasympathetic system). The origin of the innervation is probably the sacral segments of the spinal cord because the vagus nerve probably does not extend that far caudal.

The neurophysiologic basis for orgasm is even less well understood, but there are indications from a few studies that the functioning of the S_2-S_5 segments is important for achieving orgasm. It has been suggested that sensations, and thus cerebral involvement, related to orgasm in patients with SCI above T_6 are mediated either by autonomous fibers in the spinal cord that were preserved [127], or by the vagus nerve [143]. That the vagus nerve is involved in sexual experience is plausible in view

of the extensive central connections of the vagus nerve, including connections to nuclei of the limbic system such as those of the amygdala
[18].

The involvement of the autonomic nervous system has been debated.
One study has shown that the sensory experience of orgasm is mediated
by the autonomic nervous system and does not require cerebral initiation
or involvement [128]. There are most likely many other factors that are
involved in the complex mechanisms of sexual functions.

Other studies have found that sacral reflexes must be intact for experiencing orgasm elicited by direct stimulation of genitalia [128]. These
reflexes are presumed to be mediated by the pudendal nerve. Sacral segments of the spinal cord must also be intact for other autonomic sensations such as those associated with bowel distention [34], and it is
consequently important to be aware of that matter when doing sacral
rhizotomy for spasticity [133]. It should be remembered that parasympathetic innervation through the pudendal nerve originates in the sacral
spinal cord and not the vagus nerve, which probably does not extend
that far caudally.

Sexual attraction is perhaps even less well understood than that of
sexual arousal and orgasm. It has been suggested that pheromones may
be involved in a non-conscious way [94].

More knowledge about the basic physiology of sexual functions would
facilitate treatment of frequent disorders affecting sexual function, the
treatment of which now falls under several specialties of medicine and
psychology.

5.3   Pathophysiology of movement disorders

Expression of neural plasticity often occurs in connection with injuries
or other disorders of the motor system, and it has been shown in many studies
that functional re-organization of the motor system can contribute to symptoms
and signs of injuries to the spinal cord, as well as the brain [44, 109]. There is
evidence that expression of neural plasticity may contribute to movement disorders such as spasms, spasticity and other forms of dystonia. It has been known
for many years that the synaptic efficacy of afferents to alpha motoneurons is
plastic [21, 68, 109]. It is well known that changes in sensory input to one segment of the spinal cord can affect the excitability of neighboring segments [141].
Expression of neural plasticity occurs normally in response to pathologies such
as reduced sensory input, but also in response to reduced motor utilization
or reduced capabilities. Expression of neural plasticity induced by (electrical)
stimulation of specific neural structures, or by exercise and training, is used
to alleviate symptoms and signs of neurologic disorders such as pain, and for
restoration of movements in movement disorders.

In this section, we will first discuss the pathophysiology of paresis and paralysis caused by disorders that affect muscles, motor nerves and alpha motoneurons. Paresis and paralysis caused by disorders that affect structures located centrally to alpha motoneurons are often associated with movement disorders such as hypokinesia and hyperkinesia. The pathophysiology of such disorders will be discussed later in this chapter.

5.3.1   Spinal cord and brainstem disorders

Spinal cord and brainstem disorders can be divided into disorders that affect alpha motoneurons selectively, and disorders that affect the spinal cord or brainstem in general. Disorders that affect structures that are rostral to the α motoneuron normally cause more complex signs and symptoms such as hypokinesia and hyperkinesia, in addition to paresis and paralysis.

SCI can cause paresis and paralysis, but disorders and injuries that affect the spinal cord in general usually also present with symptoms and signs of other movement disorders such as hypokinesia and hyperkinesia. The cause of movement disorders of the spinal cord and the brainstem are often complex. The symptoms and signs are often the result of the initiation of a chain of events that involves many parts of the central nervous system (CNS), involving expression of neural plasticity.

Lower motor neuron disorders

ALS is a degenerative progressive disorder closely associated with the degeneration of alpha motoneurons in the spinal cord or in the brainstem, but it also includes the degeneration of motor fiber tracts and pyramidal cells in the motor cortex. Other neural systems do not seem to be involved. It typically affects both spinal and lower cranial nerve motoneurons. The disorder is progressive from onset, and from the time of diagnosis respiratory failure ensues within 6 months to 10 years with a mean of 2 years. No therapy has been effective. The pathophysiology is unknown, but familial ALS is associated with mutations of a gene that controls synthesis of SOD (superoxidize dismuthase).

5.3.2   Dyskinesia (hypokinesia and hyperkinesia)

Hypokinesia and hyperkinesia can result from injuries and other causes that result in morphological changes such as destruction of CNS tissue or ischemia. Altered function of the motor system may also occur because of reorganization of the nervous system. Morphological changes include interruption of pathways and alterations of the function of gray matter involved in processing of movement commands and initiation of movement.

Altered or absent central input to spinal segmental gray matter can alter processing either by itself or through the expression of neural plasticity. Changes in facilitatory and inhibitory input from supraspinal sources also cause symptoms of dyskinesia. Inhibitory input originates mainly from the dorsal reticulospinal tract (see p. 261). This is important in SCI where supraspinal (and rostral segmental) input to an injured part of the spinal cord is altered or absent. Since normal function depends on a correct balance between excitatory and inhibitory input, malfunction will occur when either excitatory or inhibitory input is lost or altered. Many of the symptoms and signs of SCI may be explained by the altered relationship between excitatory or inhibitory supraspinal input to segmental spinal reflex circuits, and by changes in the relationship between excitatory and inhibitory input to the spinal cord from supraspinal sources. The corticospinal and rubrospinal tracts are important in this respect because they provide excitatory input to the spinal cord.

Changes in the balance between inhibition and excitation can cause movement disorders. Rostral structures normally supply complex input to the spinal segment that is both inhibitory and excitatory on motor neurons. Altered sensory input to the spinal cord also plays a role in producing symptoms of dyskinesia.

It is assumed that many movement disorders are caused by defective utilization of input to the CPG and reflexes in the spinal cord together with misdirected or incorrect compensatory processes. All these components are plastic and subject to change from injuries and deprivation of input, but their function can also be molded and corrected by expression of neural plasticity that is evoked by training and other means such as electrical stimulation of peripheral structures (TENS) or the cerebral cortex.

Evidence of re-organization has been presented regarding the cerebral cortex, the brainstem and the spinal cord at segmental levels. Deprivation of input is the strongest promoter of neural plasticity, and injuries that cause interruption of pathways may thus (immediately or later) cause changes in function that are not directly a cause of the original morphological changes. Changes in the function of peripheral structures – including motor nerves and proprioceptive input – may promote such expression of neural plasticity. The changes in function are normally not accompanied by any detectable abnormality in morphology. Even changes in muscles and motor nerves may affect CNS structures [63, 66, 117]. The symptoms from altered function of CNS structures may change over time. Expression of neural plasticity may involve the unmasking of dormant synapses, formation or elimination of synapses, sprouting of axons and changing of synaptic efficacy (see Chapter 1). Hyperactivity, which can cause spasticity and tremor, may result from increased synaptic efficacy in excitatory neural circuits or decrease in synaptic efficacy in inhibitory circuits. Changes in the balance between inhibition and excitation is a common outcome of expression of neural plasticity that involves altered synaptic efficacy.

Loss of dexterity is the primary sign of corticospinal tract interruption. Injury to the corticospinal tract also causes abnormal posture, abnormal reflexes (spasticity) and abnormal cutaneous reflexes [27]. More of the fibers of the corticospinal tract terminate on interneurons than on motoneurons, and influence the motoneurons through their effects on reflexes that involve the interneurons on which they terminate. Changes in the function of local circuits in the spinal cord therefore play an important role in creating the symptoms and signs that are experienced after interruption of supraspinal input to spinal segmental circuits, such as occurs in SCI. For example, the cutaneous reflexes are often diminished in individuals with upper motor neuron lesions while the deep tendon reflexes are increased; again, yet another sign of the complexity of motor control.

Spasticity

Disorders and injuries affecting the spinal cord can cause spasticity. The pathophysiology of spasticity is complex and poorly understood. The anatomical location of the physiological abnormalities that cause spasticity may be local circuits at the segmental level of the spinal cord that innervate the muscles that function abnormally. The abnormality may be located in supraspinal structures. It is more likely, however, that the symptoms are caused by a complex interplay of physiological and morphological abnormalities, with several different anatomical locations being involved.

The signs of spasticity have been explained by abnormalities of spinal reflexes, mainly affecting the stretch reflex [27]. Spasticity is characterized by hyperreflexia that is more pronounced when stretching a muscle at a fast rate. The term spasticity is used to describe increased resistance against rapid stretching of muscles and increased stretch reflexes. The resistance against slow, passive stretching of muscles is less abnormal in individuals with spasticity.

The increased excitability and hyperactivity of the monosynaptic stretch reflex [27, 122] that is characteristic of spasticity can be caused either by increased excitatory input or by decreased inhibitory input to alpha motoneurons, either directly or by presynaptic modulation. Understanding how the excitability of alpha motoneurons and spinal reflexes are regulated is therefore important for understanding the pathophysiological signs of spasticity. As was discussed above (p. 271), the excitability of the monosynaptic stretch reflex can be modulated from supraspinal levels, as well as from segmental levels. The axo-axonic synapses that are involved are GABAergic, and this may explain why GABA agonists such as baclofen and benzodiazepines affect the excitability of the stretch reflex and are effective in the treatment of spasticity.

Expression of neural plasticity plays an important role in creating symptoms and signs of spasticity. Since the neural circuits in the spinal cord gray matter are not "hard-wired," their connections and functions are task dependent and can be modified by expression of neural plasticity. This can establish new connections and change synaptic efficacy in response to changing demands, or in response to loss of function through injuries or diseases.

The role of neural plasticity is probably best known from the somatosensory system [92] and pain [141], but similar reorganization can occur in the circuits that are involved in motor functions [59, 109]. Extensive reorganization probably occurs after SCI, and such re-organization may have beneficial as well as non-beneficial effects.

Many of the signs of spasticity that develop after SCI, or as a result of disorders of supraspinal origin (for instance, cerebral palsy), may be regarded as a natural compensatory response to restore normal excitability of alpha motoneurons after loss of supraspinal excitatory input by increasing the gain of spinal reflexes. This compensatory function from expression of neural plasticity can have side effects, which can produce some of the signs of spasticity.

Expression of neural plasticity in spasticity may be caused by deprivation of supraspinal input, or from changes within one or a few spinal segments. The decreased supraspinal input may cause hyperactivity of neurons at the segmental level. Increased excitability can also be caused by decreased inhibitory input from local (segmental) or from supraspinal sources, or it may be caused by increased synaptic efficacy of the motor neurons themselves. The increased excitability of spinal reflexes may be seen as an attempt to compensate for the reduced excitability of alpha motoneurons that are caused by injury.

While it has generally been assumed that the excitability of alpha motoneurons is altered in spasticity, there is little direct evidence for this [122]. Hyperactivity of the gamma system causing increased fusimotor activity [116] could cause abnormalities in the stretch reflex, and exaggerated tendon reflexes. It was earlier assumed that the increased excitability that is typical for spasticity was caused by increased gamma motor activity, but more recent studies have not shown an increased firing frequency of Ia neurons. Fusimotor overactivity cannot produce spasticity by itself [27], but evidence has been presented that the hyperreflexia in spasticity instead is caused by a disturbance in reflex circuits in the spinal cord, which in turn increases the excitability of alpha motoneurons. This does not mean, however, that the function of the motoneurons themselves is altered.

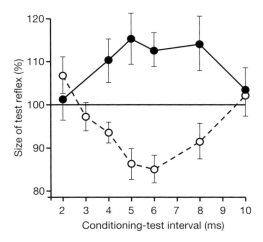

Fig. 5.31 Illustration of the effect of Ib inhibition from stimulation of the gastrocnemius nerve on the soleus H reflex in a hemiplegic individual. Open circles indicate the relative amplitude of the H reflex on the normal side as an illustration of the normal effect of Ib inhibition. Filled circles indicate the change in the amplitude of the H reflex on the side with spasticity (data from Delwaide, *et al.* 1988) [41].

Hagbarth and co-workers showed no increase in muscle spindle sensitivity in (two) spastic individuals [58], or abnormal excitability of spinal segmental and intersegmental interneurons caused by loss of supraspinal (inhibitory and excitatory) input. Changes in the properties of muscles may contribute to some of the signs of spasticity [122].

It is now generally assumed that the characteristic signs of spasticity are a result of abnormally active monosynaptic reflexes together with weaker, long-latency stretch reflexes [1, 27]. Long-term reduction in inhibition at segmental levels also seems to be involved in spasticity. Changes in the function of Ia and Ib interneurons and of Renshaw inhibition – which are all modulated by supraspinal input (see p. 279 and Fig. 5.16) – are viable candidates for explaining the physiological abnormality that causes the signs of spasticity. Some studies have presented evidence that the inhibition of alpha motoneurons by the Ib interneurons is lost in spasticity [41] (see Fig. 5.31 [122]). Abnormalities of the reciprocal inhibition of extensor contractions that normally occur in the voluntary contraction of flexors may also contribute to the signs of spasticity.

The abnormal muscle tone in spasticity may be a result of either an increased excitability or decreased inhibition. Normal muscle tone is mainly dependent on the balance between inhibitory influences on the monosynaptic stretch reflex

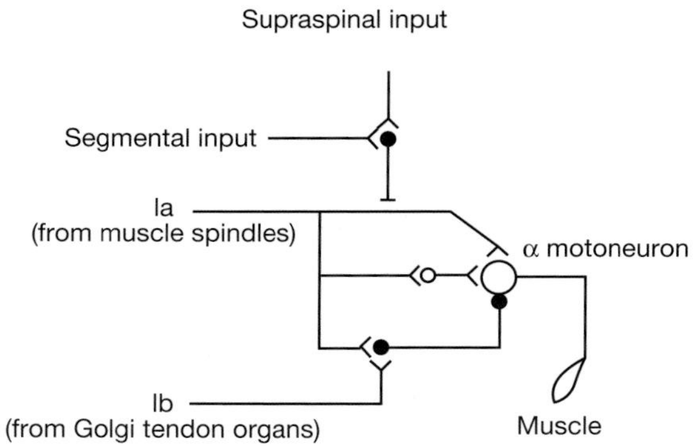

Supraspinal input

Fig. 5.32 Schematic drawing of the input onto a motoneuron pool. The supraspinal excitatory input from corticospinal fibers and their interneurons are not shown [27].

from the reticulospinal tract and excitatory input. The dorsal reticulospinal tract mediates inhibitory influence while the medial reticulospinal tract mediates facilitatory influence, mainly on extensor muscles [24].

It is known that demyelinating lesions mainly affect the lateral funiculi [104]. Lesions of the lateral funiculus lead to hypertonia and hyperreflexia. Lesions of the lateral funiculus could therefore explain the hyperreflexia in spasticity, but spasticity is reduced if the vestibulospinal tracts are also severed. These results using lesions were mainly derived from studies in monkeys; results in humans are few and are often not supported by histological controls. There are indications that the influence of the vestibulospinal tract on motor excitability may be less pronounced in humans than in animals [24].

The abnormal response to stretching a muscle is characteristic for spasticity but the reflex circuits in the spinal cord that are activated by stretching a muscle are complex (Fig. 5.32) [27] and the reflex involves excitatory (monosynaptic) input to alpha motoneurons from muscle spindles (Ia fibers), as well as inhibitory input from Ia and Ib fibers. The output of the receptors in the muscle spindles connect through fast conducting Ia fibers to the homonymous and synergistic motoneuron pool through both monosynaptic and oligosynaptic connections in the spinal cord (see p. 271). The stretch reflex can be modulated from other segmental structures (oligosynaptic reflexes etc.), and from supraspinal sources.

Modulation of the monosynaptic stretch reflex by supraspinal descending activity contributes to spasticity. This modulation is mediated through presynaptic inhibition on the Ia fibers controlling the Ia input to the alpha motoneuron [27] (Fig. 5.32), and it has been hypothesized that depression of this presynaptic inhibition of the monosynaptic reflex may play an important role in creating spasticity [27]. Both supraspinal and segmental input contribute to this presynaptic inhibition. Vibration of a muscle can produce such presynaptic inhibition that can decrease the monosynaptic reflex, as indicated by its reduction of the H reflex response. Disturbance of the reciprocal (disynaptic) Ia inhibition (Fig. 5.14 [27]) may also be involved in creating the signs of spasticity [109] (p. 205).

Changes in proprioception and the input from skin receptors can also alter the symptoms and signs of spasticity. One form of treatment of spasticity consists of severing fascicles of dorsal roots, thus decreasing proprioceptive input [126]. However, this does not mean that the proprioceptive input is altered in spasticity. The recurrent (Renshaw) inhibition provides a short loop feedback to alpha motoneurons that is basically inhibitory, but this reflex is normally modulated by input from supraspinal structures [109]. If this modulation is altered because of SCI or strokes, it can affect motor functions.

Spasticity has similarities with decerebrate rigidity seen in animals after transection of the brainstem below the red nucleus, which is associated with increased extensor tone, supporting the hypothesis that reduced inhibitory input from supraspinal sources contributes to the signs of spasticity. Electrical stimulation of the spinal portion of the cerebellum, which supplies inhibitory input to the spinal cord via vestibular nuclei, can eliminate decerebrate rigidity [22], thus supporting the hypothesis that decreased inhibitory input from supraspinal sources may be a contributing factor to some forms of spasticity.

That the response is greater to rapid extension of muscles in spasticity implies the activation of fast adapting reflex systems. There is normally a balance between velocity-dependent excitation and position- (or length-) dependent suppression of reflex activity [26, 27], but this balance is shifted towards velocity-dependent excitation in spasticity. This velocity-dependent hyperreflexia contributes to hypertonia, and contributes to the exaggerated tendon jerk reflex.

Other observations seem to reveal that reduced supraspinal input can have two opposite effects on alpha motoneurons. The presumed reduction in supraspinal input that normally occurs during sleep [118] and anesthesia [130] reduces the excitability of alpha motoneurons, while decerebration and SCI that presumably also decreases supraspinal input increases the excitability of alpha motoneurons, and increases excitability of the monosynaptic stretch reflex. These signs can be explained by the existence of both inhibitory and excitatory supraspinal input to neurons in the spinal cord (such as through the reticulospinal system (see p. 261).

Treatment of spasticity

Treatment of spasticity has taught us much about the pathophysiology of spasticity. We will therefore review some of the treatments used to alleviate the symptoms of spasticity. Many of these treatments have been found effective, although the physiological basis for their effectiveness was not completely known at the time they were introduced, and the basis for many of the different kinds of treatments that are in current use are still not completely understood.

Studies that have shown that electrical stimulation can alleviate some of the signs of spasticity indicate that the symptoms of spasticity are caused by a change in the state of the spinal cord induced by changes in (lack of) rostral input. Electrical stimulation of the skin [35, 42] or of the pudendal nerve at the rectum can immediately reduce the exaggerated monosynaptic reflex and thereby alleviate the clearest signs of spasticity. Electrical stimulation of the rectum that induces ejaculation or orgasm in patients with SCI is effective in reducing the hyperexcitability of the monosynaptic reflex characteristic of spasticity [60, 61, 128], and the effect lasts many hours after cessation of the stimulation [60, 132]. The stimulation of the pudendal nerve itself may have the effect shown in these studies, or it could be the various processes elicited during orgasm or ejaculation that cause the observed effects on the signs of spasticity. The anal canal is also innervated by visceral afferents, which are stimulated by the electrical stimulation used in these studies and that could also contribute to the observed effect.

In one study, electrical stimulation was applied through electrodes placed on the skin over the biceps or the triceps brachii muscle and stimulated at 20 pps with an intensity of only 60–80% of that which could evoke muscle activity. Such stimulation for 10 minutes reduced the subsequent reflex by 30% regarding peak joint torque, and the amplitude of the EMG potentials recorded from the muscles was also reduced [35]. In some subjects, the spasticity was reduced as much as 70%, but in other subjects, the reduction was only 5%.

In a study of the effect of anal stimulation, all 6 males and 3 females with SCI [61] experienced a decrease in spasticity lasting 4–10 hours (mean) after each treatment. This study also showed that rectal stimulation in itself caused long-lasting relief without ejaculation, and that this treatment was more effective than antispasticity medication. All subjects experienced an increase in spasticity during the stimulation, which consisted of one-second-long stimulations over 5–10 minutes [61]. The side effect was dysreflexia and increased blood pressure in people with injuries above T_6. The patients in this study were therefore treated for this with nitroglycerine and or nifedipine [61]. These authors did not mention if the stimulation elicited pain, but in view of the strength that was used (7–15 volts and 150–575 mA of 60 cycles sine waves for 1 second), it would seem a painful procedure if used in individuals with preserved pain sensation in that region of the body.

The mechanism of action of the electrical stimulation of the skin or the pudendal nerve that relieves spasticity is unknown, but it seems reasonable to assume that it may substitute for the normal central input to the spinal cord gray matter that was lost because of injury. The pudendal nerve has a rich innervation of neurons in the dorsal horns at several segments of the lower (sacral) spinal cord, and its effect on larger parts of the spinal cord can be explained by the extensive connections that exist between segments of the spinal cord, covering many segments.

The effect of electrical stimulation of the skin [35, 42] is more difficult to explain. Severing of dorsal roots has a beneficial effect on spasticity, which would seem to have the opposite effect of electrical stimulation of the skin because stimulation of the skin causes increased activity in the fibers of the dorsal roots [125, 126], whereas severing of dorsal roots decreases the sensory input to the spinal cord.

The fact that the decrease in spasticity occurs with a very short delay after electrical stimulation means that the effect cannot be caused by any morphological changes, and the most likely cause seems to be expression of neural plasticity in one form or another. In addition, the fact that electrical stimulation used to elicit orgasm in itself increased the spasticity might indicate that alleviation of the spasticity is not caused by the stimulation but rather by the orgasm, which would mean influence from high CNS centers causing the effect. Studies of the effect of masturbation seem to support that assumption [128].

Surgical treatment of spasticity consisting of severance of dorsal roots of the spinal cord to treat spasticity was inspired by animal studies of decerebrate rigidity. Sherrington demonstrated in 1898 that the rigidity in a decerebrated animal could be abolished by section of dorsal spinal roots. This observation was taken as a sign that sensory input to the spinal cord facilitates the monosynaptic stretch reflex as well as the polysynaptic withdrawal reflex.

The results of these studies support the hypothesis that signs of spasticity (increased stretch reflex) are reversible, and that the abnormalities depend on changes (increase) in synaptic efficacy and/or lowering of synaptic thresholds. The results also support the hypothesis that the increased stretch reflex is a misdirected reaction to injury that is aimed at compensating for the reduction in motor activity caused by the injury.

Operations using severance of dorsal roots to correct spasticity were performed by Foerster in 1908 [126]. Such operations have been continued in patients in whom other treatments have failed. Dorsal root partial rhizotomies have had good effects in children with cerebral palsy [126].

Selective dorsal root rhizotomy (SDR) [1] was introduced in the USA by Peacock for cerebral palsy spasticity [105] and based on the work by Fasano, 1988 [50]. DeCandia [38] had shown in animal experiments that electrical stimulation of dorsal roots showed adaptation in such a way that the second of a train of impulses elicited a smaller response than the first if the rate of stimulation was higher than 15 pps in the normal spinal cord. This depression did not occur in upper motoneuron injury. Fasano, 1988 [50] used this information in children with spasticity and found that sensory root fibers behaved differently; some behaved normally and showed adaptation, while others did not even respond when stimulated at rates of 30–50 pps. Furthermore, he cut the abnormally responding rootlets. Peacock and others [1, 105, 126] improved the safety, while Deletis [39] developed an intraoperative mapping technique that could identify rootlets that were involved in micturition and should be spared. The response to dorsal root stimulation was studied by recording compound muscle action potentials (CMAP), and the ratio between the first and second response was used as a measure of the excitability of a particular fascicule of a dorsal root.

Surgery in the dorsal root entry zone (DREZ) (mainly removing the substantia gelatinosa) was introduced for treatment of pain, but was found to also reduce the muscle tone in disorders such as MS [126] and for treating spasticity in paraplegia [125].

That surgical section of dorsal root fibers can alleviate some of the signs of spasticity does not mean that spasticity is caused by abnormal and excessive sensory input, and this treatment does not affect the cause of spasticity. Moreover, the success of dorsal rhizotomy lies in the reduction of excitatory sensory input to systems that are hyperexcitable. The hyperexcitability is most likely caused by reduced inhibitory input to spinal cord structures caused by trauma that caused the disorder.

Administration of GABA$_A$ agonists (benzodiazepines/Valium) and GABA$_B$ receptor agonists (baclofen/Lioresal) are effective in alleviating some of the symptoms of spasticity, and this supports the hypothesis that inhibition in the CNS is reduced in spasticity. Additionally, local application of baclofen on the spinal cord (by intrathecal infusion using implantable pumps) has been found to be effective in treating many forms of spasticity such as those from SCI and cerebral palsy, where supraspinal input is diminished, altered or absent. Other agents such as tizanadine (Zanaflex), which is an alpha-2 agonist, have had positive effects. It is a sign of the complexity of the phenomenon of spasticity that agents such as dantrolene, which inhibits calcium influx in peripheral muscles, and botulinum toxin, which works at the neuromuscular junction, are also effective in treating spasticity. These drugs have no known effect on the CNS, and their efficiency in alleviating symptoms of spasticity may be related to effects of plasticity that were evoked by reduced muscle activity.

5.3.3   Disorders of brainstem control of motor function

The power of brainstem mechanisms in blocking descending motor pathways is evident from the fact that skeletal muscles are paralyzed during rapid eye movement (REM) sleep (paradoxical sleep). The observation that some individuals occasionally experience waking up paralyzed for a few seconds (sleep paralysis), indicates that the normal reversal of the blockage of descending activity was delayed after the end of REM sleep (waking up). Some (few) individuals have an abnormal, or absent, blockage of descending motor activity during REM sleep [103]. This disorder is known as the "rapid eye movement sleep behavior disorder" (RBD). Individuals with RBD often make extensive body movements during sleep, sometimes live in their violent dreams physically, and perform violent activity unconsciously, sometimes even injuring other people [118, 119]. The disorder occurs most often in men and it is often associated with other neurodegenerative disorders. Individuals with RBD also have a higher risk of acquiring PD [20].

> In a recent study, 57% of RDB patients had other neurological disorders all of which (except 14%), were PD, dementia without parkinsonism, and multiple system atrophy (MSA) [20, 103]. These investigators concluded that RBD may be the first manifestation of other disorders such as PD [103].

Absence of normal paralysis during REM sleep could be caused by the failure of brainstem neurons to block the facilitatory descending activity (see p. 261) to α motoneurons, which is necessary for normal muscle activity and which normally makes those neurons excitable from supraspinal sources in the awake individual. Some studies have associated the central nucleus of the amygdala with abnormalities of sleep [95]. This hypothesis is supported by the finding that fear conditioning reduced REM sleep [95]. Benzodiazepine (Clonazepam) was effective in treating RBD [103], thus supporting the hypothesis that decreased efficacy of $GABA_A$ receptors plays a role in this disorder.

> Narcolepsy, daytime somnolence, is regarded as a disorder of REM sleep. It has a strong genetic component [57], and a prevalence of approximately 1%. Disturbances in dopaminergic, adrenergic and cholinergic modulation of expression of REM sleep are believed to be involved in causing the symptoms [5].

5.3.4   Basal ganglia, cerebellum and cerebral cortex

Movement disorders caused by physiological abnormalities in the basal ganglia and in the cerebral cortex are more complex than those where the anatomical location of the abnormality is located more caudally. Abnormal movements (hypokinesia and hyperkinesia) often occur together with paresis and paralysis, such as can be seen in cerebral palsy. Some of the disorders of the cortex and basal ganglia are inherited congenital disorders. Acquired disorders of these structures are from injuries (accident or iatrogenic), and from strokes and intracranial bleeding.

Disorders in which the basal ganglia are implicated were earlier known as extrapyramidal disorders. In the 1960s, when the anatomy became better known, it became apparent that the main output of the basal ganglia projected to the motor cortex via the thalamus. This means that the basal ganglia more accurately should be regarded as "pre-pyramidal" than extrapyramidal. Although the distinction between pyramidal and extrapyramidal motor systems is no longer valid, the terms pyramidal and extrapyramidal signs are still in use, especially in clinical connections.

Parkinson's and Huntington's diseases

Many of the disorders that are associated with the basal ganglia are age-related. The two most characteristic age-related disorders are PD and HD [19]. The incidence of PD increases with age while the incidence of HD is highest in the fourth decade of life. These two disorders are both chronic neurodegenerative disorders, which have certain commonalities and characteristic differences. The basal ganglia are the primary anatomical location of the degeneration that causes the signs and symptoms of both PD and HD, but different nuclei are affected in these two disorders.

Parkinson's disease

The typical symptoms of PD, slow movements, rigidity and low-frequency tremor are assumed to be caused by selective degeneration of dopamine-producing cells in the SNc. The motor symptoms of PD also include "freezing" reactions in many patients. The cause of these signs is not completely understood, but there is evidence that multiple factors are involved, such as hereditary factors, oxidative stress, and in particular age, which is the major risk factor. PD includes other typical age-related changes.

The motor symptoms and signs that are typical for PD are assumed to be caused by deficits in the neurotransmitter dopamine produced by cells in the substantia nigra. The cause of the decrease in production of dopamine is not known, but general degenerative, inflammatory, chemical or environmental exposure may be involved. There is evidence that mitochondrial defects, oxidative stress, degenerative and inflammatory, together with age-related, changes are involved [17]. Neurotoxicity by the neurotransmitter glutamate most likely contributes to the development of the disease [19].

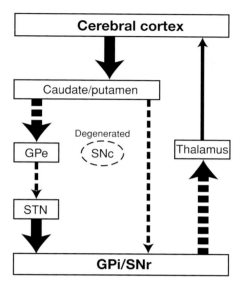

Fig. 5.33 Schematic diagram showing changes in the basal ganglia in PD causing hypokinesis. Black arrows show excitation and dashed arrows show inhibition. Thick arrows show increased activity, thin arrows show decreased activity.

Exposure to environmental factors may induce similar symptoms to PD. The fact that administration of MPTP can cause similar symptoms and signs to PD shows that specific chemicals can induce symptoms and signs of PD. It has been suggested that similar chemicals may be present in the environment, and that such exposure can contribute to the development of PD. Symptoms of PD may be induced by dopamine receptor antagonists as seen in many psychoactive drugs used to control psychotic behaviors.

PD is more complex than just the lack of dopamine, and the motor signs are often accompanied by other age-related degenerative changes such as cognitive deficits, dementia and depression. Movement deficits of PD have attracted most of the research and treatment has been focused on the movement deficits of the disease. It should not be disregarded, however, that other functions are affected.

The reduced function of the substantia nigra in PD causes both the inhibitory and the excitatory input to the striatum from the SNc to become decreased (Fig. 5.33). It is also believed that increased inhibitory influence from the striatum on the lateral segment of globus pallidus (LGP) and increased excitation from the STN to SNr and the medial segment of the globus pallidus (MGP) contribute to the symptoms of PD. Inhibitory input to the thalamus from SNr and the MGP is also supposed to be increased in patients with PD while the input from the striatum to the MGP is slightly excitatory from being inhibitory in the normal basal ganglia. The inhibitory input to the thalamus from SNr and MGP is increased and the excitatory output from the thalamus to the MI is decreased [19].

The role of possible abnormalities in proprioception as a contributing factor to the motor signs of PD has been considered. It has been suggested that at least some of the motor deficits are caused by impaired sensory function. This would agree with the finding that most neurons in SNc might not play an important role in planning motor activity. In primates, the neurons in SNc respond best to sensory stimuli [135]. In addition, neurons in the caudate nucleus, putamen and pallidum within humans and animals have been shown to respond to sensory stimuli [111]. Sensory input to nuclei of the basal ganglia is important for sensory-motor interaction and defective utilization of somatic proprioceptive input can affect many basic motor functions such as postural reflexes and initiation of movements.

> Indications that proprioception is affected and probably involved in generating the motor signs in PD comes from a study that showed impaired ability to perceive the extent of movements to a target away from the body when an individual with PD had to rely on proprioceptive feedback as guidance [70, 75]. Other tests on the same patients showed normal finger identification, graphesthesia (tactual ability to recognize writing on the skin) and localization of tactile stimuli when compared with age-matched non-PD individuals. Further support for the hypothesis that proprioception plays a role in the movement signs of PD comes from another study showing that the tremor in PD patients (assessed by EMG recordings) is affected by electrical stimulation of the median nerve [131]. Some investigators have found signs of deficits in sensory functions such as two-point discrimination threshold in patients with PD [121].
>
> Another study indicates that administering levodopa and dopamine agonists causes impairment of proprioception in PD patients [102]. The results of this study emphasize the general difficulties in interpreting research results obtained in patients who are medicated with potent neuroactive drugs, and it shows the difficulties in differentiating between the effect of the medication and the effect of the disease.

Research regarding the motor deficits in PD has benefited from studies of animal models developed by administration of the substance MPTP, which causes degeneration of dopamine producing neurons in the substantia nigra in monkeys. The discovery that MPTP causes similar neural degeneration as occurs in PD also suggests that environmental toxins may be implicated in the development of PD.

Studies of the pathophysiology of PD have focused on the changes in the functions that are caused by the morphological changes, which mostly involve the SNc. However, the functional changes that these pathologies cause can also evoke expression of neural plasticity aimed at compensating for the deficits resulting from these morphological changes. The involvement of neural plasticity has been mostly ignored in forming hypotheses about the pathologies of PD. The fact that training of various kinds is beneficial in reducing the symptoms and signs of PD indicates that expression of neural plasticity is involved in creating the symptoms and signs of PD.

Treatment of Parkinson's disease Before the advent of L-dopa for treating PD, surgical lesions were made in the basal ganglia, mostly in the pallidus (pallidotomy). This was discovered empirically by a surgeon who accidentally ligated the artery supplying the globus pallidus in a patient with PD while performing another operation on the patient [30]. Surgical treatment of PD almost fell out of use after the introduction of L-dopa in 1967, but has recently been re-introduced because of the decreasing efficacy of L-dopa that arises from continual treatment. Earlier, lesions were mainly made in the globus pallidus (pallidotomy), and later replaced by thalamotomy. Now, surgical lesions have largely been replaced through chronic electrical stimulation by implanted electrodes (DBS). The targets for implantation of electrodes for permanent stimulation are the GPi, STN and the ventral intermediary nucleus of the thalamus (Vim). The substitution of surgical lesions with DBS has assumed that DBS causes inactivation of nerve cells, which is similar to that of lesions, but reversible.

Electrical stimulation of brain tissue can have two effects: it can activate nerve cells or fiber tracts, or inactivate nerve cells by constantly depolarizing cells. It has been found that stimulation must occur at a high rate to be effective (100–250 pulses per second). It has been suggested that such high frequency stimulation exerts its effect by inhibiting [46] neural structures. Other hypotheses assume that the high-frequency stimulation constantly depolarizes cells and thereby inactivates the cells (similar to depolarizing muscle relaxants such as succenylcholine). However, electrical stimulation also stimulates fiber tracts, and fibers may be able to follow the high-frequency stimulation. This means that DBS is likely to have complex effects on the function of the structures that are subjected to such stimulation.

DBS has largely replaced making permanent lesions for movement disorders (as well as for pain, see Chapter 4). DBS has several advantages over lesioning. It is reversible and it is adjustable, and the risk of permanent morbidity is lower than making permanent lesions [113]. Some of the first stereotaxic placements of stimulating electrodes in subcortical structures for relief of movement symptoms in PD were made in the thalamus (the Vim). Such stimulation effectively suppressed tremor in PD. Later stimulation of the STN was found effective in

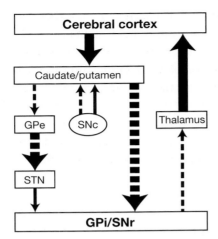

Fig. 5.34 Schematic diagram showing change in the basal ganglia in HD causing hyperkinesis (same explanations as in Fig. 5.33)

reducing movement signs of PD. Electrical stimulation of structures of globus pallidus followed and showed great benefit in treatment of PD.

The observed tolerance effect is an obstacle in the use of this technique [113]. It seems likely that the tolerance that gradually made the stimulation less effective may have to do with functional changes (expression of neural plasticity). DBS is an abnormal stimulation of specific brain tissue and many studies have shown that such stimulation causes the expression of neural plasticity (or the kindling phenomenon [54, 140] as it has been called).

Physical therapy and exercise play critical roles in rehabilitation of patients with PD, thus another example of the importance of activating neural plasticity in treatment of deficits and abnormal functions of motor systems.

Huntington's disease

As mentioned above the symptoms of HD have many similarities with those of PD and it is believed the anatomical location of the abnormalities that give rise to the motor symptoms is mainly the basal ganglia (Fig. 5.34). HD is a progressive disease that primarily affects the caudate nucleus and the putamen, but other areas of the CNS become affected as the disease progresses. While the SNc is the most affected nucleus in PD, the major abnormalities in patients with HD occur in the caudate nucleus and the putamen, which show massive degeneration. In addition, the globus pallidus is often affected in HD and there is neuronal loss in the cerebral cortex, mainly affecting layers III, V and VI.

The functional abnormalities in HD are also different from those of PD. The inhibitory and excitatory input to the striatum from the SNc is unaffected in HD, but inhibition from the striatum onto the LGP is decreased, while the inhibition on the STN from LGP is increased. The excitation from the STN to SNr and to MGP is decreased in HD while increased in PD. The inhibition on the thalamus from MGP and SNr is decreased in HD while it is increased in PD. The excitation from the thalamus to the cortex, which was decreased in PD, is increased in HD [19]. It is believed that this increase in thalamic excitation of the cortex is the cause of the increased and often inappropriate motor activity in HD [40].

Other forms of dystonia

There are numerous other forms of dystonia, but they are rare disorders and their pathophysiology is generally unknown. Many of the disorders related to the basal ganglia are congenital or hereditary and the movement disorders are often accompanied by other CNS abnormalities. Many of these other forms of dystonia include hyperkinesia and display a wide spectrum of movement disorders from tremor to spasm and various forms of chorea.

Tremor can be inherited, caused by systemic diseases such as thyroid disorders, drugs, or age-related changes. Tremor can be associated with other symptoms and signs. Chorea is a part of the symptoms of HD, but chorea is also a typical sign of other disorders of the basal ganglia. Chorea often occurs together with mental disorders. Involuntary sound production, ranging from nonverbal sounds to obscenities (coprolalia), also occurs.

Gilles de la Tourette syndrome [67] is a movement disorder (dystonia) that is characterized by sudden, rapid, recurrent movements that often include production of odd sounds. It begins in childhood, and it can be either less pronounced with age or worse. The anatomical location of the physiological abnormalities producing these symptoms are supposed to be within the cortico-striato-palido-thalamic circuit and recently treatment using DBS (bilateral thalamic stimulation) has been shown to be effective in reversing these symptoms [136]. The fact that individuals with Tourette's syndrome have cognitive deficits supports the hypothesis that other systems are affected, or that the function of the basal ganglia is not limited to motor function. In addition, patients with these disorders benefit from physical therapy and other forms of training; again, an example of the important role of neural plasticity in treatment of disorders of the nervous system.

Wilson's disease is interesting because it has motor, behavioral and psychiatric signs. It is also known as hepatolenticular degeneration. It is an autosomal recessive disorder of copper metabolism associated with reduced amounts of the copper-binding protein ceruloplasmin, and the symptoms are assumed to be caused by excess accumulation of copper in the brain and the liver. It occurs in approximately 1 in 40,000 people. In adults, these movement disorders resemble that of PD, and include tremor, dystonia, postural instability and ataxia. In addition to hepatic dysfunction, more or less pronounced psychiatric symptoms occur. Other typical findings are Kaiser-Fleischer rings in the cornea, representing depositions of copper. Common to all these disorders is that the cause is poorly understood, and even the anatomical location of the physiological abnormality is incompletely known. Therapy rests on the use of agents that inhibit copper absorption (such as zinc) and which facilitate removal of copper by chelation.

Ataxia

Ataxia is an inability to coordinate movements – especially walking – which become jerky. Involuntary movements are not included in the term ataxia. Ataxia is a general term that describes the lack of motor coordination. Ataxia may occur because of various lesions to the motor system (motor ataxia) or sensory deficits (sensory ataxia). Motor ataxia is often caused by disorders of the cerebellum, but disorders of other supraspinal structures can also cause motor ataxia. The most common cause of ataxia is from ingestion of alcohol and other hypnotic drugs. Such drugs also cause ataxia in animals including insects.

Gait and balance disturbances

Gait and balance disturbances are common and their incidence rate increases with age. Control of posture is complex and many disorders of the motor system affect the control of posture. Control of posture depends on proper function of the motor system and correct proprioceptive input from the vestibular system, together with input from receptors in joints, tendons, muscles and the skin. Visual input is important and can substitute for loss of vestibular input. The most obvious consequences of balance disturbance are falls. Falls are a frequent cause of injuries – including head injuries – which result in disabilities and deaths.

The pathophysiology of gait and balance disturbances is complex and poorly understood. There are many anatomical locations of abnormalities that can cause gait and balance disturbances. Failure to control posture can be caused by either motor dysfunction of sensory (proprioceptive) or vestibular dysfunction. These two different causes of balance and posture control can be distinguished by the Romberg test[11], which is said to be positive for sensory causes.

The ventral spinocerebellar tracts are often involved in causing motor ataxia. Sensory ataxia can be caused by faulty proprioceptive input, especially from the vestibular system. Ataxia can affect limbs, trunk, eye and other bulbar musculature. Gaze evoked nystagmus is a form of ataxia.

Little is known about the involvement of neural plasticity in these disorders. The fact that treatment such as training and exercise have beneficial effects on these disorders indicates that expression of neural plasticity may be involved in generating some of the symptoms. Resistance to medical treatment may also be caused by expression of neural plasticity in an attempt to compensate for the changes caused by the treatment. This means that the beneficial medically induced effects decrease.

> While the symptoms and signs of movement disorders are often caused by damage to motor pathways, strokes that affect sensory systems may produce signs of movement disorders because the normal sensory feedback is affected. Any damage to proprioception may affect the ability to control posture and control voluntary movements.

5.3.5 Disorders of the cerebral cortex

Movement disorders of the cerebral cortex can be caused by cell destruction or ischemia resulting from vascular incidents and other forms of trauma. Cerebral palsy is the most common disorder of the motor cortex that presents with symptoms of paresis, paralysis, and hypo- and hyperactive movement disorders of various kinds. It is a non-progressive disorder that can be caused by many different forms of insults such as asphyxia, trauma, vascular events, congenital abnormalities and kernicterus[12] [55]. Many factors that lead to these diffuse symptoms and signs are difficult to identify. The pathophysiology is poorly understood.

Other disorders that are related to the cerebral motor cortex may be induced through the expression of neural plasticity that can cause reorganization of the cerebral cortex.

---

[11] Romberg test: The patient stands steady with feet together, first with eyes open, then with eyes closed. Patients with motor ataxia may or may not be unsteady in this position, but their unsteadiness is not affected by having their eyes open or closed (negative Romberg sign). Patients with sensory ataxia become unsteady with closed eyes (positive Romberg sign). Otolaryngologists often use a more difficult version of the test, where the patient places his/her feet ahead of each other instead of together.

[12] Kernicterus: Jaundice associated with high levels of unconjugated bilirubin, or in small premature infants with more modest degrees of bilirubinemia.

Reorganization of motor cortex

Severing of a peripheral nerve in adult rats causes a reorganization of the MI [66]. The cortical areas adjacent to those represented by the muscles innervated by the severed nerve expands into the territory of the severed nerve. This is similar to what occurs in the sensory system after sensory deprivation (see pp. 87, 112), and it means that cortical motor maps are not stable in adult animals as had been assumed earlier. Within a few hours after transection of a peripheral nerve, stimulation of the affected cortical area elicits contraction of muscles that normally were represented by adjacent areas of the MI. The rapid change in responsiveness indicates that existing synaptic connections have altered their efficacy rather than new connections (spouting) causing these changes. These investigators [66] found evidence that this re-organization was caused by release of tonic inhibition that normally exists in the cortical interconnections, and they could create similar re-organization by pharmacological means applied to the MI using bicuculine ((-)bicuculine methobromide), a $GABA_A$ receptor antagonist to cause a release of GABAergic inhibition.

It is not known in which way such reorganization of the motor cortex affects control of movement, but it seems logical to assume that some of the unexplained symptoms and signs from motor nerve injuries may be related to such cortical re-organization.

Complex CNS disturbances

Complex consequences of disorders of the cerebral cortex may be involved in the cause of several disorders. Sensory motor interaction is observed in reaching and it has been hypothesized that the primary motor cortex is involved in somatosensory processing. What is normally regarded as motor deficits may therefore be partly due to sensory deficits of failed connections between sensory and motor systems [100]. For example, visual feedback in processing of movement commands is important, especially for hand movements such as reaching. The visual processing follows some of the principles of stream segregation, and visual processing in the dorsal stream is important for control of movements such as reaching.

An example of a complex effect of strokes on voluntary movements can be caused by deficits of the visual system. Strokes that cause damage to one of the two visual pathways in the association cortices affect processing of spatial and object information independently. Mel Goodale and his co-workers have shown that visual information that guides grasping is processed within different areas of the association cortices from that where a "stream" which is involved in perception of form is processed. Individuals with strokes in these regions may have selective deficits in

Table 5.2 *Characteristics of the M, H and F*

Response	Latency	Amplitude dependence	Variability	Affected by Anesthesia
M	Short	Amplitude saturates after threshold	Minimal	Minimal
H	Long	Response peaks at intermediate stimuli	Small	Large
F	Long	Maximal at larger stimuli	Large	Large

either grasping or in visual perception [96]. An individual with a stroke that affects the dorsal stream may lose the ability to use vision to guide motion, whereas another stroke victim in whom the ventral stream is affected may be able to guide hand motion using vision while unable to recognize the form of objects.

There are indications that the symptoms and signs of Williams disease are not a result of deficits in processing of movement information in the dorsal stream of the visual association cortices, but rather a selective dysfunction of three-dimensional form perception in the visual system [98].

Balient's syndrome, which is characterized by optic ataxia and simultagnosia[13], is another example of a complex cortical disturbance that is usually due to damage to the superior temporal-occipital areas in both hemispheres.

5.4   The role of neural plasticity in rehabilitation

This chapter has provided examples of disorders where expression of neural plasticity has contributed to the symptoms and signs of disorders of the motor system. Neural plasticity also plays an important role in alleviating symptoms and signs. Injuries and abnormal function are prominent factors in causing expression of neural plasticity that provide compensation for abnormal function and reduced or absent function. Physical therapy is the most used means to facilitate expression of neural plasticity for the purpose of compensating for deficits and correcting malfunction of the motor system. The mechanisms behind such promotion of expression of neural plasticity for recovery (or replacement) of function in brain injuries such as from strokes have been studied in animal (rat [71] and monkey) models.

Studies of the reorganization of cortical areas that are adjacent to the destroyed regions have been studied for the purpose of designing methods to

---

[13] Simultagnosia is an inability to recognize multiple elements in a visual presentation while single objects or elements can be appreciated.

enhance expression of neural plasticity for recovering function [53]. These studies have resulted in introduction of methods to facilitate expression of neural plasticity that can compensate for deficits suffered by stroke victims. Electrical stimulation of the cerebral cortex using implanted electrodes has been developed for that purpose in animal experiments (rats [2] and monkeys [108]). The technique has been tried in a few studies on humans, with good results [23].

Individual differences in motor cortex organization is considerable, and it may therefore be necessary to map the motor cortex of individual stroke victims in order to instigate effective treatment [33].

References

1. Abbott, R., Sensory Rhizotomy for the Treatment of Childhood Spasticity, in *Neurophysiology in Neurosurgery*, V. Deletis and J. L. Shils, Editors. 2002, Academic Press: Amsterdam. pp. 219–230.
2. Adkins-Muir, D. L. and T. A. Jones, Cortical Electrical Stimulation Combined with Rehabilitative Training: Enhanced Functional Recovery and Dendritic Plasticity Following Focal Cortical Ischemia in Rats. *Neurol. Res.*, 2003. **25**: pp. 780–788.
3. Albe-Fessard, D., G. Sarfel, G. Guiot, P. Derome, E. Hertzog, G. Vourc'h, H. Brown, P. Alleonard, J. Herrand De La, and J. C. Trigo, Electrophysiological Studies of Some Deep Cerebral Structures in Man. *J. Neuro. Sci.*, 1966. **3**: pp. 37–51.
4. Albin, R. L., A. B. Young, and J. B. Penney, The Functional Anatomy of Basal Ganglia Origin. *Trends Neurosci.*, 1989. **12**: pp. 366–375.
5. Aldrich, M. S., Z. Hollingsworth, and J. B. Penney, Dopamine Receptor Autoradiography of Human Narcoleptic Brain. *Neurology*, 1992. **42**: pp. 410–5.
6. Alexander, G. E. and M. D. Crutcher, Functional Architecture of Basal Ganglia Circuits: Neural Substrate of Parallel Processing. *Trends Neurosci.*, 1990(13): pp. 266–71.
7. Alexander, G. E., M. D. Crutcher, and M. R. Delong, Basal Ganglia-Thalamocortical Circuits: Parallel Substrates for Motor, Oculomotor, "Prefrontal" and "Limbic" Functions. *Progr. Brain Res.*, 1990. **85**: pp. 119–146.
8. Alstermark, B., M. Pinter, and S. Sasaki, Brainstem Relay of Disynaptic Pyramidal Epsps to Neck Motoneurons in the Cat. *Brain Res.*, 1983. **259**: pp. 147–150.
9. Amassian, V. E., M. Stewart, G. J. Quirk, and J. L. Rosenthal, Physiologic Basis of Motor Effects of a Transient Stimulus to Cerebral Cortex. *Neurosurg.*, 1987. **20**: pp. 74–93.
10. Amassian, V. E., R. Q. Cracco, and P. J. Maccabee, Focal Stimulation of Human Cerebral Cortex with the Magnetic Coil: A Comparison with Electrical Stimulation. *Electroenceph. Clin. Neurophys.*, 1989. **74**: pp. 401–416.
11. Amassian, V. E., G. J. Quirk, and M. Stewart, A Comparison of Corticospinal Activation by Magnetic Coil and Electrical Stimulation of Monkey Motor Cortex. *Electroenceph. Clin. Neurophys.*, 1990. **77**: pp. 390–401.

12. Amassian, V. E., Animal and Human Motor System Neurophysiology Related to Intraoperative Monitoring, in *Neurophysiology in Neurosurgery*, V. Deletis and J. L. Shils, Editors. 2002, Academic Press: Amsterdam. pp. 3–23.

13. Andersen, P., P. J. Hagan, C. G. Phillips, and T. P. S. Powell, Mapping by Microstimulation of Overlapping Projections from Area 4 to Motor Units of the Baboon's Hand. *Proc. R. Soc. London ser B.*, 1975. **188**: pp. 31–60.

14. Ashby, P. and M. Wiens, Reciprocal Inhibition Following Lesions of the Spinal Cord in Man. *J. Physiol.*, 1989. **414**: pp. 145–57.

15. Baldisera, F., H. Hultborn, and M. Illert, Integration of Spinal Neuronal Systems, in *Handbook of Physiology – The Nervous System II*, J. M. Brookhart and V. B. Mountcastle, Editors. 1981, American Physiological Society: Bethesda, MD. pp. 509–595.

16. Barker, A. T., R. Jalinous, and I. L. Freeston, Non-Invasive Magnetic Stimulation of the Human Motor Cortex. *Lancet*, 1985: pp. 1106–1107.

17. Bennett, D. A., L. A. Beckett, A. M. Murray, and E. Al., Prevalence of Parkinsonian Signs and Associated Mortality in a Community Population of Older People. *N. Eng. J. Med.*, 1996. **334**: pp. 71–76.

18. Berthoud, H. R. and W. L. Neuhuber, Functional and Chemical Anatomy of the Afferent Vagal System. *Autonomic Neurosci.*, 2000. **85**(1–3): pp. 1–17.

19. Blandini, F., C. Tassorelli, and J. T. Greenamyre, Movement Disorders, in *Principles of Neural Aging*, S. U. Dani, A. Hori, and G. F. Walter, Editors. 1997, Elsevier: Amsterdam.

20. Boeve, B. F., M. H. Silber, T. J. Ferman, J. A. Lucas, and J. E. Parisi, Association of REM Sleep Behavior Disorder and Neurodegenerative Disease May Reflect an Underlying Synucleinopathy. *Movement Disorders*, 2001. **16**(4): pp. 622–30.

21. Brink, E., P. J. Harrison, E. Jankowska, D. A. McCrea, and B. Skoog, Post-Synaptic Potentials in a Population of Motoneurons Following Activity of Single Interneurons in the Cat. *J. Physiol.*, 1983. **343**: pp. 341–359.

22. Brodal, P., *The Central Nervous System*. 1998, Oxford University Press: New York.

23. Brown, J. A., H. L. Lutsep, S. C. Cramer, and M. Weinand, Motor Cortex Stimulation for Enhancement of Recovery after Stroke: Case Report. *Neurol. Res.*, 2003. **25**: pp. 815–818.

24. Brown, P., Pathophysiology of Spasticity. *J. Neurol. Neurosurg. Psychiatry*, 1994. **57**: pp. 773–777.

25. Brown, R. H. and C. L. Nash, Current Status of Spinal Cord Monitoring. *Spine*, 1979. **4**: pp. 466–478.

26. Burke, D. and J. W. Lance, Studies of the Reflex Effects of Primary and Secondary Spindle Endings in Spasticity, in *New Developments in Electromyography and Clinical Neurophysiology*, J. E. Desmedt Editor. 1973, Karger: Basel. pp. 475–495.

27. Burke, D., Spasticity as an Adaptation to Pyramidal Tract Injury, in *Functional Recovery in Neurological Disease*, S. G. Waxman, Editor. 1988, Raven Press: New York.

28. Caspary, D. M., A. Raza, Lawhorn, B. A. Armour, J. Pippin, and S. P. Arneric, Immunocytochemical and Neurochemical Evidence for Age-Related Loss of

GABA in the Inferior Colliculus: Implications for Neural Presbycusis. *J. Neurosci.*, 1990. **10**: pp. 2363–2372.

29. Caspary, D. M., J. C. Milbrandt, and R. H. Helfert, Central Auditory Aging: GABA Changes in the Inferior Colliculus. *Exp. Gerontol.*, 1995. **30**: pp. 349–360.

30. Cooper, I. S., Ligation of the Anterior Choroidal Artery for Involuntary Movements in Parkinsonism. *Psychiatry*, 1953. **27**: pp. 317–319.

31. Courchesne, E., J. Townsend, N. A. Akshoomof, O. Saitoh, R. Yeung-Courchesne, A. J. Lincoln, H. E. James, R. H. L. Schreibman, and L. Lau, Impairment in Shifting Attention in Autistic and Cerebellar Patients. *Behav. Neurosci.*, 1994. **108**: pp. 848–865.

32. Crago, A., J. C. Houk, and W. Z. Rymer, Sampling of Total Muscle Force by Tendon Organs. *J. Neurophys.*, 1982. **47**: pp. 1069–1083.

33. Cramer, S. C., R. R. Nbenson, V. C. Burra, D. Himes, K. R. Crafton, J. S. Janowsky, J. A. Brown, and H. L. Lutsep, Mapping Individual Brains to Guide Restorative Therapy after Stroke: Rationale and Pilot Studies. *Neurol Res*, 2003(25): pp. 811–814.

34. Creasey, G. H., Restoration of Bladder, Bowel, and Sexual Function. *Topics Spinal Cord Inj. Rehabil.*, 1999. **5**: pp. 21–32.

35. Daly, J. J., E. B. Marsolais, L. M. Mendell, W. Z. Rymer, A. Stefanovska, J. R. Wolpaw, and C. Kantor, Therapeutic Neural Effects of Electrical Stimulation. *IEEE Trans. Rehab. Eng.*, 1996. **4**(4): pp. 218–230.

36. Davis, M., D. S. Gendelman, M. D. Tischler, and P. M. Gendelman, A Primary Acoustic Startle Circuit-Lesion and Stimulation Studies. *J. Neurosci.*, 1982. **2**: pp. 791–805.

37. Davis, M., The Role of the Amygdala in Fear and Anxiety. *Ann. Rev. Neurosci*, 1992. **15**: pp. 353–375.

38. Decandia, M., L. Provini, and H. Taborikova, Mechanisms of the Reflex Discharge Depression in Spinal Motoneurone During Repetitive Orthodromic Stimulation. *Brain Res.*, 1967. **4**: pp. 284–291.

39. Deletis, V., Intraoperative Neurophysiology and Methodologies Used to Monitor the Functional Integrity of the Motor System, in *Neurophysiology in Neurosurgery*, V. Deletis and J. L. Shils, Editors. 2002, Academic Press: Amsterdam. pp. 25–51.

40. Delong, M. R., Primate Models of Movement Disorders of Basal Ganglia Origin. *Trends Neurosci.*, 1990. **13**: pp. 281–85.

41. Delwaide, P. J. and E. Oliver, Short Latency Autogenic Inhibition (Ib Inhibition) in Human Spasticity. *J. Neurol. Neurosurg. Psych.*, 1988. **51**: pp. 1548–50.

42. Dewald, J. P., J. D. Given, and W. Z. Rymer, Long-Lasting Reductions of Spasticity Induced by Skin Electric Al Stimulation. *IEEE Trans. Rehab. Eng.*, 1996. **4**(4): pp. 231–242.

43. Dietz, V., Spinal Cord Pattern Generators for Locomotion. *Clin. Neurophysiol.*, 2003. **114**(8): pp. 1379–89.

44. Dimitrijevic, M. R., Model for the Study of Plasticity of the Human Nervous System: Features of Residual Spinal Cord Motor Activity Resulting from Established Post-Traumatic Injury, in *Plasticity of the Neuromuscular System (Ciba Foundation Symposium 138)*. 1988, Wiley: Chichester. pp. 227–239.

45. Donoghue, J. P., S. Suner, and J. N. Sanes, Dynamic Organization of Primary Motor Cortex Output to Target Muscles in Adult Rats. II. Rapid Reorganization Following Motor Nerve Lesions. *Exp. Brain Res.*, 1990. **79**(3): pp. 492–503.

46. Dostrovsky, J. O. and A. M. Lozano, Mechanisms of Deep Brain Stimulation. *Movement Disorders*, 2002. **17**(Suppl. 3): pp. S63–68.

47. Eccles, J. C., Plasticity at Its Simplest Level, in *Centennial Lectures of E. E. Squibb & Son*. 1959, Putnam & Sons: New York. pp. 217–244.

48. Edgeley, S. A., J. A. Eyre, R. Lemon, and S. Miller, Excitation of the Corticospinal Tract by Electromagnetic and Electrical Stimulation of the Scalp in the Macaque Monkey. *J. Physiol. (Lond.)*, 1990. **425**: pp. 301–320.

49. Elbert, T., C. Pantev, C. Wienbruch, B. Rockstroh, and E. Taub, Increased Cortical Representation of the Fingers of the Left Hand in String Players. *Science*, 1995. **270**(5234): pp. 305–7.

50. Fasano, V. A., G. Broggi, and S. Zeme, Intraoperative Electrical Stimulation for Functional Posterior Rhizotomy. *Scand. J. Rehab. Med.*, 1988. **17**: pp. 149–54.

51. Fetz, E. E., K. Toyama, and W. Smith, Synaptic Interaction between Cortical Neurons, in *Cerebral Cortex*, E. G. Jones and A. Peters, Editors. 1990, Plenum: New York. pp. 1–47.

52. Flament, D., P. A. Fortier, and E. E. Fetz, Response Patterns and Post-Spike Effects of Peripheral Afferents in Dorsal Root Ganglia of Behaving Monkeys. *J. Neurophysiol.*, 1992. **67**: pp. 875–889.

53. Frost, S. B., S. Barbay, K. M. Friel, E. J. Plautz, and R. J. Nudo, Reorganization of Remote Cortical Regions after Ischemic Brain Injury: A Potential Substrate for Stroke Recovery. *J. Neurophysiol.*, 2003. **89**(6): pp. 3205–14.

54. Goddard, G. V., Amygdaloid Stimulation and Learning in the Rat. *J. Comp. Physiol. Psychol.*, 1964. **58**: pp. 23–30.

55. Goetz, C. G. and E. J. Pappert, Textbook of Clinical Neurology. 1999, W. B. Saunders Company: Philadelphia.

56. Gordon, T., J. Hegedus, and S. L. Tam, Adaptive and Maladaptive Motor Axonal Sprouting in Aging and Motoneuron Disese. *Neurol. Res.*, 2004. **26**: pp. 174–85.

57. Guilleminault, C., E. Mignot, and F. C. Grumet, Familial Patterns of Narcolepsy. *Lancet*, 1989. **2**: pp. 1376–9.

58. Hagbarth, K. E., G. Wallin, and L. Lofstedt, Muscle Spindle Responses to Stretch in Normal and Spastic Subjects. *Scand. J. Rehab. Med.*, 1973. **5**: pp. 156–159.

59. Hall, E. J., D. Flament, C. Fraser, and R. Lemon, Non-Invasive Brain Stimulation Reveals Reorganized Cortical Outputs in Amputees. *Neurosci. Lett.*, 1990. **116**: pp. 379–386.

60. Halstead, L. S. and S. W. J. Seager, The Effects of Rectal Probe Electrostimulation on Spinal Cord Injury Spasticity. *Paraplegia*, 1991. **29**: pp. 43–47.

61. Halstead, L. S., S. W. J. Seager, J. M. Houston, K. Whitsell, M. Dennis, and P. W. Nance, Relief of Spasticity in Sci Men and Women Using Rectal Probe Electrostimulation. *Paraplegia*, 1993. **31**: pp. 715–721.

62. Hiersemenzel, L., A. Curt, and V. Dietz, From Spinal Shock to Spasticity: Neuronal Adaptations to a Spinal Cord Injury. *Neurology*, 2000. **54**(8): pp. 1574–82.

63. Hoheisel, U., G. Beylich, and S. Mense, Effects of an Acute Muscle Nerve Section on Excitability of Dorsal Horn Neurons in the Rat. *Pain*, 1995. **60**(22): pp. 151–158.

64. Hulliger, M., The Mammalian Muscle Spindle and Its Central Control. *Rev. Physiol. Biochem. Pharmacol.*, 1984. **101**: pp. 1–110.

65. Humphrey, D. R. and W. S. Corrie, Properties of Pyramidal Tract Neuron System within Functionally Defined Subregion of Primate Motor Cortex. *J. Neurophys.*, 1978. **41**: pp. 216–243.

66. Jacobs, K. M. and J. P. Donoghue, Reshaping the Cortical Motor Map by Unmasking Latent Intracortical Connections. *Science*, 1991. **251**: pp. 944–947.

67. Jankovic, J., Tics in Other Neurological Disorders, in *Handbook of Tourette's Syndrome and Related Tic and Behavioral Disorders*, R. Kurlan, Editor. 1993, Marcel Dekker: New York. pp. 167–182.

68. Jankowska, E. and W. J. Roberts, Synaptic Actions of Single Interneurons Mediating Reciprocal Ia Inhibition to Motoneurons. *J. Physiol.*, 1972. **222**: pp. 623–642.

69. Jankowska, E. and A. Lundberg, Interneurons in the Spinal Cord. *Trends Neurosci.*, 1981. **4**: pp. 230–233.

70. Jobst, E. E., M. E. Melnick, N. N. Byl, G. A. Dowling, and M. J. Aminoff, *Sensory Perception in Parkinson Disease*. Arch. Neurol., 1997. **54**: pp. 450–4.

71. Jones, T. A., S. D. Bury, D. L. Adkins-Muir, L. M. Luke, R. P. Allred, and J. T. Sakata, Importance of Behavioral Manipulations and Measures in Rat Models of Brain Damage and Brain Repair. *Ilar Journal*, 2003. **44**(2): pp. 144–52.

72. Joodaki, M. R., G. R. Olyaei, and H. Bagheri, The Effects of Electrical Nerve Stimulation of the Lower Extremity on H-Reflex and F-Wave Parameters. *Electromyography Clin. Neurophysiol.*, 2001. **41**(1): pp. 23–8.

73. Kaneko, K., S. Kawai, F. Y., H. Morieta, and A. Ofuji, The Effect of Current Direction Induced by Transcranial Magnetic Stimulation on Corticospinal Excitability in Human Brain. *Electroenceph Clin Neurophys*, 1966. **101**: pp. 478–482.

74. Khaslavskaia, S., M. Ladouceur, and T. Sinkjaer, Increase in Tibialis Anterior Motor Cortex Excitability Following Repetitive Electrical Stimulation of the Common Peroneal Nerve. *Exp. Brain Res.*, 2002. **143**(3): pp. 309–315.

75. Khudados, E., F. W. J. Cody, and J. O'Boyle, Proprioceptive Regulation of Voluntary Ankle Movements, Demonstrated Using Muscle Vibration, Is Impaired by Parkinson's Disease. *J. Neurol. Neurosurg. Psychiatry*, 1999. **67**: pp. 504–510.

76. Kitagawa, H. and A. R. Møller, Conduction Pathways and Generators of Magnetic Evoked Spinal Cord Potentials: A Study in Monkeys. *Electroenceph. Clin. Neurophys.*, 1994. **93**: pp. 57–67.

77. Kothbauer, K. F., Motor Evoked Potential Monitoring for Intramedullary Spinal Cord Tumor Surgery, in *Neurophysiology in Neurosurgery*, V. Deletis and J. L. Shils, Editors. 2002, Academic Press: Amsterdam. pp. 73–92.

78. Kuypers, H. G. J. M., Anatomy of the Descending Pathways, in *Handbook of Physiology – the Nervous System*, J. M. Brookhart and V. B. Mountcastle, Editors. 1981, American Physiological Society: Bethesda, MD. pp. 597–666.

79. Lazzaro Di, V., A. Oliviero, F. Pilato, P. Mazzone, A. Insola, F. Ranieri, and P. A. Tonali, Corticospinal Volleys Evoked by Transcranial Stimulation of the Brain in Concious Humans. *Neurol. Res.*, 2003. **25**: pp. 143–150.

80. Lenz, F. A., J. O. Dostrovsky, H. C. Kwan, R. R. Tasker, K. Yamashiro, and J. T. Murphy, Methods for Microstimulation and Recording of Single Neurons and Evoked Potentials in the Human Central Nervous System. *J. Neurosurg.* 1988. **68**(4): pp. 630–4.

81. Lenz, F. A., J. O. Dostrovsky, R. R. Tasker, K. Yamashiro, H. C. Kwan, and J. T. Murphy, Single-Unit Analysis of the Human Ventral Thalamic Nuclear Group: Somatosensory Responses. *J. Neurophysiol.*, 1988. **59**(2): pp. 299–316.

82. Lenz, F. A., R. R. Tasker, H. C. Kwan, S. Schnider, R. Kwong, Y. Murayama, J. O. Dostrovsky, and J. T. Murphy, Single Unit Analysis of the Human Ventral Thalamic Nuclear Group: Correlation of Thalamic "Tremor Cells" with the 3–6 Hz Component of Parkinsonian Tremor. *J. Neurosci.*, 1988. **8**(3): pp. 754–64.

83. Lenz, F. A., H. C. Kwan, J. O. Dostrovsky, and R. R. Tasker, Characteristics of the Bursting Pattern of Action Potentials That Occurs in the Thalamus of Patients with Central Pain. *Brain Res.*, 1989. **496**(1–2): pp. 357–60.

84. Lenz, F. A., H. C. Kwan, J. O. Dostrovsky, R. R. Tasker, J. T. Murphy, and Y. E. Lenz, Single Unit Analysis of the Human Ventral Thalamic Nuclear Group. Activity Correlated with Movement. *Brain*, 1990. **113**(Pt 6): pp. 1795–1821.

85. Lenz, F. A., R. Martin, H. C. Kwan, R. R. Tasker, and J. O. Dostrovsky, Thalamic Single-Unit Activity Occurring in Patients with Hemidystonia. *Stereotact. Funct. Neurosurg.*, 1990. **54–55**: pp. 159–62.

86. Lenz, F. A., C. J. Jaeger, M. S. Seike, Y. C. Lin, S. G. Reich, M. R. Delong, and J. L. Vitek, Thalamic Single Neuron Activity in Patients with Dystonia: Dystonia-Related Activity and Somatic Sensory Reorganization. *J. Neurophysiol.*, 1999. **82**(5): pp. 2372–92.

87. Lindstrom, S., Recurrent Control from Motor Axon Collaterals on Ia Inhibitory Pathways in the Spinal Cord of the Cat. *Acta Physiol. Scand. Suppl.*, 1973. **392**: pp. 1–43.

88. Lundberg, A. and P. Voorhoeve, Effects from Pyramidal Tract on Spinal Reflex Arcs. *Acta Physiol. Scand.*, 1962. **56**: pp. 201–219.

89. Lundberg, A., Multisensory Control of Spinal Reflex Pathways. *Prog. Brain Res.*, 1979. **50**: pp. 11–28.

90. McCrea, D. A., Spinal Circuitry of Sensorimotor Control of Locomotion. *J. Physiol.*, 2001. **533**(1): pp. 41–50.

91. Merton, P. A. and H. B. Morton, Electrical Stimulation of Human Motor and Visual Cortex through the Scalp. *J. Physiol.*, 1980. **305**: pp. 9–10P.

92. Merzenich, M. M., J. H. Kaas, J. Wall, R. J. Nelson, M. Sur, and D. Felleman, Topographic Reorganization of Somatosensory Cortical Areas 3b and 1 in

Adult Monkeys Following Restricted Deafferentiation. *Neuroscience*, 1983. **8**(1): pp. 3–55.

93. Møller, A. R., Cranial Nerve Dysfunction Syndromes: Pathophysiology of Microvascular Compression, in *Neurosurgical Topics Book 13, 'Surgery of Cranial Nerves of the Posterior Fossa,' Chapter 2*, D. L. Barrow, Editor. 1993, American Association of Neurological Surgeons: Park Ridge. IL. pp. 105–129.

94. Møller, A. R., *Sensory Systems: Anatomy and Physiology*. 2003, Academic Press: Amsterdam.

95. Morrison, A. R., L. D. Sanford, and R. J. Ross, The Amygdala: A Critical Modulator of Sensory Influence on Sleep. *Biological Signals & Receptors*, 2000. **9**(6): pp. 283–96.

96. Munhall, K. G., P. Servos, A. Santi, and M. A. J. A. Goodale, 2002, Dynamic Visual Speech Perception in a Patient with Visual Form Agnosia. *NeuroReport*, 2002. **13**(14): pp. 1793–6.

97. Naito, A., Y. J. Sun, and Y. Yanagidaira, Electromyographic (Emg) Study of Cold Shivering in the Chronic Spinal Dog. *Jap. J. Physiol.*, 1997. **47**(1): pp. 81–6.

98. Nakamura, M., Y. Kaneoke, K. Watanabe, and R. Kakigi, Visual Information Process in Williams Syndrome: Intact Motion Detection Accompanied by Typical Visuospatial Dysfunctions. *European Journal of Neuroscience*, 2002. **16**: pp. 1810–1818.

99. Nicolas, G., V. Marchand-Pauvert, D. Burke, and E. Pierrot-Deseilligny, Corticospinal Excitation of Presumed Cervical Propriospinal Neurons and Its Reversal to Inhibition in Humans. *J. Physiol.*, 2001. **533**(3): pp. 903–19.

100. Nudo, R. J., K. Friel, and S. W. Delia, Role of Sensory Deficits in Motor Impairments after Injury to Primary Motor Cortex. *Neuropharmacol.*, 2000. **39**(5): pp. 733–42.

101. Nuwer, M. R., Use of Somatosensory Evoked Potentials for Intraoperative Monitoring of Cerebral and Spinal Cord Function. *Neurologic Clinics*, 1988. **6**(4): pp. 881–97.

102. O'Suilleabhain, P., J. Bullard, and R. B. Dewey, Proprioception in Parkinson's Disease Is Acutely Depressed by Dopamine Medications. *J. Neurol Neurosurg Psychiatry*, 2001. **71**: pp. 607–10.

103. Olson, E. J., B. F. Boeve, and M. H. Silber, Rapid Eye Movement Sleep Behaviour Disorder: Demographic, Clinical and Laboratory Findings in 93 Cases. *Brain*, 2000. **123**(2): pp. 231–239.

104. Oppenheimer, D. R., The Cervical Cord in Multiple Sclerosis. *Neuropath. Appl. Neurobiol.*, 1978. **4**(151–162).

105. Peacock, W. J., L. J. Arens, and B. Berman, Cerebral Palsy Spasticity: Selective Posterior Rhizotomy. *Pediatr. Neurosci.*, 1987. **13**: pp. 61–66.

106. Pierrot-Deseilligny, E., Peripheral and Descending Control of Neurones Mediating Non-Monosynaptic Ia Excitation to Motoneurons: A Presumed Propriospinal System in Man. *Prog. Brain Res.*, 1989. **80**: pp. 305–314.

107. Pierrot-Deseilligny, E., Propriospinal Transmission of Part of the Corticospinal Excitation in Humans. *Muscle & Nerve.*, 2002. **26**(2): pp. 155–72.

108. Plautz, E. J., S. Barbay, S. B. Frost, K. M. Friel, N. Dancause, E. V. Zoubina, A. M. Stowe, B. M. Quaney, and R. J. Nudo, Post-Infarct Cortical Plasticity and Behavioral Recovery Using Concurrent Cortical Stimulation and Rehabilitative Training: A Feasibility Study in Primates. *Neurol. Res.*, 2003. **25**: pp. 801–810.

109. Porter, R. and R. Lemon, *Cortical Function and Voluntary Movement*. 1993, Clarendon Press: Oxford.

110. Ralston, D. D. and H. J. Ralston, The Termination of the Corticospinal Tract Axons in the Macaque Monkey. *J. Comp. Neurol.*, 1985. **242**: pp. 325–337.

111. Reale, R. A. and T. J. Imig, Auditory Cortical Field Projections to the Basal Ganglia of the Cat. *Neurosci.*, 1983. **8**(1): pp. 67–86.

112. Rosen, J. B., J. M. Hitchcock, C. Sananes, M. J. D. Miscrendino, and M. Davis, A Direct Projection from the Central Nucleus of the Amygdala to the Acoustic Startle Pathway: Anterograde and Retrograde Tracing Studies. *Behav. Neurosci.*, 1991. **105**: pp. 817–25.

113. Rosenow, J. M., A. Y. Mogilner, A. Ahmed, and A. R. Rezai, Deep Brain Stimulation for Movement Disorders. *Neurol. Res.*, 2004. **26**: pp. 9–20.

114. Rösler, K. M., Transcranial Magnetic Brain Stimulation: A Tool to Investigate Central Motor Pathways. *News Physiol. Sci.*, 2001. **16**: pp. 297–302.

115. Rudomin, P., Presynaptic Control of Synaptic Effectiveness of Muscle Spindle and Tendon Organ Afferents in the Mammalian Spinal Cord, in *The Segmental Motor System*, M. D. Binder and L. M. Mendell, Editors. 1990, Oxford University Press: Oxford. pp. 349–380.

116. Rushworth, G., Some Aspects of the Pathophysiology of Spasticity and Rigidity. *Clin. Pharmacol. Therapeutics*, 1964. **6**: pp. 828–36.

117. Sanes, J. N., S. Suner, and J. P. Donoghue, Dynamic Organization of Primary Motor Cortex Output to Target Muscles in Adult Rat. I. Long Term Patterns of Reorganization Following Motor or Mixed Peripheral Nerve Lesions. *Exp. Brain Res.*, 1990. **79**: pp. 479–491.

118. Schenck, C. H., M. W. Mahowald, S. W. Kim, K. A. O'Conner, and T. D. Hurwitz, Prominent Eye Movements During NREM Sleep and REM Sleep Behavior Disorder Associated with Fuoxetine Treatment of Depression and Obsessive-Compulsive Disorder. *Sleep*, 1992. **15**(3): pp. 226–35.

119. Schenck, C. H., J. L. Boyd, and M. W. Mahowald, A Parasomnia Overlap Disorder Involving Sleepwalking, Sleep Terrors, and REM Sleep Behavior Disorder in 33 Polysomnographically Confirmed Cases. *Sleep*, 1997. **20**(11): pp. 972–81.

120. Schieppati, M., The Hoffman Reflex: A Means of Assessing Spinal Reflex Excitability and Its Descending Control in Man. *Prog. Neurobiol.*, 1987. **28**: pp. 345–376.

121. Schneider, J. S., S. G. Diamond, and C. H. Markham, Parkinson's Disease: Sensory and Motor Problems in Arms and Hands. *Neurology*, 1987. **37**: pp. 951–6.

122. Sehgal, N. and J. R. McGuire, Beyond Ashworth: Electrophysiologic Quantification of Spasticity. *Physical Medicine and Rehabilitation Clinics of North America*, 1998. **9**(4): pp. 949–979.

123. Sie, K. C. Y. and E. W. Rubel, Rapid Changes in Protein Synthesis and Cell Size in the Cochlear Nucleus Following Eighth Nerve Activity Blockade and Cochlea Ablation. *J. Comp. Neurol.*, 1992. **320**: pp. 501–508.

124. Simons, D. G. and S. Mense, Understanding and Measurement of Muscle Tone as Related to Clinical Muscle Pain. *Pain*, 1998. **75(1)**(1): pp. 1–17.

125. Sindou, M. and D. Jeanmonod, Microsurgical-Drez-Otomy for Treatment of Spasticity and Pain in the Lower Limbs. *Neurosurgery*, 1989. **24**: pp. 655–670.

126. Sindou, M. and P. Mertens, Selective Spinal Cord Procedures for Spasticity and Pain, in *Neurophysiology in Neurosurgery*, V. Deletis and J. L. Shils, Editors. 2002, Academic Press: Amsterdam. pp. 93–117.

127. Sipski, M. L., C. J. Alexander, and R. C. Rosen, Orgasm in Women with Spinal Cord Injuries: A Laboratory-Based Assessment. *Arch. Phys. Med. Rehabil.*, 1995. **76**: pp. 1097–1102.

128. Sipski, M. L., C. J. Alexander, and R. R. Rosen, Sexual Arousal and Orgasm in Women: Effects of Spinal Cord Injury. *Ann. Neurol.*, 2001. **49**(1): pp. 35–44.

129. Sloan, T. and D. Angell, Differential Effect of Isoflurane on Motor Evoked Potentials Elicited by Transcortical Electric or Magnetic Stimulation, in *Handbook of Spinal Cord Monitoring*, S. S. Jones, *et al.*, Editors. 1993, Kluver Academic Publishers: Hingham, MA. pp. 362–367.

130. Sloan, T., Anesthesia and Motor Evoked Potential Monitoring, in *Neurophysiology in Neurosurgery*, V. Deletis and J. L. Shils, Editors. 2002, Academic Press: Amsterdam. pp. 451–474.

131. Spiegel, J., G. Fuss, C. Krick, K. Schimrigk, and U. Dillmann, Influence of Proprioceptive Input on Parkinsonian Tremor. *J. Clin. Neurophysiol.*, 2002. **19**(1): pp. 84–9.

132. Stein, R., Letter to the Editor. *Paraplegia*, 1991. **29**: pp. 495–497.

133. Sun, W. M., R. Macdonagh, D. Forster, and E. Al., Anorectal Function in Patients with Complete Spinal Transection before and after Sacral Posterior Rhizotomy. *Gastroenterology*, 1994. **108**: pp. 990–998.

134. Tamaki, T., H. Takano, and K. Takakuwa, Spinal Cord Monitoring: Basic Principles and Experimental Aspects. *Cent. Nerv. Syst. Trauma*, 1985. **2**: pp. 137–149.

135. Tatton, W. G., M. J. Eastman, W. Bedingham, M. C. Verrier, and I. C. Bruce, Defective Utilization of Sensory Input as the Basis of Bradykinesia, Rigidity, and Decreased Movement Repertoire in Parkinson's Disease: A Hypothesis. *Can. J. Neurol. Sci.*, 1984. **11**: pp. 136–43.

136. Temel, Y. and V. Visser-Vandewalle, Surgery in Tourette Syndrome. *Mov. Disord.*, 2004. **19**(1): pp. 3–14.

137. Topka, H., L. G. Cohen, R. A. Cole, and M. Hallett, Reorganization of Corticospinal Pathways Following Spinal Cord Injury. *Neurology*, 1991. **41**(8): pp. 1276–1283.

138. Vitek, J. L., R. A. E. Bakay, T. Hashimoto, Y. Kaneoke, K. Mewes, J. Y. Zhang, D. B. Rye, P. Starr, M. S. Baron, R. Turner, and M. R. Delong, Microelectrode-Guided Pallidotomy: Technical Approach and Application for Treatment of Medically Intractable Parkinson's Disease. *J. Neurosurg.*, 1998. **88**: pp. 1027–43.

139. Vitek, J. L., V. Chockkan, J. Y. Zhang, Y. Kaneoke, M. Evatt, M. R. Delong, S. Triche, K. Mewes, T. Hashimoto, and R. A. Bakay, Neuronal Activity in the Basal Ganglia in Patients with Generalized Dystonia and Hemiballismus. *Ann. Neurol.*, 1999. **46**(1): pp. 22–35.

140. Wada, J. A., *Kindling 2.* 1981, Raven Press: New York.

141. Wall, P. D., The Presence of Ineffective Synapses and Circumstances which Unmask Them. *Phil. Trans. Royal Soc. (Lond.)*, 1977. **278**: pp. 361–372.

142. Walsh, E. G., *Muscles, Masses and Motion: The Physiology of Normality, Hypotonicity, Spasticity and Rigidity.* 1992, Blackwell: Oxford.

143. Whipple, B., C. A. Gerdes, and B. R. Komisaruk, Sexual Response to Self-Stimulation in Women with Complete Spinal Cord Injury. *J. Sex. Res.*, 1996. **33**: pp. 231–240.

144. White, S. R. and R. S. Neuman, Facilitation of Spinal Motoneuron by 5-Hydroxytryptamine and Noradrenaline. *Brain Res.*, 1980. **185**: pp. 1–9.

145. Wiesendanger, M., The Pyramidal Tract. Its Structure and Function, in *Handbook of Behavioral Neurobiology*, A. L. Towe and E. S. Luschei, Editors. 1981, Plenum: New York. pp. 401–490.

146. Wolpaw, J. R. and J. A. O'Keefe, Adaptive Plasticity in the Primate Spinal Stretch Reflex: Evidence of a Two-Phase Process. *J. Neuro. Sci.*, 1984. **4**: pp. 2718–24.

147. Yoshida, M., A. Rabin, and A. Anderson, Monosynaptic Inhibition of Pallidal Neurons by Axon Collaterals of Caudatonigral Fibers. *Exp. Brain Res*, 1972. **15**: pp. 33–347.

6

___

Cranial nerves and neurotology

Introduction

This chapter concerns disorders of cranial nerves and the vestibular system. Disorders of cranial nerves include paresis and paralysis of motor nerves such as facial palsy, and hyperactivity of motor nerves such as hemifacial spasm (HFS). Trigeminal and glossopharyngeal neuralgia[1] (TGN and GPN) are hyperactivity of sensory systems that results in pain (neuralgia). Disorders of cranial nerves such as HFS, TGN and GPN are known as "vascular compression disorders" because they can be effectively cured by moving a blood vessel off the respective cranial nerve root (microvascular decompression[2] (MVD) [109, 111]. The pathophysiology of HFS is discussed in detail in this chapter because it serves as a model of other hyperkinetic disorders. The pathophysiologies of other disorders that can be cured by MVD are also discussed. Other disorders of nerves such as those that are caused by inflammation and injuries of nerves are discussed in Chapter 2.

The vestibular system provides proprioceptive input to the motor system via the vestibulospinal tract, and this input aids in voluntary body movements as well as in automatic functions like keeping posture, as was discussed in Chapter 5. In this chapter, we will discuss disorders that are associated with the vestibular system such as benign paroxysmal vertigo (BPPV). A disorder of the vestibular system that is associated with vascular compression of the vestibular

___

[1] The term neuralgia is used to describe a severe and sharp shooting pain that is perceived in the distribution of a nerve (see Chapter 4).

[2] In MVD operations, a blood vessel is moved off the root of a cranial nerve. This operation is performed mostly on the root of CN V for TGN, on the root of CN VII for HFS and on CN IX for GPN (see Chapter 4) but also on CN VIII for disabling positional vertigo (DPV) and severe tinnitus.

nerve (DPV) will also be discussed in this chapter. Ménière's disease affects both the vestibular and the auditory system. The vestibular component of Ménière's disease is discussed in this chapter and the auditory components are discussed in Chapter 3 (p. 106). We will also discuss schwannoma of cranial nerves in this chapter.

6.1   Symptoms and signs of disorders of cranial nerves

Cranial nerve motoneurons are involved in movement disorders similar to those of the spinal cord producing hyperactive disorders such as spasm and synkinesis. Symptoms from sensory nerves are pain and paresthesia. Facial nerve palsy and abducens paresis are the most common forms of paresis and paralysis of cranial nerves. Pain affects mostly CN V (TGN) and the CN IX (GPN). HFS is the best known of motor disorders that can be cured by MVD operations (cure rate approximately 85%) [10]. Patients with spasmodic torticollis have been treated by MVD [37, 124, 159] but the results of such operations are not as good as the results of MVD to treat TGN and HFS. Disorders associated with similar pathology of sensory nerves such as TGN and GPN have similar high cure rates [11, 85].

Diagnosis of some cranial nerve disorders is challenging because the symptoms and signs of disorders of cranial nerves are not only different because of the diverse function of the affected nerves, but similar pathologies of different cranial nerves can produce many different symptoms and signs.

Physicians in specialties such as neuro-ophthalmology and neurotology often treat disorders of the optic, auditory and vestibular nerves. Other health care professionals, like audiologists, speech therapists and optometrists can also diagnose disorders of these cranial nerves. Some cranial nerve disorders such as TGN and DPV can be treated effectively both by medicine and by surgical operations. The choice between treatments often depends on the specialty to which the patient's physician belongs. The subtle and often conflicting symptoms and signs of rare disorders such as the vascular decompression disorders, often cause patients to be shuttled between physicians of different specialties, and often offered different kinds of treatments.

6.1.1   Motor disorders

Disorders of cranial motor nerves cause paralysis, paresis, synkinesis and hyperactivity. The most common paralysis of cranial motor nerves is facial paralysis. Idiopathic facial paralysis is known as Bell's palsy. Paralysis can also occur because of trauma and from iatrogenic causes. Abducens paresis is not uncommon and prevents movement of the eye in a lateral direction from a mid position.

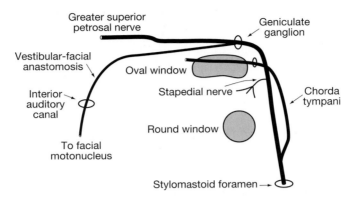

Fig. 6.1 Anatomy of the facial nerve.

Bell's palsy [139] is a typical example of a disorder that usually causes total paralysis of the mimic muscles on one side of the face [145]. Bell's palsy presents with rapidly increasing facial weakness that usually turns into total paralysis within hours. Bell's palsy has a high rate of spontaneous recovery, but the mimic muscles in some few patients remain total paralyzed for the rest of their life. The etiology of Bell's palsy is not completely known, but many authors assume that it is caused by viral inflammation [2] [4]. It is assumed that the nerve is swollen somewhere within its (long) bony canal (Fallopian (or facial) canal). There are others who have found evidence that the paralysis is caused by nerve entrapment of an unknown cause [140]. Therefore, some surgeons perform decompression operations of the facial nerve to treat Bell's palsy [141].

Recovery from Bell's palsy is often accompanied by synkinesis (see p. 358). It has been inferred that the "Mona Lisa smile" (Gioconda smile) may be a result of synkinesis that has developed after Bell's palsy [3]. It has been shown that oral synkinesis can be reduced (or relieved) by training [18].

The complexity of disorders of the facial nerve such as Bell's palsy is partly caused by the long and intricate course of the facial nerve from the facial motonucleus to the nerve's emergence from the stylomastoid foramen (Fig. 6.1).

Surgically induced trauma to the facial nerve is decreasing because of improved surgical methods such as microneurosurgery, and the introduction of intraoperative neurophysiologic monitoring at the beginning of the 1980s [105, 106, 110, 185, 186]. Earlier, surgical damage to the intracranial portions of motor nerves such as the facial nerve occurred frequently in operations in the cerebello-pontine angle (CPA) such as in operations for vestibular schwannoma [110, 186] (for a review see Jackler 1994 [62]). Other cranial motor nerves such as CN III, IV, VI, and XII may be damaged in operations for other skull base tumors. Such complications have been significantly reduced after the introduction of intraoperative neurophysiologic monitoring [103, 154] as well as by improvements of surgical techniques – aided by the advent of technologies such as the operating microscope [143], and now more recently the use of endoscopes (minimally invasive surgery).

The peripheral part of the facial nerve can be injured during operations on the face such as cosmetic operations (facelift) and in operations for temporomandibular joint (TMJ) disorders. In addition to causing paresis or paralysis, trauma to motor nerves often causes synkinesis (which is a result of expression of neural plasticity, see pp. 15, 358). Synkinesis (involuntary muscle activity that accompanies voluntary movements), often occurs after recovery from paralysis.

Unilateral hyperactive motor disorders of cranial nerves include HFS, oculomotor spasm and trigeminal spasm. These disorders are also known as "vascular compression" disorders and will be discussed below. Bilateral motor disorders that are related to cranial motor nerves (blepharospasm, spasmodic torticollis, spasmodic dysphonia) are probably disorders of central motor systems such as the basal ganglia, and these disorders are discussed in Chapter 5.

6.1.2   Sensory disorders

Sensory disorders of cranial nerves are loss or reduced function, and paresthesia and other phantom symptoms including pain. Neuritis of cranial nerves such as that of the vestibular portion of CN VIII produces violent symptoms from the vestibular system consisting of vertigo (feeling the world is spinning), vomiting and dizziness. Neuronitis of the auditory portion of the CN VIII usually results in deafness that is sometimes accompanied by tinnitus that can be severe. Auditory and vestibular neuronitis is usually unilateral.

Sensory cranial nerves can be damaged during neurosurgical operations [110]. The auditory-vestibular nerve is especially vulnerable, because approximately 1 cm of this nerve has central myelin and thus lacks the supportive tissue found in the peripheral portion of the nerve [86, 88, 164, 165] (see Chapter 2). Surgically induced injuries to the CN VIII can result in vertigo, tinnitus and hearing loss. Introduction of intraoperative neurophysiologic monitoring has reduced such iatrogenic injuries, most noticeably for the auditory nerve [53, 106, 110], but also markedly for the vestibular nerve [155].

TGN and GPN are sensory disorders of cranial nerves that belong to the group of vascular compression disorders that are discussed below. Rare disorders such as anesthesia dolorosa of the face is discussed in Chapter 4.

Little is known about the pathophysiology of other neuralgias of cranial nerves such as those related to the Herpes zoster virus (shingles, Ramsey-Hunt syndrome, etc.), except that viral infection is assumed to cause inflammation that causes abnormal firing of axons of peripheral nerves. It seems likely that changes in the central processing of pain signals may be altered in these types of nerve pain, in a similar way to that which occurs in TGN (see Chapters 3 and 4).

6.1.3   *The vascular compression syndrome*

Vascular compression disorders is a group of disorders that is related to specific cranial nerves, and which can be cured by moving a blood vessel off the respective cranial nerve [10, 11] (for a review, see [111]). The best-known disorders are HFS and TGN, where the symptoms are abnormal muscle activity (spasm and synkinesis) and pain, respectively (for a review, see [109, 112]). GPN [85, 109, 162], some forms of vestibular and auditory disorders (DPV) [15, 121, 122] and tinnitus [117, 121, 149] (discussed in Chapter 3), and possibly some forms of spasmodic torticollis [37, 138] also belong to this group. Intermedius neuralgia (geniculate neuralgia) [90, 142, 148] may also have a similar pathology. The symptoms of these disorders reflect hyperactivity and altered function and expression of neural plasticity is most likely involved in generation of the symptoms.

Hemifacial spasm

HFS is a progressive disorder that is characterized by periods of spasm of facial muscles on one side of the face [34, 109]. HFS is a rare disease (incidence: 0.74 per 100,000 in white men and 0.81 per 100,000 in white women) [6] that has its onset relatively late in life. In between attacks, the function of the facial (mimic) musculature is normal. In most individuals, the spasm begins around one eye and extends to other facial muscles on the same side of the face. After many (10–20) years, the spasm may even involve the platysma; however, the muscles above the eyes are rarely involved (perhaps related to the different innervation of the muscles of the forehead compared with other mimic muscles, see p. 347). Most patients with HFS also experience synkinesis, but only few experience facial muscle weakness. HFS can be cured by moving a blood vessel off the intracranial portion of the facial nerve (MVD operation) [47, 111] and the cure rate is 85–95% [10, 104].

> The synkinesis of face muscles in individuals with HFS can be demonstrated by recording of the R_1 component of the blink reflex (see p. 348) [128], which normally only involves the orbicularis oculi muscles [83]. In patients with HFS other facial muscles such as the orbicularis oris and the mental muscles also contract as part of the blink reflex [34, 128]. The R_1 component of the blink reflex in patients with HFS can also be recorded on the affected side under general anesthesia such as in patients undergoing MVD operations for HFS (but not on the unaffected side) [100, 109].
>
> Patients with HFS have an abnormal muscle response [33, 59, 100, 107] (also known as the lateral spread response [97]) that can be elicited

by electrical stimulation of a branch of the facial nerve, while the electromyographic (EMG) response is recorded from muscles that are innervated by a different branch of the facial nerve [59, 100, 107] (Figs. 6.2, 6.3, 6.4). In individuals who do not have HFS, such stimulation does not produce any measurable EMG activity in muscles that are innervated by other branches of the facial nerve. The latency of the initial component of the abnormal muscle response in patients with HFS is approximately 10 msec (Fig. 6.4). The abnormal muscle response is assumed to be similar to the F-response and it thus reflects an abnormally high excitability of the facial motonucleus (see p. 271). The initial response to electrical stimulation of a peripheral branch of the facial nerve is followed by EMG potentials that may last several 100 msec (Fig. 6.4). The prolonged response reflects repetitive firings of motoneurons that produce repetitive muscle contractions (spasm).

Considering the similarities in the pathophysiology of HFS and TGN, one would expect that similar medical treatment as is effective in treating TGN (carbamazepine, phenytoin and baclofen) would also be effective in treating HFS. These drugs, however, have low efficacy in treating HFS [132, 152]. Other treatments of HFS have consisted of selective severing of the branch of the facial nerve that innervate muscles around the eye [94] (summarized recently by Dobie and Fisch, 1986 [32]). Surgically induced damage to the facial nerve in the middle ear has been used as treatment of HFS [187]. These treatments, however, do not have the same efficacy as MVD and are associated with facial weakness or paresis. More recently, patients with HFS have been treated with injections of Botulinum toxin (Botox) in the facial muscles that are affected by the spasm [91, 132, 176].

Hyperkinetic disorders of other cranial nerves

Spasm of the mastication muscles is very rare. Auger reported 3 patients [7], and Thompson reported one case of "hemimasticatory spasm" [172]. One case of spasm in connection with hemiatrophy of face muscle has been described [72]. Another rare disorder that affects muscles innervated by cranial nerves is cyclic oculomotor spasm [79]. This disease has similarities with HFS but affects the third cranial nerve [109].

Spasmodic torticollis is related to the eleventh cranial nerve and is characterized by involuntary head movements [138]. Spasmodic torticollis occurs in two forms: one that affects the neck muscles bilaterally, and one that has a distinct unilateral pattern [61, 16, 76, 151]. The bilateral form may be caused by supranuclear pathology (such as basal ganglia). Spasmodic torticollis is troublesome because patients cannot keep their head steady, but most complaints are because of pain from the muscles that are constantly contracting and relaxing.

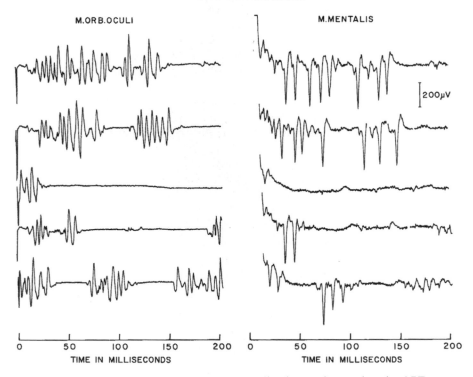

Fig. 6.2 Abnormal muscle response recording in a patient undergoing MVD operation for HFS shown on a long time scale (from Møller and Jannetta 1985 [101]). Reprinted from *Exp. Neurol.* 93, pp. 110–119, with permission from Elsevier.

Treatment with MVD has had some success, but at a lower rate than the treatment of TGN and HFS [37]. MVD seems to be more successful in the unilateral form than in the bilateral form [125].

Trigeminal neuralgia

Trigeminal neuralgia (TGN) or tic douloureux is a typical mononeuropathy. It is a progressive disorder that has been studied extensively, and it is one of the best-known neuralgias of cranial nerves [43, 179]. TGN occurs with an incidence of 5.9 per 100,000 in women and 3.4 per 100,000 in men (in a white population in the USA) [71]. TGN seems to occur spontaneously with no known cause.

The symptoms are attacks of lacerating pain in specific areas of the face and head. The pain from TGN is referred to specific areas of the face, most commonly

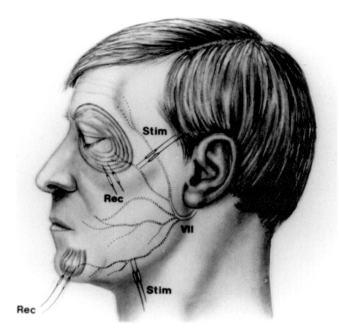

Fig. 6.3 Placement of recording and stimulating electrodes for recording of the abnormal muscle contraction [99]. Reprinted from *Experientia* vol. 41, pp. 415–417, 1985, with permission from Birkhäuser Verlag AG, Switzerland.

to the second or third division of the trigeminal nerve and inside the mouth. TGN usually has distinct trigger points[3], which are well-defined regions of the face or inside the mouth where sensory stimulation by touch or cold can trigger attacks of pain [43] (see Chapter 4). Eating or exposure to cold winds can often elicit pain attacks. The trigger points may be located away from the region of pain. Anesthetizing the trigger point can often relieve the pain. Severe TGN that is not effectively treated may lead to suicide.

TGN is one of only a few pain disorders that is well defined, and for which several effective and well-defined treatments are in use [5, 11, 39, 55, 89]. The pathophysiology of the disorder is also better understood than that of many other pain disorders [40, 42, 43] (see p. 189). TGN can be treated with a high degree of success by several methods: by medicine (carbamazepine, phenytoin and/or baclofen, or gabapentin) [39, 170], or surgically by microvascular decompression (MVD) operation of the intracranial portion of CN V [11, 44, 162], or by

---

[3] Trigger points are locations on the skin (or in the mouth) where sensory stimulation (touch, cold or warmth) can elicit an attack of pain. Many forms of pain have distinct trigger points from which pain can be elicited or from which attacks of pain can be initiated.

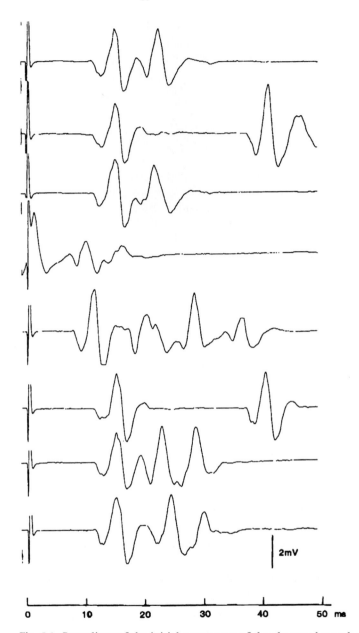

Fig. 6.4 Recordings of the initial component of the abnormal muscle response in a patient undergoing a MVD operation for HFS. (Reprinted from Møller and Jannetta, 1987 [104], *J. Neurosurg.*, vol. 66, 681–685, 1987 with permission.)

partial trigeminal rhizotomy [5, 166]. Injection of glycerol near the trigeminal ganglion is also an effective treatment [55]. The cure rate by the MVD operation for TGN is approximately 85% [11]. Similar cure rates are achieved by other methods such as partial section of the trigeminal nerve root [166] or by glycerol injection in the trigeminal ganglion [55]. Medical treatment using carbamazepine, baclofen or gabapentin also has high cure rates [39] especially in the early phases of the disease (for an overview of results of treatments, see [108, 111]). More recently, gamma radiation has been used to treat TGN [81].

> Although the neurosurgeon Walter Dandy reported he had seen vessels in close contact with the trigeminal nerve root, he was not the first to make use of the finding in treatment of TGN [111] but continued to perform partial sectioning of the root of CN V to treat TGN. Gardner [44] was the first to point to the possibility that vascular compression might be involved in the creation of the symptoms of TGN, and he and his co-worker showed that MVD operations were effective in treating the disorder. The treatment of TGN using MVD was popularized by Jannetta [67] (see [111]).

Atypical trigeminal neuralgia is a pain condition of the face that is different from those of TGN. Atypical trigeminal neuralgia [51] is characterized by constant pain that is often poorly localized and without trigger points. Atypical face pain does not respond to the same treatments as TGN and GPN. However, atypical face pain is often not distinguished from TGN when diagnosis of pain of the face is made.

Neuralgias of other cranial nerves

Two other cranial nerves are associated with neuralgias namely CN IX (GPN) and the intermedius nerve (Wriesberg's nerve) (geniculate neuralgia). GPN is characterized by pain in the throat and sides of the neck, while nervous intermedius neuralgia gives pain deep in the ear. Typically, the frequency of pain attacks in these disorders increases with time as the intensity of the pain increases.

GPN [25, 85] is a rare disorder with an unknown incidence rate. The symptoms are attacks of pain similar to those of TGN but referred to the throat area. It can be treated successfully by MVD of the root of CN IX [67, 162] and medically by carbamazepine. Earlier, section of parts of CN IX was performed to treat the disorder, but MVD of CN IX is as effective in relieving the pain.

Nervus intermedius neuralgia is a little known rare unilateral disorder that is also known as geniculate neuralgia. It is characterized by attacks of sharp pain that is localized deep in the ear. It can be successfully treated by moving a blood vessel off the nervus intermedius or by sectioning of some fascicles of the nervus intermedius intracranially [90, 142, 148], and probably by medical treatment with carbamazepine (Tegretol) as well.

Tinnitus

Tinnitus has many forms and many causes (tinnitus is discussed in detail in Chapter 3). Some forms of tinnitus can be alleviated by MVD of the auditory nerve indicating that tinnitus in a few individuals is related to vascular contact with the auditory nerve [116, 119, 121, 122, 153].

Tic convulsif

Cushing [24] coined the term "tic convulsif" to describe a combination of TGN and HFS. It is a very rare disorder and there is considerable disagreement about how this disorder should be defined, and whether it exists at all. It is possible that the brief facial muscle twitches that often occur in patients with TGN in connection with attacks of pain may appear in the same way as the spasm in HFS in some patients and that this is what has been interpreted as a separate disease and named tic convulsif [136]. Some investigators [184] have defined tic convulsif as a combination of HFS and geniculate neuralgia (nervus intermedius neuralgia) (see p. 339).

6.1.4   Bilateral cranial nerve disorders

Blepharospasm [13] is characterized by bilateral involuntary contraction of the muscles around the eyes causing forceful closure of the eyes. Since it is bilateral, it is assumed to involve supranuclear structures, probably including the basal ganglia. Blepharospasm usually only affects muscles around the eyes and it occurs mostly in elderly individuals.

Spasmodic dysphonia is caused by a dysfunction of the larynx that can affect adductor and abductor muscles, or the vocal cords, the former being the most common [173, 180]. Spasmodic dysphonia is related to CN X but since the vocal cords are affected bilaterally the anatomical location of the physiologic abnormalities that cause the spasm is probably central to the motonucleus of CN X. Little is known about its pathophysiology but it seems likely that it has central causes such as dysfunction of the basal ganglia [173, 180].

Tics are complex stereotyped movements that may occur in patients with neurologic injury but can also be seen in individuals suffering from obsessive-compulsive disorders (OCD) [49]. Tics can often be suppressed voluntarily. Tourette's syndrome is manifested by the presence of tics and the symptoms typically begin in childhood. All these disorders may involve the basal ganglia, but little is known about what causes these disorders. Neuroleptic agents that block central dopaminergic activity can reduce the severity of the tics.

Amyotrophic lateral sclerosis (ALS) is a progressive degenerative disorder of alpha motoneurons (see p. 245) and cortical motoneurons that often affects CN IX and XII in early stages of the disease, causing difficulties in speaking. In the beginning of the development of the disease the speech deficits resemble those caused by intoxication. As the disorder progresses, the difficulties in speaking increase and other muscle groups become involved (see p. 299).

6.2   Vestibular disorders

Two different kinds of vestibular disorders can be identified: One kind disturbs balance and interferes with walking (ataxia). The other kind produces symptoms such as vertigo, lightheadedness, faintness and nausea, and often spontaneous eye movements (nystagmus). These two kinds of vestibular disorders may occur simultaneously. Some vestibular disorders are associated with vertigo and nausea that are initiated by head movements [9, 116], while others produce similar symptoms that occur spontaneously (without body movements).

Symptoms of vestibular disorders can be caused by disorders of the vestibular apparatus in the inner ear, the vestibular portion of the CN VIII (such as vestibular neuronitis) and by re-organization of the vestibular central nervous system through the expression of neural plasticity. The best-known endorgan disorders are Ménière's disease and BPPV. Ménière's disease has attracted much attention, and many vestibular disorders are often erroneously labeled Ménière's disease. The same occurs for BPPV, just as an indication of the power of having names of disorders.

6.2.1   Balance disturbances

The vestibular apparatus provides information about head movements to motor systems of the CNS. Decreased vestibular function makes it difficult to keep the balance and coordinate movements (ataxia) such as those for walking. However, the function of the vestibular system can be substituted by other senses through expression of neural plasticity. Vision and proprioception from receptors in joints, muscles and the skin can take over the functions that normally belong to the vestibular system. Sudden loss of vestibular function causes severe balance disturbances but these symptoms decrease with time as other systems take over the lost function. The time it takes to complete the changes in the nervous system to transfer vestibular tasks to other senses depends on the age of the individual. A child may regain near normal function within a few weeks after loss of vestibular function, a young individual can regain function in a few months, but a person over 60 years of age may improve after loss of vestibular function but never regain normal posture and the ability to walk normally.

6.2.2   *Vertigo, nausea and lightheadedness*

The information from the vestibular system normally does not elicit any conscious perceptions. The activation of the vestibular system through head movements normally occurs without any conscious perceptual awareness like that of other proprioceptive inputs but disorders that affect the vestibular receptor organ in the inner ear or the vestibular nerve such as vestibular neuritis can result in awareness of activation of the vestibular system. Individuals with vestibular disorders often perceive head movements as a spinning sensation, or causing autonomic reactions such as vomiting. This means that the information from the balance organ in the inner ear is re-directed to other parts of the CNS than those normally reached by such information. Abnormal eye movements (nystagmus) are often present in disorders of the vestibular system, either spontaneously or evoked by head movements. Individuals with vestibular disorders may also have a spinning sensation without head movements (vertigo) indicating that some CNS structures have become hyperactive.

Similar reactions as those seen in vestibular disorders may occur in response to abnormal activation of the vestibular system or immediately after such head movements. Excessive motion and, in particular where the supporting structures of the body move, such as on a boat, can cause an incorrect feeling of motion with vertigo and autonomic symptoms such as vomiting even in the absence of vestibular disorders.

These symptoms and signs of vestibular disorders indicate that the vestibular system has a great ability to change its function through expression of neural plasticity. Likewise, the redirection of information from the vestibular organ to regions of the brain that are normally not activated by head movements, may occur.

6.2.3   *Specific vestibular disorders*

The two most common vestibular disorders are BPPV and Ménière's disease. DPV is a rare disorder [15, 70, 116, 122].

Benign paroxysmal positional vertigo

BPPV is a non-progressive self-limiting disorder that is characterized by nystagmus and episodes of vertigo from head movements. BPPV (sometimes known as benign paroxysmal positional nystagmus BPPN) [9] is the cause of

20% of all incidences of balance symptoms. The most common cause of BPPV in people under the age of 50 is head injury, but BPPV is also associated with migraine [60]. Like many other diseases of sensory organs, the incidence of BPPV increases with age [38] and reaches 50% of all forms of vestibular disorders in older people, thus being the most common vestibular disorder in elderly individuals. Specific head movement exercise has been used successfully to treat BPPV [19] (Epley maneuver [135]).

Ménière's disease

Ménière's disease is a progressive disease that is defined as a triad of symptoms: attacks of vertigo, fluctuating hearing loss and tinnitus. The auditory symptoms are discussed in Chapter 3, and the vestibular symptoms are discussed in this chapter. Ménière's disease occurs in attacks between which the individual is relatively free of vestibular symptoms. The symptoms last for 1–2 days and can reoccur in a few days or in a few months. The treatments are diuretics, low-salt diets, etc.

Disabling positional vertigo

DPV is characterized by constant vertigo and nausea [118]. DPV is a progressive disorder and is often incapacitating. Patients with DPV may over time be bedridden most of the time, or at least unable to work or maintain normal daily activity [120, 122]. Individuals with DPV experience discomfort from any head movement, and they often spend most of their time sitting or in bed because this is the body position in which they feel the least uncomfortable [116]. The disorder can be treated by MVD of the vestibular nerve root [70] (success rate of approximately 80% [116, 120, 122]).

6.2.4   Tumors of cranial nerves

The most frequent and best-known tumor of cranial nerves is the vestibular schwannoma. Tumors of the trigeminal nerve are also common.

Vestibular schwannoma

Vestibular schwannoma[4] [62, 130] are slow growing benign tumors that may not grow at all, or may decrease in size, or vanish totally [12, 22].

---

[4] Vestibular schwannoma were earlier known as acoustic tumors. The reason for the name acoustic tumor was that the most pronounced symptoms and signs arose from the auditory system. When it became clear that these tumors most frequently grow from the (superior) vestibular nerves, and the fact that these tumors are the result of excessive growth of Schwann cells, attempts were made to change the name to vestibular schwannoma. However, the compliance with the change of name has been slow.

Vestibular schwannoma occurs with an incidence of approximately 1 in 100,000, but autopsies show an incidence of 2.4% (sic) [12], indicating that the occurrence of Vestibular schwannoma without symptoms is common. Many tumors therefore never become diagnosed (some investigators [156] have found these numbers to be exaggerated). Investigators, however, agree that most of the small tumors that are detected by imaging methods are slow growing; many are stable and some even regress over time [22, 161]. This information is important for treatment because it has been the routine to treat acoustic tumors surgically whenever detected. The findings that tumors in fact may decrease in size and in many cases pose no health threat have hopefully changed the approach to treatment [57]. The risks of complications in such operations have also been re-evaluated [114, 129].

Vestibular schwannoma have been assumed to begin to grow from the Obersteiner-Redlich zone (glial margin) but recent studies have shown that some tumors begin to grow from sites of CN VIII that are peripheral to the Obersteiner-Redlich zone (see chapter on peripheral nerves) [183].

Vestibular schwannoma cause symptoms from the auditory and vestibular systems such as hearing deficits and reduced vestibular function, and hyperactive symptoms such as tinnitus and vertigo are often present. In fact, the first symptom of vestibular schwannoma is tinnitus and if the tumor grows slowly, tinnitus and hearing loss may be the only symptoms. Tinnitus from other causes is common, and the occurrence of tinnitus alone is therefore not a valuable sign in the diagnosis of a vestibular schwannoma. Asymmetric hearing loss, vestibular symptoms and elevated threshold and poor growth of the acoustic middle ear reflex response and abnormal auditory brainstem responses, are all important signs and symptoms of a vestibular schwannoma.

The tinnitus may increase after treatment of the tumor (surgical removal [58] or gamma radiation). Patients with small tumors who are operated while they still have vestibular function may experience vestibular symptoms after tumor removal because of the surgical destruction of the vestibular nerve.

Trigeminal nerve tumors

Most trigeminal nerve tumors are benign (schwannoma) and grow slowly. They can attain large sizes without giving any symptoms and they therefore often become large skull base tumors before they are detected [154].

6.3   Anatomy and physiology of cranial nerves

Cranial nerves are similar in many ways to peripheral spinal nerves but they have much greater variation in their functions, and their fiber types are more varied. They do not have distinctly different roots for sensory and motor parts except CN V, which consists of a separate sensory division (portio major) and a motor and proprioceptive division (portio minor). Other cranial nerves that contain different kinds of fibers enter or exit the CNS as mixed sensory, motor, autonome and visceral nerves.

Sensory nerve fibers that innervate receptors in the ear, eye, nose and tongue enter the central nervous system as parts of cranial nerves VIII, II, I, and VII respectively. The sensory portion of the fifth cranial nerve, which enters the brainstem, innervates receptors in the skin of the face and the mouth. The cranial nerves VII and IX also carry some sensory fibers.

Some cranial nerves are exclusively sensory (CN I, CN II and CN VIII) and some are exclusively motor nerves (CN IV, CN VI, CN XI and CN XII). Some cranial nerves such as CN III, CN VII, CN IX and CN X also contain fibers that belong to the autonomic nervous system, while some contain sensory fibers from the viscera [182].

The cell bodies of sensory nerve fibers are located in ganglia, such as the Gasserian ganglion for the CN V. The fibers of the auditory and vestibular nerve (CN VIII) are also bipolar cells, with their cell bodies located in the spiral ganglion and the vestibular (Scarpa's) ganglion respectively. The sensory division of CN V contains fibers that innervate sensory receptors in the skin of the face and in the mouth. Pain receptors in the same regions of the head also travel in the fifth cranial nerve, which additionally contains fibers that innervate the dura mater and cranial and intracranial blood vessels. Cranial nerve IX also carries some somatic sensory fibers that innervate the pharynx and the ear canal. Some sensory fibers in CN X innervate the ear canal. For details about the anatomy of cranial nerves see Wilson-Pauwels, 1988 [182] or Brodal [20].

Parasympathetic innervation of the body is supplied by CN X (except for parts of the rectum, bladder, uterus and prostate gland that enter the spinal cord at S_{3-4} segments, see Chapter 4, p. 168 and Fig 4.10). CN III containsparasympathetic fibers to the eye. The greater petrosal nerve of CN VII carries parasympathetic fibers to nasal, palatal, lacrimal, submandibular, and sublingual glands. CN IX carries parasympathetic fibers to the parotid gland (Fig 3.7). The afferent sympathetic fibers of the cranial nerves terminate in the solitary nucleus in the medulla.

Sympathetic innervation of the head involves the superior cervical ganglion, the fibers of which follow the internal carotid artery to innervate the dura and some intracranial arteries. Sympathetic fibers that innervate other structures of the head follow cranial nerves from the superior cervical ganglion. Sympathetic fibers that innervate other structures of the head follow cranial nerves from the superior cervical ganglion. Sympathetic fibers from cells in the stellate ganglion innervate the heart and the lungs. Fibers from the cells in the superior cervical ganglion travel through the stellate ganglion and join fibers from that ganglion to enter the spinal cord at the T_1 level.

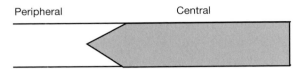

Fig. 6.5A   Schematic drawing of the transition zone between peripheral and central nerves.

The motor fibers of cranial nerves have cell bodies in the motonuclei of the respective cranial nerves.

6.3.1   Cranial nerve roots

The disorders that can be cured by MVD operations have focused on the structure of cranial nerve roots. The transition zone between peripheral and central myelin is known as the "root exit or entry zone," (REZ) or the Obersteiner-Redlich zone. It has a cone-shaped formation ("glial dome" [14, 146, 165, 181], Fig. 6.5A) where the central portion contains oligodendrocytes and astrocytes, and the axons have thin myelin that is generated by oligodendrocytes [146, 169]. The glial dome is penetrated by axons at a node of Ranvier. This change in structure from the peripheral to the central parts of nerves is evident from electron micrographs when examining a cross-section of cranial nerves (Fig. 6.5B), but visual observation of an exposed nerve reveals no difference between the peripheral and the central portion of cranial nerves. This transitional zone can only be visualized microscopically. It has a length of 1–3 mm, being longer in sensory nerves than in motor nerves [1]. The transition between central and peripheral myelin occurs at a distance from the entrance or exit of a nerve that is different for the different cranial nerve (Fig. 6.6B).

The transition zone between peripheral and central myelin has been assumed to play a role in vascular compression disorders [56, 111]. Vestibular schwannoma (and trigeminal nerve tumors) are assumed to start to grow from the transition zone although that assumption has been questioned recently [183].

6.3.2   Brainstem motonuclei

The organization of cranial nerve motonuclei is similar to the organization of the motonuclei of the ventral horns of the spinal cord, but less is known about the neural circuitry in cranial nerve motonuclei than what is known about the organization of the ventral horn of the spinal cord (see Chapter 5).

Sensory nerves terminate in nuclei on the same side, and motor nerves generally originate in motonuclei on the same side. The facial motoneurons are exceptions because the muscles of the upper part of the face (forehead) receive bilateral innervation from the facial motor cortex, whereas the motoneurons

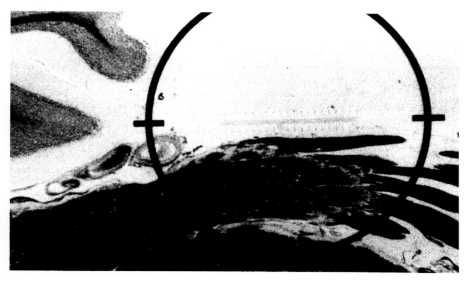

Fig. 6.5B Photomicrograph of a section of the trigeminal sensory root showing the REZ, the junction between central and peripheral myelin. The scale is 2 mm [1]. Reprinted from C. B. T. Adams, 1993. The Physiology and Pathophysiology of Posterior Fossa Cranial Nerve Dysfunction Syndromes: Non Microvascular Perspective. In D. L. Barrow (Ed.), *Neurosurgical Topics* Book 13, *Surgery of Cranial Nerves of the Posterior Fossa*. American Association of Neurological Surgeons: Park Ridge, Illinois, pp. 131–154, with permission.

innervating muscles of the lower part of the face only receive unilateral (crossed) innervation.

Facial expressions are important in communication between individuals. Facial expressions are complex and several different types of expression can be discerned. The facial motonucleus receives separate input from limbic structures and the motor cortex. Often, emotional smiling can be evoked either voluntarily from the motor cortex or involuntarily through input from limbic structures (amygdala) to the facial motoneurons [29]. The smile evoked by command from limbic structures is distinctly different from those coming from the primary motor cortex (MI). A genuine smile cannot be produced on command. Lesions of the tract between the MI and the facial motonucleus do not prevent spontaneous facial expressions, and patients with such lesions can smile in response to a good joke but cannot produce a polite social smile. Central pareses such as capsular hemiplegia are often associated with exaggerated emotional facial expressions (smiling or crying) that the individual cannot suppress. Patients with disorders of the basal ganglia such as Parkinson's disease (PD) lack the ability of spontaneous emotional facial expressions, whereas voluntary, social smiling is possible.

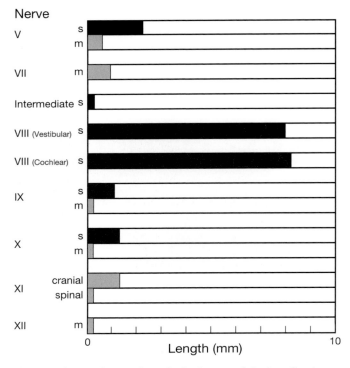

Fig. 6.6 Distance in mm from the brainstem of the interface between the peripheral and the central myelin for the lower cranial nerves (s: sensory; m: motor portions) [56, 169].

Signs of the complexity of cranial nerve motonuclei comes from animal studies of the facial motonucleus, which have shown the existence of dormant synapses that make interconnections between facial motoneurons that innervate different groups of facial muscles [150]. These studies showed that repeated electrical stimulation of the facial nerve caused the development of synkinesis of facial muscles similar to the abnormal muscle response that can be observed in patients with HFS. It was concluded that these changes were caused by expression of neural plasticity that unmasked dormant synapses that connected different motoneurons in the facial motonucleus [150].

6.3.3   Brainstem reflexes

Some of the cranial motor systems include reflexes that are similar to spinal reflexes, whereas other cranial nerve reflexes are different. For example, several of the muscles that are innervated by cranial nerves lack muscle spindles and therefore lack the monosynaptic stretch reflex. The trigeminal system plays

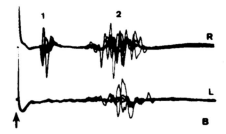

Fig. 6.7 Blink reflex response elicited by electrical stimulation of the supraorbital nerve. Note that the R_1 component is unilateral while the R_2 component is bilateral. The time base is 100 msec [50]. Reprinted from *Electrodiagnosis of neuromuscular disease*, Williams and Wilkins: Baltimore, 1983, reprinted with permission.

a similar role for the facial motor system as proprioceptive feedback in spinal motor systems. The mimic muscles of the face do not seem to have muscle spindles to provide such feedback.

Blink reflex

The blink reflex is one of several trigeminal-facial reflexes. The blink reflex is a reflex for protecting the eye. It is normally elicited by activating skin receptors in the region around the eye, including the eyelid and the cornea. The reflex causes contraction of the orbicularis oculi muscles and closes the eyelid. The blink reflex would be equivalent to the H-response (p. 27) that can be recorded from spinal nerves but instead of muscle spindles supplying information about the length of the muscles, the feedback about contractions of facial muscles is provided by the trigeminal sensory system.

The blink reflex is an important test used in neurologic examinations [76]. For this purpose, the reflex is elicited by electrical stimulation of the supraorbital nerve and EMG potentials are recorded from the orbicularis oculi muscles. When elicited by electrical stimulation the supraorbital nerve has two distinct components, known as the R_1 and R_2 components [83]. The earliest component (R_1) has a latency of approximately 10 msec, while the second response (R_2) has a latency of approximately 30 msec (Fig. 6.7). The unilateral R_1 response has less variability than the R_2 response, which is bilateral.

The earliest response (R_1) is caused by a disynaptic reflex; one synapse is in the trigeminal sensory nucleus, and from there neurons connect to facial motoneurons where the second synapse is located. The R_2 component is bilateral and is a polysynaptic reflex. The R_2 component is sensitive to hypnotics while

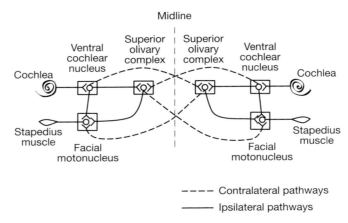

Midline

Fig. 6.8 Reflex arc of the acoustic middle ear reflex for the ipsilateral and contralateral stapedius reflex [113].

the R_1 reflex response is less affected by hypnotics, but it is abolished during surgical anesthesia (except in patients with HFS [100], see p. 334).

Normally, only muscles that are innervated by the zygomatic branch of the facial nerve are activated by electrical stimulation of the supraorbital nerve, but in certain pathological conditions other muscles of the face may also be involved (synkinesis). Synkinesis of the blink reflex may be present in patients with HFS [100, 128, 174] (see p. 334) and after injuries to the facial nerve.

Jaw reflex

Sudden stretching of the muscles that are innervated by the motor portion of the trigeminal nerve (portio minor) causes a reflex response similar to the stretch reflex of skeletal muscles. Electrical stimulation of the nerve innervating the masseter muscle causes a muscle response [133] that is a monosynaptic reflex similar to the H reflex of muscles that are innervated by the spinal cord. This shows that the muscles that are innervated by the motor portion of the CN V have proprioceptors (muscle spindles) unlike those of muscles innervated by CN VII.

Acoustic middle ear reflex

In humans, the acoustic middle ear reflex causes contraction of the stapedius muscle (innervated by the facial nerve) in response to a strong sound (see [113]). The threshold is approximately 85 dB above the threshold of hearing. The reflex arc for the ipsilateral reflex includes the cochlear receptors (hair cells), the cochlear nucleus and the facial motonucleus (Fig. 6.8). A parallel pathway includes a nucleus in the superior olivary complex (SOC). The contralateral reflex arc always involves the SOC (Fig. 6.8) [17, 113]. In many animals, the tensor tympani muscles (innervated by the motor portion of CN V) contracts in response to a strong sound stimulus (but probably not in humans, see [113]).

Contraction of the stapedius muscle decreases the sound transmission through the middle ear and the reflex therefore acts to regulate the sound that reaches the cochlea. Impulsive and rapidly varying sounds are not affected by the attenuation of sound by the contraction of the stapedius muscle because of the latency of the reflex and the relatively slow build up of force in the stapedius muscles. The reflex is bilateral and sound in one ear elicits a contraction of the stapedius muscle on both sides but the reflex response from the contralateral stapedius muscle is lower than that of the ipsilateral muscle [95, 113].

The threshold of the acoustic middle ear reflex is normally elevated and often completely abolished in the presence of a vestibular schwannoma. The reason for this could be that the tumor affects the function of the facial nerve, but it seems more likely that the effect is caused by injury of the auditory nerve caused by the tumor. The reason may instead be an uneven reduction of conduction velocity of fibers in the auditory nerve caused by the tumor. Such spatial dispersion (see p. 111) would make auditory stimulation less effective in activating neurons in the cochlear nucleus on which many nerve fibers converge and thereby reduce the strength of the acoustic middle ear reflex response. Other forms of injury to the auditory nerve are also associated with elevation of the threshold of the acoustic middle ear reflex and, especially, poor growth of the amplitude of the reflex response with increasing stimulus sound intensity [123] (see [113]).

6.3.4   The vestibular system

The vestibular system helps to keep an image steady on the retina during head movements by activating the extraocular muscles through the vestibular ocular reflex (VOR) (see p. 355). Together with input from the visual system and proprioceptors in the joints, tendons and muscles the vestibular system contributes to maintain posture and to create a sense of space. The vestibular system is often regarded as a part of the proprioceptive system because activation of the vestibular system does not normally evoke any sensation. These functions are important, yet the vestibular system can be non-functional without any noticeable symptoms and most of its functions can be taken over by other systems such as proprioception and vision through plastic changes in the nervous system.

Vestibular sensory organs

The sensory organs of the vestibular system are located in the inner ear and consist of three anatomically distinct parts: the three semicircular canals,

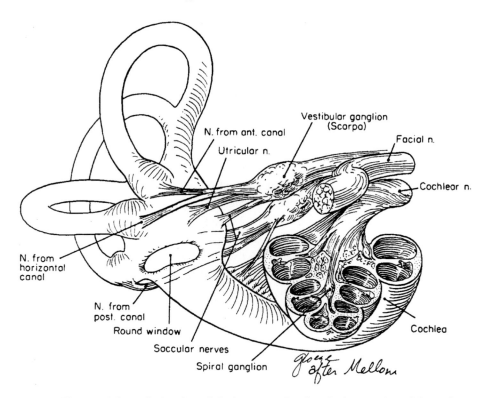

Fig. 6.9 Schematic drawing of the inner ear showing the innervation of the various parts of the vestibular apparatus.

the utricle and the saccula (Fig. 6.9). The three semicircular canals sense angular motion of the head in three planes and the utricle and the saccula provide static information about head (and thereby body) position. The sensory cells of the horizontal, anterior, and posterior semicircular canals are located in the ampullae (cristae), which are enlargements of the semicircular canals. Similar sensory cells are located in the maculae of the utricle and saccula. The sensory cells in all three parts of the vestibular system are known as hair cells, which are similar to those in the cochlea (see Chapter 3) with the difference that the kinocilium is preserved in the vestibular hair cells (Fig. 6.10 [77, 178]). Similar to the sensory cells in the cochlea, two types of vestibular hair cells are found in all three parts of the vestibular system: Type I and Type II (Fig. 6.10). Type I is flask shaped with a large calyx-like nerve terminal surrounding the base of the cell. Type II sensory cells are cylindrical in shape with efferent synapses located on the cell body.

The stimuli to the vestibular hair cells in the cristae are the flow of fluid in the semicircular canals, which makes the cells respond to the velocity of head

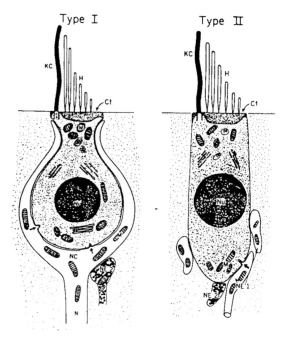

Fig. 6.10 Schematic drawing of two types of hair cells in the vestibular organ (Based on Wersäll 1956 [178].)

movement. The hair cells of the maculae are stimulated by the movement of the otoliths, which makes the utricular and saccular maculae respond to static tilt and dynamic linear acceleration. Because of the directional sensitivity and the organization of hair cells in the maculae, nerve fibers that innervate the maculae have a preferred axis of greatest sensitivity.

Innervation of vestibular sensory cells

The afferent nerve fibers of vestibular hair cells are myelinated bipolar cells with the cell bodies located in Scarpa's ganglion. The axons have diameters of up to 20 μ, which make them some of the largest mammalian nerve fibers. Efferent nerve fibers terminate on the calyx of the hair cells (Fig. 6.10). Type II vestibular hair cells are cylindrical in shape with synapse-like connections to afferent and efferent nerve fibers (Fig. 6.10).

Neural pathways

The first nuclei of the ascending vestibular pathways are the vestibular nuclei, the outputs of which form two main pathways: one to the motonuclei of the extraocular muscles through the medial longitudinal fasciculus (MLF), and

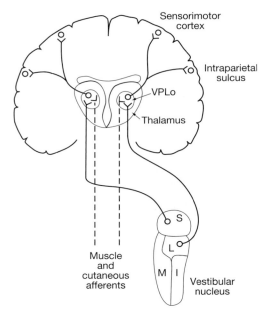

Fig. 6.11 Connections from the vestibular nuclei (S: superior nucleus; M: medial nucleus; L: lateral nucleus; I: inferior nucleus) to the thalamic nuclei (ventroposterior nucleus, pars oralis, VPLo), the sensorimotor cortex (SMC) and the intraparietal sulcus (IPS). (Based on Baloh and Honrubia [9].)

one that projects to the spinal cord (Fig. 6.11). The nerves from the semicircular canals terminate in the medial vestibular nucleus and those from the utriculus terminate (mainly) in the lateral vestibular nucleus (Deiter's nucleus).

The axons of neurons in the medial vestibular nucleus that receive input from the semicircular canals descend in the medial vestibulospinal tract. The axons of neurons in the lateral vestibular nucleus that receive input from the utriculus descend in the lateral vestibulospinal tract [20]. These spinal pathways contribute to posture (see Chapter 5, p. 255).

The neurons in the medial vestibular nucleus that project to the extraocular muscles through the MLF receive input from the semicircular canals and the utriculus (Fig. 6.11). The neurons of the superior vestibular nucleus also project to the motor nuclei of the extraocular muscles through the MLF. Some of the fibers of the MLF are crossed; others are uncrossed. Descending (efferent) fibers from neurons in the motonuclei of the extraocular muscles are inhibitory and terminate mainly on neurons in the superior vestibular nucleus. Purkinje cells in the flocculus of the cerebellum receive input from the vestibular apparatus (semicircular canals), and the same cells receive input from the visual system (the retina) via the pretectal nucleus and the inferior olive.

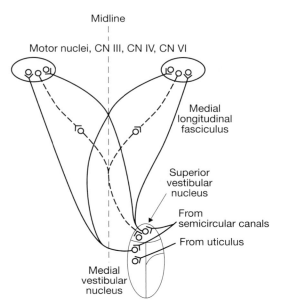

Fig. 6.12 Connections from the vestibular nuclei to the motonuclei of the extraocular muscles.

The neurons in the superior and lateral vestibular nuclei project to neurons in the posterior lateral nuclei of the thalamus. The neurons of these nuclei project to two cortical areas, the sensorimotor cortex (SMC) and the intraparietal sulcus (IPS). The SMC is a small area of the somatosensory cortex that is located close to the face area [20]. Neurons located near the junction between the insula and the IPS are also activated by stimulation of the semicircular canals and from proprioceptors around the upper cervical joint [20]. These neurons also receive input from the visual system, and it is believed that these cortical areas integrate information about body movements from the vestibular and visual systems.

Vestibular ocular reflex

The vestibular system controls eye movements through the VOR. The extraocular muscles that control the position of the eyes are also under the control of the visual system and other parts of the brain in addition to voluntary control. The VOR causes the eyes to move in response to head movements, elicited by activation of the semicircular canals of the vestibular system. The purpose is to compensate for head movements so that an image on the retina is kept steady independent of the head position.

The fibers from the vestibular nuclei project to motoneurons of cranial nerves III, IV and VI that innervate the extraocular muscles through the MLF (Fig. 6.12).

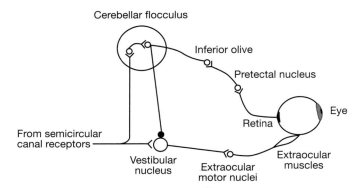

Fig. 6.13 Connections from the cerebellum to the vestibular nuclei and the VOR.

These connections are the anatomical basis for the VOR. The output of the Purkinje cells of the cerebellum has inhibitory influence on the neurons in the vestibular nucleus (Fig. 6.13). This makes it possible to adjust the gain in the VOR based on visual input and thereby keep an image steady on the retina during head movements (avoids retinal slip [20]).

If the head movement is larger than what can be compensated for by the extraocular muscles, the eyes move fast in the opposite direction to reset the eye position. Large head movements therefore cause (slow) compensatory movements of the eyes (slow pursuit) that are interrupted by fast resetting movements (saccades). This combination of slow and fast movements is known as nystagmus. Slow pursuit (slow movements of the eyes to follow a moving object) is assumed to be controlled by pontine nuclei and the cerebellar flocculus. Cortical regions are involved in smooth pursuit (parieto-temporal areas). Some of these eye movements are voluntary, such as slow pursuit, while other movements such as saccades are reflex movements. Recording of nystagmus in response to head movements is an important diagnostic tool.

Ideally, the eye should move (in the opposite direction) exactly as much as the head moves, thus a gain of 1.0 of the VOR. Differences from a gain of 1.0 are signs of disorders affecting the vestibular system. Proper movement of the eyes to keep an image steady on the retina requires that the gain of the VOR be changed when a person changes spectacles to a different strength. The gain of the VOR is extremely plastic and can change to compensate, for instance, when using eyeglasses. More dramatic changes in visual input such as occur from wearing spectacles with reversing prisms can reverse the gain from +1.0 to −1.0 thus reversing the compensatory movement of the eye [73]. After a short time, the VOR can adapt to such an extent that the person is able to play tennis while wearing reversing prisms [73]. This means that not only has the gain of the VOR changed through adaptation (expression of neural plasticity), but in fact a reversal of the VOR has occurred.

The VOR has been a frequent object of study because it lends itself to mathematical modeling using linear circuit theory. Its large adaptability is easy to study quantitatively. Testing of the VOR, including determination of the gain and phase (lag) of the VOR is useful in clinical diagnosis.

The otolith–ocular reflex is another vestibular reflex that also has a high degree of plasticity [78].

Visual control of extraocular muscles

In addition to being controlled by the vestibular system, the extraocular muscles are also under the control of the visual system. Fast movements of the eyes (saccades), are believed to be generated by cortical and subcortical structures. In the monkey, it has been shown that several cortical areas are involved in control of eye movements such as striate (visual), the posterior parietal cortex and area 8 (frontal eye field). The other cortical areas that are involved in eye movements are important for the control of slow pursuit. Lesions in the frontal eye field on one side impair voluntary saccades to the opposite side of the lesion but pursuit is intact [74, 137]. It is therefore believed that the frontal eye field is involved in initiation of saccades.

Awareness of body position

Convergence of information from the utricle, the saccula, various proprioceptive sense organs and the visual system onto the same neurons is believed to contribute to the conscious awareness of body posture and the orientation of the body in space. Either one of these two kinds of (proprioceptive or visual) input seems to be able to substitute for the other one, thus, a form of redundancy or compensatory plasticity.

6.4   Pathophysiology of cranial nerves

Trauma and diseases that affect cranial nerves produce similar symptoms and signs as that of spinal nerves, but the symptoms of injury from cranial nerves are often more complex than those from injury of spinal nerves. Neural plasticity is an important factor in creating symptoms and signs of many disorders of cranial nerves. Expression of neural plasticity is most likely involved in many forms of spasm and synkinesis that are related to cranial motonuclei. Disorders of cranial nerves often affect the function of their respective nuclei. It is therefore important to regard the cranial nerves and their nuclei as a unit. There is evidence that expression of neural plasticity is involved in pain conditions such as face pain (TGN) and other pain conditions such as GPN and nervus intermedius neuralgia (see Chapter 4). Other hyperactive disorders where neural plasticity plays an important role are some forms of tinnitus.

6.4.1   Cranial motor nerves

Bell's palsy is an example of conduction block within a cranial nerve. The pathophysiology has been discussed extensively [4]. Inflammation has been thought to be the cause of Bell's palsy [2] [4], (see p. 331) and it has been suspected of being related to viral or other causes of inflammation. Other studies have suggested other causes on the basis of the outcome of treatment [63, 140]. Bell's palsy is more prevalent in individuals with diabetes mellitus [2], supporting the theory that several factors may be involved in causing the paralysis. However, the effectiveness of any treatment for Bell's palsy is difficult to prove because spontaneous recovery is high (approximately 95%).

> That viral agents are involved in some cases of Bell's palsy is supported by the results from a study of 185 cases of Bell's palsy, which found that 12% were diagnosed as Ramsay-Hunt syndrome, while in 46 of these 185 patients (25%), the diagnosis was herpes zoster (confirmed by acute and convalescent serum titers for varicella zoster virus) [145].
>
> Other investigators have found evidence that the conduction block in the facial nerve is caused by swelling of the nerve in the bony canal. This hypothesis is supported by the finding that surgical decompression of the nerve is an effective treatment [140, 141]. Other surgeons have found the decompression operation to be controversial [4]. Histological studies of specimens from the facial nerve of patients with facial palsy show signs of Wallerian degeneration of various degrees, and it was concluded that the disorder has multiple causes of vascular, inflammatory, or degenerative changes [92].

Injury or disorders of cranial motor nerves may cause reorganization of cranial motor nerve nuclei creating hyperactive symptoms such as spasms and synkinesis. Early evidence of reorganization of cranial nerve motonuclei from injuries of their motor nerves comes from studies of the facial motonucleus [82] which demonstrated morphological changes in the facial motonucleus after section of the facial nerve. Injuries to the facial nerve also cause morphological changes in the facial nucleus [82, 171].

Injuries to cranial nerves can cause hyperactive symptoms and signs such as spasm and synkinesis. Such signs are often present when motor nerves such as the facial nerve have regenerated after injury. It was earlier believed that synkinesis was a result of misdirected outgrowth of axons so that they terminated on the wrong muscles. More recently, it has become evident that the synkinesis of facial muscles after traumatic injuries in humans can be alleviated by proper training [18]. The results of these studies indicate that the anatomical location of the physiological abnormality that causes the synkinesis is in the CNS and not due to regenerating axons missing their targets. These results indicate that synkinesis can be caused by re-organization of the facial motonucleus through the expression of neural plasticity evoked by injuries of the facial nerve. These findings support the importance of regarding cranial nerves and their nuclei as a functional unit.

Recognizing that changes in motor nerves and muscles can affect the function of the motonuclei brings up the question regarding the possible side effects of long term muscle relaxation such as that accomplished by administration of botulinum toxin (Botox).

Animal studies have shown that electrical stimulation of the facial nerve can promote cross-talk between neurons that give rise to nerve fibers of different branches of the facial nerve [150], further supporting the hypothesis that the functions of motonuclei are plastic and that their functions can be altered by abnormalities in the motor nerves.

6.4.2   Sensory nerves

While conduction block in the trigeminal nerve causes numbness the most important effect is caused by deprivation of input to the CNS, which can evoke expression of neural plasticity. For example, there is evidence that the severe pain that often is associated with trauma or other causes of conduction block in the trigeminal nerve is caused by expression of neural plasticity initiated by deprivation of sensory input. Pain may also be caused by the absence of input from $A\beta$ fibers that normally exert inhibitory influence on pain transmission in the trigeminal nucleus as it does in the dorsal horn of the spinal cord (see Chapter 4, p. 164). Injuries to the trigeminal nerve may be caused by trauma or from iatrogenic causes in connection with operations in the face or the cerebello-pontine angle.

Another cause of symptoms from injured sensory nerves that still conduct nerve impulses ("slightly injured nerves") is increased temporal dispersion of the neural activity that reaches the neurons of the first sensory nucleus. Increased temporal dispersion in a nerve that conducts information impairs the preservation of the temporal structure of the information and it may alter excitation of neurons on which many nerve fibers converge (see Chapter 2, p. 60). For example, increased temporal dispersion in the auditory nerve causes blurring of the temporal pattern of the discharges that arrive at the cochlear nucleus, resulting in the degradation of the temporal information important for speech discrimination. The importance of timing for processing of auditory information such as speech is evident from many studies. The distribution of fiber diameters and thereby the conduction velocity of fibers of the auditory nerve is unusually narrow, which means that the variation of the conduction velocity among different auditory nerve fibers is normally small and consequently the temporal dispersion of activity that arrives at its target neuron is small (see Chapter 3). Lesions of the auditory nerve broaden the distribution of conduction velocities among auditory nerve fibers and thereby causes increased temporal dispersion of the neural activity that reaches the cochlear nucleus. That is assumed to be the reason why auditory nerve lesions often cause greater degrees of impaired speech discrimination than that which occurs because of hearing loss caused by disorders of the cochlea [109] (see [113] and Chapter 3, where Fig. 3.13 shows typical results obtained before and after iatrogenic lesions of the auditory nerve that had occurred from surgical manipulations of the nerve).

The distribution of fiber diameters of the auditory nerve becomes larger with age causing increased variation conduction velocity, and that increases the temporal dispersion of the input to the cochlear nucleus. That is most likely contributing to the increased difficulties in understanding speech that many elderly individuals experience. That decrease in speech discrimination cannot be explained solely by loss of sensitivity (elevated hearing threshold) that commonly occurs with age and which has been assumed to be caused by loss of cochlear hair cells but a part of the age-related loss of speech discrimination most likely has a neural origin (see p. 104).

6.4.3   The "microvascular compression syndrome"

It became evident many years ago that disorders like TGN and HFS could be effectively cured by moving an offending vessel off the respective cranial nerve using a technique called microvascular decompression (MVD) (for review of the history of the MVD operation, see [111]). Based on this experience, it was hypothesized that "pulsatile pressure" from arteries [64, 66] caused demyelination of nerve fibers, with subsequent facilitation of direct electrical communication between individual "bare" axons (ephaptic transmission) [45, 127]. The high success rate of MVD operations of such disorders as HFS [10], TGN [11] and GPN [85] has been taken to support the hypothesis that the symptoms and the signs of these disorders were caused by the close contact of the nerve root with a blood vessel ("vascular compression"). But vascular contact with cranial nerve roots has been reported by different investigators in studies of cadavers [93, 134, 164] to occur in 50% or more of individuals who have had no symptoms of TGN or HFS. While vascular compression thus occurs commonly in non-symptomatic individuals at high rates HFS and TGN are rare disorders with reported incidence of

0.74 per 100,000 in white men and 0.81 per 100,000 in white women [6] for HFS; and 5.9 per 100,000 in women and 3.4 per 100,000 in men for TGN [71]. Observations made during MVD operations for other cranial nerve disorders also confirm that vascular contact with cranial nerves in the cerebello-pontine angle is common, and does not normally give any symptoms or signs from other cranial nerves. This contradiction between morphological findings and occurrence of "vascular compression" disorders is naturally a disturbing fact in the attempts to link vascular compression as a cause of these disorders. The fact that HFS and spasm of the mastication muscles are very rare disorders means that close contact between a blood vessel and a cranial nerve root cannot alone produce noticeable symptoms, and it has been suggested that one or more other factors is necessary for the symptoms to manifest [109].

The high incidence of vascular contact with cranial nerve roots in asymptomatic individuals shows that vascular contact is not sufficient to cause symptoms and signs [109] but the high success rate of MVD operations for HFS, TGN and GPN shows that the close contact with a blood vessel is necessary for the development and maintenance of the symptoms and signs of these disorders. There is also physiological evidence that such vascular contact is necessary for maintaining the symptoms of these disorders [98].

The fact that neither one of these factors seems to give any noticeable symptoms when they occur alone, and symptoms only manifest when these two factors occur together, explains why removal of one of these factors (vascular contact with a nerve root) can remove the symptoms and signs of the disorder and thus provide a "cure" without removing all factors that are necessary for expression of the symptoms.

The hypothesis that (at least) two different factors are necessary to cause symptoms of the vascular compression disorders is supported by the observation that noticeable anatomical deformation of the nerve root from the offending blood vessel is rarely seen from visual inspection during MVD operations. Intraoperative monitoring in operations for HFS of the abnormal muscle contraction have demonstrated that moving such small vessels off the facial nerve root causes an immediate cessation of the abnormal muscle contraction [104] (Fig. 6.14). The fact that the symptoms and signs of HFS can be relieved permanently by moving small arteries (arterioles) or even veins off the facial nerve root [69, 80] also speaks against the hypothesis that pulsatile force would cause demyelination that could enable subsequent direct communication between bare axons (ephaptic transmission). The fact that moving very small vessels – including veins – off the facial nerve root can cure HFS even in patients who have extensive contractions of their facial muscles during attacks [69, 80, 104]

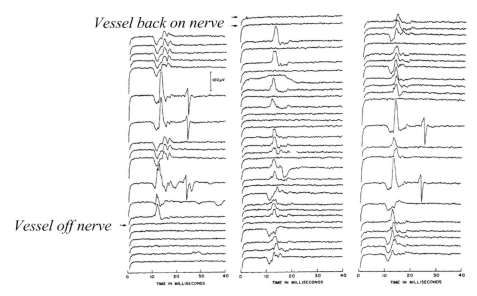

Vessel back on nerve

Vessel off nerve

Fig. 6.14 Abnormal muscle response recorded from the mentalis muscle in response to electrical stimulation of the zygomatic branch of the facial nerve in a patient undergoing an MVD operation for HFS. Consecutive recordings (beginning at the top of the left column) to stimulation at a rate of 5 pps [98]. Reprinted from *Neurosurgery*, vol. 16, 612–618; 1985, with permission.

indicates that the role of blood vessels is not mechanical as was assumed earlier [68].

> Histological studies of the facial nerve root in patients with HFS are few, and these have shown only minor changes, such as hypo- and hyper-myelination of some nerve fibers, but most nerve fibers were found to be normal in the region of vascular contact [147].
>
> A postmortem study [23] of an individual with familial HFS found signs of nerve degeneration and an increased number of corpora amy-lacea at the site of vascular compression, but there was no detectable demyelination or gliosis. It has generally been assumed that demyelina-tion is a prerequisite for ephaptic transmission. This individual had a redundant loop of the anterior inferior cerebellar artery (AICA) and a vein plexus in close contact with the facial nerve at the REZ.
>
> That slight injury of a cranial nerve can facilitate (but not cause) the development of hyperactive symptoms is supported by animal (rat) stud-ies that have shown that facial spasm and the abnormal muscle response that is typical for HFS develops after a blood vessel is brought in close contact with a peripheral branch of the facial nerve that has been injured by tying a chromic suture around the nerve [84]. Close contact with a blood vessel alone did not cause any measurable abnormalities. These

results support the hypothesis that more than one factor is necessary for creation of the symptoms and signs of HFS.

That close contact between a cranial nerve and a blood vessel may have some effect is supported by the observation that many of the patients who were operated on for DPV had slight muscle quivering around the eyes [101]. This has no resemblance to the symptoms of HFS and it could only be seen by a trained observer and was rarely noticed by the patient. Of more than 350 patients who were operated upon to relieve DPV by MVD of the eighth cranial nerve, none had HFS (M. B. Møller, personal communication, 1990). This supports the hypothesis that vascular compression in itself does not produce noticeable symptoms or signs. The observed quivering of the orbicularis oculi muscles was likely caused by irritation of the facial nerve from close contact with the blood vessel, but it did not develop into HFS. Patients with HFS sometimes have subtle auditory nerve signs as indicated by small anomalies in their audiograms [115], but these HFS patients do not have DPV, nor do they have severe tinnitus, again supporting the hypothesis that vascular compression in itself does not cause noticeable symptoms or signs. Other studies, however, have shown that patients with HFS or TGN may have measurable vestibular abnormalities [131] that may be caused by a close contact between the vestibular nerve and a blood vessel.

There is thus considerable evidence that the "vascular compression" of cranial nerves is different from the various forms of entrapment of peripheral nerves. Instead, the close contact between a cranial nerve root and a blood vessel is more likely to exert its effect by irritating the nerve in question and probably activate nerve fibers to produce abnormal firings [109, 111, 112], which then affect the nucleus of the respective cranial nerve.

Below we will discuss the pathophysiology of specific microvascular compression disorders.

Hemifacial spasm

Two hypotheses about the pathophysiology of HFS have prevailed. One explains the typical signs of HFS, namely spasm and synkinesis by assuming that ephaptic transmission[5] occurs between demyelinated (denuded) nerve fibers at the location where blood vessels are in contact with each other in the facial nerve root [45, 47, 127]. The other hypothesis claims that these signs are caused by pathology of a central origin (most likely the facial motonucleus [35, 97, 109, 112].

---

[5] Ephaptic transmission describes direct neural transmission between bare axons. It has been shown to occur for a short period in acutely injured nerves [52, 101], but it is questionable if it plays any important role in persistent neural injuries, although some studies support that hypothesis [144].

Abnormal crosstalk (synkinesis) is one of the signs of HFS. It can be demonstrated by recordings of the blink reflex ("lateral spread") [128] as well as from recordings of the abnormal muscle contractions that are typical for patients with HFS [33, 101]. The blink reflex response is normally limited to the orbicularis oculi muscles, but in patients with HFS, it also includes contractions of other face muscles – thus a sign of synkinesis [128].

The anatomical location of these physiological abnormalities is crosstalk that may occur either between axons at the facial nerve root (ephaptic transmission) or between cells in the facial motonucleus. Clinical studies of patients with HFS have questioned whether ephaptic transmission could cause the symptoms and signs of HFS [34, 174] because the signs of pathology in HFS can involve most of the facial muscles including the platysma as seen in patients who have had HFS for many years. It seems unlikely that ephaptic transmission could cause such massive contractions, because that would require that almost all facial nerve fibers were denuded and were in close contact with each other.

Results of intraoperative electrophysiological recordings in patients undergoing MVD operations for HFS have indicated that the anatomical location of the physiological abnormality that causes the crosstalk that is typical for HFS is central to the location of vascular contact [97]. The same intraoperative studies as well as animal experiments in models of HFS have supported the hypothesis that the anatomical location of the physiological abnormality is the facial motonucleus.

> Intraoperative studies have shown that the existence of an abnormal muscle contraction that is typical for HFS could not be explained by ephaptic transmission at the location of the vascular contact. Only in a single patient did such intraoperative neurophysiologic measurements show electrophysiological signs of ephaptic transmission [102]. This phenomenon lasted only a few minutes and it occurred after the facial nerve root had undergone extensive surgical manipulations and appeared to have been injured. The signs of ephaptic transmission (shortened latency of the abnormal muscle response by approximately 2 msec) was only observed in a single operation out of many hundred operations for HFS where similar intraoperative recordings were made [109]. This observation of signs of ephaptic transmission between nerve fibers is in good agreement with the early descriptions of ephaptic transmission between injured myelinated nerve fibers [52], and in spinal (dorsal) roots [144].
>
> Instead recordings from other patients showed consistent evidence that the anatomical location of the abnormality that causes the crosstalk in patients with HFS is central to the location of the vascular contact with the root of the CN VII. These studies thus supported the hypothesis that there are functional abnormalities in the facial motonucleus in patients with HFS that include establishment of connections between populations of motoneurons [97]. This is consistent with the hypothesis

that was originally proposed by Ferguson [35]. These functional connections between neurons that innervate different groups of facial muscles may be a result of unmasking of dormant synapses, which connect motoneurons that give rise to nerve fibers of different branches of the facial nerve.

The abnormal muscle response (Figs. 6.2 and 6.3) is assumed to be caused by backfiring of alpha motoneurons in response to antidromic stimulation of the motor nerve. It may thus be similar to the F-response and it is therefore an indication that the excitability of the facial motoneurons is higher than normal. The presence of the abnormal muscle response supports the hypothesis that the facial motonucleus is hyperactive in HFS [59, 97, 109].

It was hypothesized [97] that the changes in the function of the facial motoneurons are similar to those of the kindling phenomenon described by Goddard [48] who showed that novel stimulation of the amygdala nucleus could lead to hyperactivity (seizure activity) and it was later reported that novel stimulation of (or deprivation of input to) other nuclei can cause reorganization of the nuclei, causing hyperactivity and altered processing [177]. The novel stimulation that causes the facial motonucleus to become hyperactive may be generated by the irritation of the facial nerve from close contact with a blood vessel, or unknown factors.

The abnormal muscle contraction cannot be elicited after the offending vessel is moved off the facial nerve (Fig. 6.15) [54, 98, 104]. This suggests that some abnormal neural activity is generated in the facial nerve by the close contact with a blood vessel, and that this abnormal activity is necessary to maintain the hyperactivity of the facial motor nucleus.

The fact that the abnormal muscle response disappears instantaneously during operations for HFS when the offending vessel is moved off the facial nerve [98] (Fig. 6.14), indicates that the abnormal activity in the facial nerve caused by the close contact with a blood vessel is necessary in order to sustain the abnormality in the facial motonucleus.

The R_1 component of the blink reflex can be recorded during general anesthesia in patients with HFS on the affected side (Fig. 6.15) [100] but not on the unaffected side. This indicates that the suppression of the blink reflex that is normally caused by general anesthesia is counteracted by the hyperactivity of facial motoneurons in patients with HFS, thus a further indication that the facial motonucleus is hyperactive in individuals with HFS. The latency of the blink reflex elicited on the affected side during anesthesia is slightly longer than that of the normal blink reflex [100] (Fig. 6.15). (The abnormal muscle reflex is much less affected by anesthesia than the blink reflex.)

Animal studies have supported the hypotheses that the signs of HFS (spasm and synkinesis) are caused by abnormalities in the facial motonucleus. One such animal model of HFS was created by electrical stimulation of the facial nerve according to the kindling paradigm [150, 158]. Repeated electrical stimulation of the facial nerve at the stylomastoid

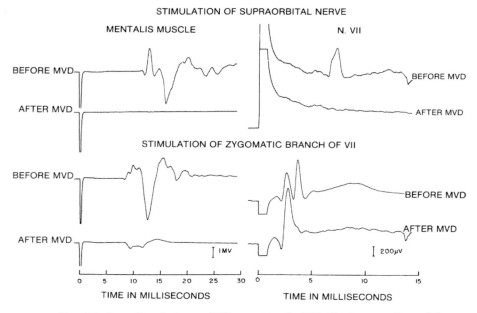

Fig. 6.15 Recording during an MVD operation for HFS. The top recordings of the synkinetic component of the R_1 component of the blink reflex (from the mentalis muscle) and the response from the exposed root of the CN VII, before and after the offending vessel have been moved off the facial nerve intracranially. Bottom recordings show the abnormal muscle response recorded from the mentalis muscle elicited from the zygomatic branch of the facial nerve and the response from the root of the CN VII, before and after the offending vessel has been moved off the facial nerve intracranially [100]. Reprinted from *J. Neurol. Sci.*, 72; 171–183, 1986, with permission.

foramen in rats caused the development of an abnormal muscle response that is similar to that which is present in individuals with HFS [158] (Fig. 6.16) after approximately 4 weeks of daily stimulation of the facial nerve.

These findings support the hypothesis that synkinesis of facial muscles can be caused by novel stimulation of the facial nerve that is presumed to cause unmasking of dormant synapses and thereby facilitating cross activation of different muscle groups.

The mass movements of facial muscles in very young children may also be a result of functional connections between different groups of facial motoneurons by synapses that later become dormant during normal postnatal development.

Spasmodic torticollis

The pathophysiology of the two forms of spasmodic torticollis, the unilateral and the bilateral forms [125], is likely to be different (cf HFS and

SINGLE RESPONSE

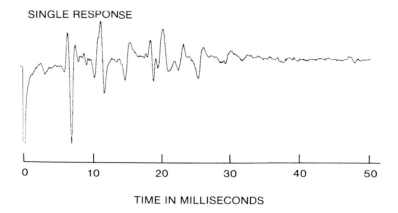

TIME IN MILLISECONDS

AVERAGE OF 256 RESPONSES

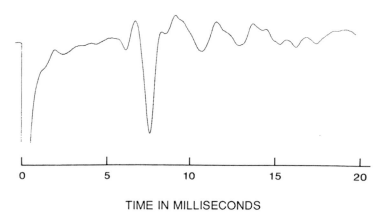

TIME IN MILLISECONDS

Fig. 6.16 Recording of the abnormal muscle response in a rat after stimulation of the facial nerve at the stylomastoid foramen daily for 4 weeks. Top recording: Response to a single stimulus. Bottom recording: Average of 256 responses [158]. Reprinted from *Exp. Neurol.*, 98; 336–349, 1987 with permission from Elsevier.

blepharospasm). The bilateral form of spasmodic torticollis may involve basal ganglia hyperactivity while the pathology of the unilateral type may be associated with the eleventh cranial nerve's motonucleus on the affected side similar to HFS.

Electrophysiological studies performed during MVD operations of patients with unilateral spasmodic torticollis have shown the presence of an abnormal muscle response similar to that which is present in HFS [151] supporting the hypothesis that the unilateral spasmodic torticollis has similarities with HFS. The bilateral form does not exhibit such abnormal muscle responses, indicating that the pathophysiology of the bilateral form of the disorder may be similar to blepharospasm.

Other studies have shown that the suppression of EMG activity in the sternocleidomastoid muscle from electrical stimulation of the supraorbital nerve is lower in patients with spasmodic torticollis than in normal individuals [126]. If reduced inhibition is the cause of spasmodic torticollis then the pathophysiology of this disorder may be similar to other forms of dystonia [13]. These investigators did not, however, differentiate between bilateral and unilateral spasmodic torticollis.

Cyclic oculomotor spasm with paresis

This disorder has similarities with HFS and it is probably caused by hyperactivity of the third cranial nerve nucleus [79] thus having similar pathophysiology as HFS. Close contact between a blood vessel and a portion of the third cranial nerve seems to be involved [79].

Spasm of mastication muscles

While the blood vessel that is in contact with the sensory root of CN V in patients with TGN (p. 337) is often also in close contact with the motor portion (portio minor) of CN V (that innervate the muscles of mastication) and spasm of these muscles occurs rarely [7, 172] (see p. 335). Even when the portio minor of CN V is deformed by the close contact with a blood vessel, symptoms from the mastication muscles are absent. This supports the hypothesis that the close contact between a cranial nerve root and a blood vessel only creates symptoms and signs when another factor (or factors) is present [109].

Trigeminal neuralgia

TGN has many similarities with HFS but also differences, one difference being that medical treatment is as efficient as MVD in TGN but no known medical treatment is effective in treating HFS. TGN can be treated with the same efficiency by partial section of the trigeminal nerve, while partial section of the facial nerve never became an established method of treatment of HFS although tried with some positive results reported [36, 187].

As for HFS, whether the symptoms of TGN are caused by pathologies of the nerve itself or its root [16, 31, 44–46] or whether they are caused by abnormal activity of specific populations of neurons in the CNS [40–42, 109, 112] has been a matter of discussion for a long time. The hypothesis that claims that pathology of the nerve root is the cause of the symptoms assumes that ectopic spikes and possibly crosstalk (ephaptic transmission) occur between fibers that are slightly injured by close contact with a blood vessel [46, 157].

It has been proposed that the hyperactivity is induced by the irritation of the trigeminal nerve root by a blood vessel causing increased and abnormal activity in the fibers of the sensory part of the trigeminal nerve (portio major). Other investigators have hypothesized that the anatomical location of the pathologies that cause the symptoms of TGN is the CNS and it has been postulated that the cause of the symptoms of TGN is impaired segmental inhibition in the trigeminal nucleus causing hyperactivity in the trigeminal sensory nucleus [42]. The fact that TGN can be treated successfully by drugs that have central action such as carbamazepine and baclofen [39] (agonist of the B receptors of gamma butyric acid; GABA$_B$) is a strong indication of central nervous system involvement in producing the pain.

> The hypothesis that decreased segmental inhibition is a factor in generating the pain of TGN is supported by findings from animal studies, which have shown that drugs such as carbamazepine (Tegretol) and phenytoin (Dilantin) that are effective in treating TGN affect segmental inhibition [40]. In these studies, carbamazepine was found to be more effective than phenytoin [170], which is in agreement with experience from clinical studies in patients with TGN that have shown that carbamazepine is more effective than phenytoin. These drugs are sodium channel blockers but they also have other actions.
>
> Baclofen, a GABA$_B$ receptor agonist, has been shown to increase segmental inhibition in the trigeminal brainstem complex [40], and this drug is likewise effective in treatment of TGN. The beneficial effect of baclofen is stereo specific and levo-baclofen ((-)-baclofen) is at least 5 times more effective than racemic baclofen in treating patients with TGN [39]. Dextro-baclofen has no known effect on segmental inhibition, and it may be the cause of the side effects of racemic baclofen.

Disabling positional vertigo

DPV can be cured by MVD of the intracranial portion of the vestibular nerve [15, 70, 116, 118, 120, 122] and it has therefore been associated with vascular compression of the vestibular nerve. As in the other vascular compression disorders, there are indications that the symptoms and signs of DPV are caused by functional changes in the CNS. The close contact between a blood vessel and the vestibular nerve root [70, 116, 153] is most likely only one of several factors that are necessary to cause development of the symptoms of DPV. The symptoms of DPV (more or less constant vertigo, lightheadedness and nausea that are aggravated by head movements) indicate that information from the vestibular organ has been re-routed in the CNS. The fact that symptoms and signs of DPV can be alleviated by administration of diazepam [118] supports the hypothesis that DPV is a disorder of the central nervous system rather than a disorder of the vestibular organ or the vestibular nerve. Other studies indicate that the symptoms of DPV are signs of vestibular hyperactivity [153] supporting the hypothesis that the anatomical location of the physiological abnormalities that cause the symptoms is the CNS.

Tinnitus

Tinnitus often occurs after acute injury to the intracranial portion of the auditory nerve, such as may occur from surgical manipulation or in connection with tumors that affect the auditory portion of the eighth cranial nerve (mostly vestibular schwannoma) [21]. The fact that tinnitus often occurs immediately after operations in the cerebello-pontine angle (such as MVD operations) where the intracranial portion of the auditory nerve has been manipulated surgically provides strong evidence that injury to the auditory nerve is involved in creating the pathological conditions that cause tinnitus [96]. However, these observations of involvement of the auditory nerve in tinnitus do not mean that the anatomical location of the physiological abnormalities that cause the tinnitus is the auditory nerve. Rather, there are several indications that the forms of tinnitus that can be cured by MVD operations are caused by changes in the function of CNS structures, thus similar to other hyperactive cranial nerve disorders.

> The complexity of the pathophysiology of tinnitus even in selected populations is evident from the results of a study of 72 individuals [121] who underwent MVD to treat severe tinnitus that showed that the success rate of MVD operations was significantly different in male and female. Using the same criteria for inclusion in the study and for evaluating the results of MVD of the auditory nerve [121], for men the success rate (for total relief or significant improvement) was 29.3% and for women was 54.8% in this group of 31 women and 41 men who were operated on using the MVD technique. There are several possible reasons for this difference. It is possible that the amount of female reproductive hormones versus testosterone plays a role but the higher incidence of noise exposure in men than in women may also have contributed to this observed difference in treatment results. The difference in treatment results of other MVD disorders (HFS and TGN) for men and women is small, and it is generally higher than that for tinnitus (80–90% [10, 11] versus average of 40% for tinnitus in men and women [121]). It is perhaps less surprising that those patients with less favorable outcome had had tinnitus for a longer period than those with better outcome [121].

Bilateral tinnitus is different from unilateral tinnitus, and MVD of the auditory nerve has a lower success rate for treatment of the bilateral form compared with the unilateral form of tinnitus [175]. Unilateral tinnitus may at least initially be caused by pathologies of the ear or the auditory nerve, but bilateral tinnitus most likely has central causes that may not primarily involve the ear or the auditory nerve (see Chapter 3).

History of the "microvascular decompression syndrome"

Microvascular compression of cranial nerves can be seen from different perspectives depending on a person's background and interests. The surgeon is interested in the exact location and course of the offending vessels and goes to great length to describe these and how they vary from patient to patient [56, 67, 87, 164]. The anatomist is interested in morphological changes that the vessel may cause to the nerve [75, 147, 165]. The physiologist and the neurologist are focused on the abnormal neural activity in the respective nerve that may be caused by the close contact with a blood vessel and how that can affect the function of more rostral neural structures [42, 109] and cause the symptoms and signs of these disorders.

> The history about "the vascular compression syndrome" of cranial nerve roots and its connection with TGN goes back to the neurosurgeon Walter Dandy (1932) who described that patients with TGN had a "vascular conflict" of the trigeminal nerve root and reported that he believed this vascular contact (compression) was the cause of tic douloureux [27, 28]. Dandy, however, did not attempt to move these blood vessels off the trigeminal nerve root in order to treat TGN. Instead, he sectioned parts of the trigeminal nerve in the cerebello-pontine angle (CPA) to treat patients with TGN [26]. Earlier, Cushing (1920) [24] had hypothesized that compression of the roots of the trigeminal and the glossopharyngeal nerves were implicated in TGN and GPN. Much later, Taarnhøj (1956) [167, 168] and Gardner and Miklos (1959) [44] were the first to describe the beneficial effect on patients with TGN from surgical decompression of the trigeminal nerve root, an operation that later became known as the MVD operation. This operation was later popularized by Jannetta [65] and further developed by other neurosurgeons [80, 162, 163] (for details about the history of the MVD operation, see [111]). Now, MVD of the trigeminal nerve root is a common treatment of TGN.
>
> Gardner and Sava reported the presence of similar vascular compression of the seventh cranial nerve root in patients with HFS in 1962 [47].

6.5   Pathophysiology of the vestibular system

Disorders that affect the receptor organ in the inner ear or the vestibular nerve can result in awareness of activation of the vestibular system. For example, vestibular nerve neuritis and disorders of the vestibular organ can make activation of the vestibular organ reach consciousness and cause symptoms and signs such as nausea, lightheadedness or vertigo in response to head movements. When head movements are felt it means that information from the balance organ in the inner ear has been re-directed to other parts of the CNS than those that are normally reached by such information. This means that symptoms from the vestibular system are clearly related to plastic changes in the nervous system. Since these symptoms can develop suddenly neural sprouting as a cause of redirection of information is less likely to be the cause, and the anomaly is most likely the result of changes in synaptic efficacy (opening of dormant synapses) in already anatomically established pathways.

Excessive motion, and head movements, in particular where the body moves such as experienced on a boat, can cause an incorrect feeling of motion (dizziness) and autonomic symptoms such as vomiting. Nausea and the feeling of unsteadiness and lightheadedness can be caused by abnormal output from the vestibular apparatus, which may elicit an abnormally high firing rate, or change the discharge pattern to burst firing.

Symptoms from the vestibular system may also be created because of incompatibility between the input from vision and body proprioceptors with that from the vestibular system. Space sickness that has achieved much attention since the beginning of space travel is another pathologic reaction in response to abnormal motions where the output from the vestibular organ is incompatible with the output of other proprioceptive systems and vision. This means that changes in the firing pattern of neurons in the vestibular nervous system may open dormant synapses (see p. 26) thus an expression of neural plasticity. Other involvements of the autonomic nervous system such as those that may occur in response to abnormal head motion do not seem to be of any benefit to the organism.

The fact that patients with some vestibular disorders perceive head movements means that the information from the balance organ in the inner ear has been re-directed to other parts of the CNS than those normally reached by such information. Such pathological re-direction of information may be more or less permanent and caused by the expression of neural plasticity that results in opening neural connections from the vestibular system to neurons in the CNS that normally do not receive input from the vestibular system. This may occur by change in the efficacy of synapses (unmasking of dormant synapses) or by morphological changes through sprouting of axons and dendrites. Change in protein synthesis can also occur because of changed input and it may change the excitability of nerve cells in the CNS [160].

It is believed that symptoms that can be alleviated by moving a blood vessel off the vestibular nerve root (DPV) are in fact caused by reorganization of the central vestibular nervous system (DPV was discussed above, p. 339).

Disorders of the vestibular system are often manifest by abnormalities of the VOR that controls the external eye muscles and serves to keep an image steady on the retina during head movements (see p. 354). Anomalies of the VOR are signs of expression of neural plasticity.

6.5.1   *Benign paroxysmal positional vertigo*

Contemporary theories about the pathophysiology of BPPV suggest that it is caused by a mechanical disorder of the vestibular organ that stimulates the receptors in an abnormal way in response to head movements. Basophilic deposits in the posterior semicircular canal are supposed to cause the anomalies. The novel output of the vestibular organ that reaches higher CNS centers is assumed to cause the symptoms of BPPV. The efficiency of a treatment that makes use of head movement exercises, known as the Epley maneuver [135], supports the hypothesis that the symptoms are caused by abnormalities in the vestibular apparatus in the inner ear. It is possible that such abnormal activity can cause abnormal neural activity in the vestibular nerve that can open synapses that are normally dormant (unmasking of ineffective synapses) in the vestibular nuclei and thereby establish connections to brain regions that normally do not receive information from the vestibular organ.

However, there are many vestibular disorders that are diagnosed as BPPV but which have no known cause. It is estimated that half of the cases of BPPV have no known cause. Others may be caused by virus, strokes and in connection with Ménière's disease (misdiagnosis!).

6.5.2   *Ménière's disease*

Ménière's disease is characterized by symptoms from both the auditory and the vestibular system (with episodes of fluctuating hearing loss, tinnitus and vertigo). The symptoms and signs of Ménière's disease have been assumed to be caused by imbalance in the fluid pressure (or rather fluid volume) in the inner ear. Consequently, treatments have been aimed at reducing fluid volume, by diet and diuretics. Recently, however, it has been shown that a treatment using air puffs that are applied to the middle ear cavity [30] is effective in alleviating symptoms of the disease. This treatment stimulates receptors in the inner ear (auditory and vestibular) and the fact that such treatment can alleviate the vestibular symptoms of Ménière's disease indicates that the pathophysiology of the disease is more complex than earlier believed and that the anatomical location of the physiological abnormality that causes the symptoms and signs of Ménière's disease may be the CNS. Such stimulation of the vestibular system by air puffs may cause expression of neural plasticity in a similar way to electrical stimulation of the skin (TENS, see p. 32) that is used in treatment of neuropathic pain (see p. 221).

6.5.3   *Other disorders of the vestibular nerve and nervous system*

Disorders of the vestibular nerve such as vestibular schwannoma and vestibular neuritis that cause reduced or absent vestibular function were discussed above. The functional adaptation to vestibular deficits that occurs in these disorders involves re-routing of information by expression of neural plasticity evoked by deprivation of input. That process of compensation for lack of vestibular input takes time as is evident from the fact that vestibular deficits that occur rapidly, for example from inflammation of the vestibular nerve, cause violent symptoms and disruption of posture whereas slow destruction of the vestibular nerve such as happens during the growths of vestibular schwannoma may cause few or no signs from the vestibular system. The fact that recovery from vestibular deficits varies greatly with the age of the individual is a sign of decreasing reserves with age.

6.5.4   *Nystagmus*

Since the vestibular system controls the position of the eyes through the VOR, disturbances in vestibular function can cause abnormal movements of the eyes known as nystagmus. Nystagmus (involuntary movements of the eyes) that may occur spontaneously or because of head movements is an important clinical sign of vestibular disturbances [8, 9]. Recording of eye movements (nystagmus) is used in testing of disturbances in vestibular function (electronystagmography, ENG). Rhythmic movements of the eyes (nystagmus) can be produced by abnormal activation of the vestibular system. Various disorders are associated with nystagmus and recording nystagmus is an important clinical test [8, 9].

Spontaneous eye movements (spontaneous nystagmus) is a sign that occurs in many different disorders but it can also be congenital and individuals with this abnormality have normal vision – again a sign of the remarkable adaptability of the vestibulo-ocular system.

6.6   Treatment benefits from knowing pathophysiology

As our understanding of the pathophysiology of disorders that are related to cranial nerves improves, treatments also improve. Earlier treatments were directed at correcting presumed morphological abnormalities. The evidence from recent studies that have shown that the symptoms of many disorders that are related to cranial nerves are caused by functional changes of the nervous system has changed the focus of treatment and brought new treatments into use. Such functional changes in the nervous system can be treated by appropriate stimulation of the sensory organ in question or by electrical stimulation of the structures of the nervous system. Even vestibular disorders such as Ménière's disease may be caused by functional changes in the nervous system and that has focused treatment from the (possible) morphological changes in the inner ear to changes in the function of the central nervous system.

References

1. Adams, C. B. T., The Physiology and Pathophysiology of Posterior Fossa Cranial Nerve Dysfunction Syndromes: Non Microvascular Perspective, in *Neurosurgical Topics Book 13, 'Surgery of Cranial Nerves of the Posterior Fossa,'* D. L. Barrow, Editor. 1993, American Association of Neurological Surgeons: Park Ridge, Illinois. pp. 131–154.

2. Adour, K. K., J. Wingerd, and H. E. Doty, Prevalence of Concurrent Diabetes Mellitus and Idiopathic Facial Paralysis (Bell's Palsy). *Diabetes*, 1975. **24**(5): pp. 449–51.

3. Adour, K. K., Mona Lisa Syndrome: Solving the Enigma of the Gioconda Smile. *Ann. Otol. Rhinol. Laryngol.*, 1989. **98**(3): pp. 196–9.

4. Adour, K. K., Decompression for Bell's Palsy: Why I Don't Do It. *European Arch. Oto-Rhino-Laryngol.*, 2002. **259**(1): pp. 40–7.

5. Apfelbaum, R. I., A Comparison of Percutaneous Radiofrequency Trigeminal Neurolysis and Microvascular Decompression of the Trigeminal Nerve for Treatment of Tic Douloureux. *Neurosurgery*, 1977(1): pp. 16–21.

6. Auger, R. G. and J. P. Whisnant, Hemifacial Spasm in Rochester and Olmsted County, Minnesota, 1960 to 1984. *Arch. Neurol.*, 1990(47): pp. 1233–1234.

7. Auger, R. G., W. J. Litchy, T. L. Cascino, and J. E. J. A. N. Ahlskog, Hemimasticatory Spasm: Clinical and Electrophysiologic Observations. *Neurology*, 1992. **42**(12): pp. 2263–6.

8. Baloh, R. W., *Dizziness, Hearing Loss, and Tinnitus: Essentials of Neurology*. 1984, F. A. Davis: Philadelphia.

9. Baloh, R. W. and V. Honrubia, *Clinical Neurophysiology of the Vestibular System*. 1990, F. A. Davis Company: Philadelphia.

10. Barker, F. G., P. J. Jannetta, D. J. Bissonette, P. T. Shields, and M. V. Larkins, Microvascular Decompression for Hemifacial Spasm. *J. Neurosurg.*, 1995. **82**: pp. 201–210.

11. Barker, F. G., P. J. Jannetta, D. J. Bissonette, M. V. Larkins, and H. D. Jho, The Long-Term Outcome of Microvascular Decompression for Trigeminal Neuralgia. *N. Eng. J. Med.*, 1996. **334**: pp. 1077–1083.

12. Beenstock, M., Predicting the Stability and Growth of Acoustic Neuromas. *Otol. Neurotol.*, 2002. **23**: pp. 542–49.

13. Berardelli, A., J. C. Rothwell, B. L. Day, and C. D. Marsden, Pathophysiology of Blepharospasm and Oromandibular Dystonia. *Brain*, 1985. **108**: pp. 593–608.

14. Berthold, C. H. and T. Carlstedt, Observations on the Morphology at the Transition Between the Peripheral and the Central Nervous System in the Cat. II General Organization of the Transitional Region in S1 Dorsal Rootlets. *Acta Physiol. Scand*, 1977. **Suppl. 446**: pp. 23–42.

15. Bertrand, R. A., P. Molina, and J. D. Hardy, Vestibular Syndrome and Vascular Anomaly in the Cerebello-Pontine Angle. *Acta Otolaryngol. (Stockh)*, 1977(3): pp. 187–194.

16. Boivie, J., Central Pain, in *Textbook of Pain*, P. D. Wall and R. Melzack, Editors. 1999, Churchill Livingstone: Edinburgh. pp. 879–914.

17. Borg, E., On the Neuronal Organization of the Acoustic Middle Ear Reflex. A Physiological and Anatomical Study. *Brain Res*, 1973. **49**: pp. 101–123.

18. Brach, J. S., J. M. Van Swearingen, J. Lenert, and P. C. Johnson, Facial Neuromuscular Retraining for Oral Synkinesis. *Plastic and Reconstructive Surgery*, 1997. **99**(7): pp. 1922–1931.

19. Brandt, T., S. Steddin, and R. B. Daroff, Therapy for Benign Paroxysmal Positioning Vertigo, Revisted. *Neurology*, 1994. **44**: pp. 796–800.

20. Brodal, P., *The Central Nervous System*. 1998, Oxford University Press: New York.

21. Cacace, A. T., T. J. Lovely, D. J. McFarland, S. M. Parnes, and D. F. Winter, Anomalous Cross-Modal Plasticity Following Posterior Fossa Surgery: Some Speculations on Gaze-Evoked Tinnitus. *Hear. Res.*, 1994. **81**: pp. 22–32.

22. Charabi, S., J. Thomsen, M. Tos, B. Charabi, M. Mantoni, and S. E. Børgesen, Acoustic Neuroma/Vestibular Schwannoma Growth: Past, Present and Future. *Acta Otolaryngol. (Stockh)*, 1998. **118**: pp. 327–32.

23. Coad, J. E., J. D. Wirtschafter, S. J. Haines, R. C. Heros, and T. Perrone, Familial Hemifacial Spasm Associated with Arterial Compression of the Facial Nerve. *J. Neurosurg.*, 1991. **74**(290–296).

24. Cushing, H., The Major Trigeminal Neuralgias and Their Surgical Treatment Based on Experience with 332 Gasserian Operations. *Am. J. Med. Sci.*, 1920(160): pp. 158–184.

25. Dandy, W., Glossopharyngeal Neuralgia (Tic Douloureux) Its Diagnosis and Treatment. *Arch Surg*, 1927(15): pp. 198–214.

26. Dandy, W., An Operation for the Cure of Tic Douloureux. Partial Section of the Sensory Root at the Pons. *Arch Surg*, 1929(18): pp. 687–734.

27. Dandy, W., The Treatment of Trigeminal Neuralgia by the Cerebellar Route. *Ann Surg*, 1932(96): pp. 787–795.

28. Dandy, W., Concerning the Cause of Trigeminal Neuralgia. *Am. J. Surg.*, 1934(24): pp. 447–455.

29. Davis, M., The Role of the Amygdala in Fear and Anxiety. *Ann. Rev. Neurosci*, 1992. **15**: pp. 353–375.

30. Densert, B. and K. Sass, Control of Symptoms in Patients with Ménière's Disease Using Middle Ear Pressure Applications: Two Years Follow-Up. *Acta Otolaryng. (Stockh.)*, 2001. **121**: pp. 616–621.

31. Devor, M., The Pathophysiology of Damaged Peripheral Nerves, in *Textbook of Pain*, P. D. Wall and R. Melzack, Editors. 1994, Churchill Livingstone: Edinburgh. pp. 79–100.

32. Dobie, R. and U. Fisch, Primary and Revision Surgery (Selective Neurectomy) for Facial Hyperkinesis. *Arch. Otolaryngol. Head Neck Surg.*, 1986(112): pp. 154–163.

33. Esslen, E., Der Spasmus Facialis – Eine Parabioserscheinung: Elektrophysiologische Untersuchnungen Zum Enstehungsmechanismus Des Facialisspasmus. *Dtsch. Z. Nervenheil.*, 1957. **176**: pp. 149–172.

34. Esteban, A. and P. Molina-Negro, Primary Hemifacial Spasm: A Neurophysiological Study. *J. Neurol. Neurosurg. Psych.*, 1986. **49**: pp. 58–63.

35. Ferguson, J. H., Hemifacial Spasm and the Facial Nucleus. *Ann. Neurol.*, 1978. **4**: pp. 97–103.

36. Fisch, U. and E. Esslen, The Surgical Treatment of Facial Hyperkinesis. *Arch Otolaryngol Head Neck Surg*, 1972(5): pp. 400–405.

37. Freckmann, N., R. Hagenah, H. D. Herrmann, and D. Muller, Treatment of Neurogenic Torticollis by Microvascular Lysis of the Accessory Nerve Roots: Indication, Technique, and First Results. *Acta Neurochir. (Wien)*, 1981(59): pp. 167–175.

38. Froehling, D. A., M. D. Silverstein, D. N. Mohr, C. W. Beatty, K. Offord, and D. J. Ballard, Benign Positional Vertigo: Incidence and Prognosis in a Population-Based Study in Olmsted County, Minnesota. *Mayo Clinic Proceedings*, 1991. **66**(6): pp. 596–601.

39. Fromm, G., Medical Treatment of Patients with Trigeminal Neuralgia, in *Trigeminal Neuralgia*. G. H. Fromm and B. J. Sessle, Editors. 1991, Butterworth-Heinemann: Boston. pp. 133–144.

40. Fromm, G. H., A. S. Chattha, C. F. Terrence, and J. D. Glass, Role of Inhibitory Mechanisms in Trigeminal Neuralgia. *Neurology*, 1981. **31**: pp. 683–687.

41. Fromm, G. H., Effects of Different Classes of Antiepileptic Drugs on Brain-Stem Pathways. *Fed. Proc.*, 1985. **44**: pp. 2432–2435.

42. Fromm, G. H., Pathophysiology of Trigeminal Neuralgia, in *Trigeminal Neuralgia*, G. H. Fromm and B. J. Sessle, Editors. 1991, Butterworth-Heinemann: Boston. pp. 105–130.

43. Fromm, G. H. and B. J. Sessle, *Trigeminal Neuralgia*. 1991, Butterworth-Heinemann: Boston.

44. Gardner, W. and M. Miklos, Response of Trigeminal Neuralgia to "Decompression" of Sensory Root. *JAMA*, 1959(170): pp. 1773–1776.

45. Gardner, W., Crosstalk – the Paradoxical Transmission of a Nerve Impulse. *Arch. Neurol.*, 1966(14): pp. 149–156.

46. Gardner, W. J., Concerning the Mechanism of Trigeminal Neuralgia and Hemifacial Spasm. *J. Neurosurg.*, 1962(19): pp. 947–958.

47. Gardner, W. J. and G. A. Sava, Hemifacial Spasm – a Reversible Pathophysiologic State. *J. Neurosurg.*, 1962(19): pp. 240–247.

48. Goddard, G. V., Amygdaloid Stimulation and Learning in the Rat. *J. Comp. Physiol. Psychol.*, 1964. **58**: pp. 23–30.

49. Goetz, C. G. and E. J. Pappert, *Textbook of Clinical Neurology*. 1999, W. B. Saunders Company: Philadelphia.

50. Goodgold, J. and A. Evberstein, *Electrodiagnosis of Neuromuscular Diseases*. 1983, Williams & Wilkins: Baltimore.

51. Gouda, J. J. and J. A. Brown, Atypical Facial Pain and Other Pain Syndromes. *Neurosurgery Clinics of North America*, 1997. **8**(1): pp. 87–100.

52. Granit, R., L. Leksell, and C. R. Skoglund, Fibre Interaction in Injured or Compressed Region of Nerve. *Brain*, 1944(67): pp. 125–140.

53. Grundy, B., Evoked Potentials Monitoring, in *Monitoring in Anesthesia and Critical Care Medicine.*, C. Blitt, Editor. 1985, Churchill-Livingstone: New York. pp. 345–411.

54. Haines, S. J. and F. Torres, Intraoperative Monitoring of the Facial Nerve During Decompressive Surgery for Hemifacial Spasm. *J. Neurosurg.*, 1991(74): pp. 254–257.

55. Hakanson, S., Trigeminal Neuralgia Treated by Injection of Glycerol into the Trigeminal Cistern. *Neurosurgery*, 1981(9): pp. 638–646.

56. Hamlyn, P. J., *Neurovascular Compression of the Lower Cranial Nerves.* 1999, Elsevier: Amsterdam.

57. Hoistad, D. L., G. Melnik, B. Mamikoglu, R. Battista, C. A. O'Connor, and R. J. Wiet, Update on Conservative Management of Acoustic Neuroma. *Otol. Neurotol.*, 2001. **22**: pp. 682–685.

58. House, J. W. and D. E. Brackmann, Tinnitus: Surgical Treatment, in *Tinnitus (Ciba Foundation Symposium 85)*. 1981, Pitman Books Ltd.: London.

59. Ishikawa, M., T. Ohira, J. Namiki, M. Kobayashi, M. Takase, T. Kawase, and S. Toya, Electrophysiological Investigation of Hemifacial Spasm after Microvascular Decompression: F Waves of the Facial Muscles, Blink Reflexes, and Abnormal Muscle Responses. *J. Neurosurg.*, 1997. **86**: pp. 654–661.

60. Ishiyama, A., K. M. Jacobson, and R. W. Baloh, Migraine and Benign Positional Vertigo. *Ann. Otol. Rhinol. Laryngol.*, 2000. **109**: pp. 377–80.

61. Itagaki, S., S. Saito, and O. Nakai, Electrophysiological Study on Hemifacial Spasm – Usefulness in Etiological Diagnosis and Pathophysiological Mechanism. *Brain Nerve (Tokyo)*, 1989. **41**: pp. 1005–1011.

62. Jackler, R. K., Acoustic Neuroma (Vestibular Schwannoma), in *Neurotology*, R. K. Jackler and D. Brackmann, Editors. 1994, Mosby: St. Louis. pp. 729–785.

63. Jannetta, P. and D. Bissonette, Bell's Palsy: A Theory as to Etiology. Observations in Six Patients Treated by Microsurgical Relief of Neurovascular Compression. *Laryngoscope*, 1978. **88**(5): pp. 849–854.

64. Jannetta, P. J., Arterial Compression of the Trigeminal Nerve at the Pons in Patients with Trigeminal Neuralgia. *J. Neurosurg.*, 1967. **26**: pp. 169–162.

65. Jannetta, P. J., Microsurgical Exploration and Decompression of the Facial Nerve in Hemifacial Spasm. *Curr. Top. Surg. Res.*, 1970(2): pp. 217–222.

66. Jannetta, P. J., Neurovascular Cross Compression in Patients with Hyperactive Dysfunction Symptoms of the Eighth Cranial Nerve. *Surg. Forum*, 1975. **26**: pp. 467–469.

67. Jannetta, P. J., Observations on the Etiology of Trigeminal Neuralgia, Hemifacial Spasm, Acoustic Nerve Dysfunction and Glossopharyngeal Neuralgia. Definitive Microsurgical Treatment and Results in 117 Patients. *Neurochir. (Stuttg)*, 1977(20): pp. 145–154.

68. Jannetta, P. J., Neurovascular Compression in Cranial Nerve and Systemic Disease. *Ann. Surg.*, 1980(192): pp. 518–525.

69. Jannetta, P. J., Hemifacial Spasm Caused by a Venule: Case Report. *Neurosurg.*, 1984. **14**: pp. 89–92.

70. Jannetta, P. J., M. B. Møller, and A. R. Møller, Disabling Positional Vertigo. *New Engl. J. Med.*, 1984(310): pp. 1700–1705.

71. Katusic, S., C. Beard, E. Bergstralh, and L. Kurland, Incidence and Clinical Features of Trigeminal Neuralgia, Rochester, Minnesota 1945–1984. *Ann Neurol*, 1990(27): pp. 89–95.

72. Kaufmann, M. D., Masticatory Spasm in Facial Hemiatrophy. *Ann. Neurol.*, 1980. **7**: pp. 585–587.

73. Keller, E. L. and W. Precht, Adaptive Modification of Central Vestibular Neurons in Response to Visual Stimulation through Reversing Prisms. *J. Neurophys.*, 1979. **42**(3): pp. 896–911.

74. Keller, E. L. and S. J. Heinen, Generation of Smooth-Pursuit Eye Movements: Neuronal Mechanisms and Pathways. *Neurosci. Res.*, 1991. **11**(2): pp. 79–107.

75. Kerr, F. W., Evidence of a Peripheral Etiology of Trigeminal Neuralgia. *J. Neurosurg.*, 1967. **26**(1): pp. 168–74.

76. Kimura, J., *Electrodiagnosis in Diseases of Nerve and Muscle: Principles and Practice.* 1989, F. A. Davis Company: Philadelphia.

77. King, R. B., J. N. Meagher, and J. C. Barnett, Studies of Trigeminal Nerve Potentials in Normal Compared to Abnormal Experimental Preparations. *J. Neurosurg.*, 1956(13): pp. 176–183.

78. Koizuka, I., Adaptive Plasticity in the Otolith-Ocular Reflex. *Auris, Nasus, Larynx.*, 2003. **30**(Suppl): pp. 3–6.

79. Kommerell, G., E. Mehdorn, U. P. Ketelsen, and C. Vollrath-Junger, Oculomotor Palsy with Cyclic Spasms: Electromyographic and Electron Microscopic Evidence of Chronic Peripheral Neuronal Involvement. *Neuro-Ophthalmol.*, 1988. **8**: pp. 9–21.

80. Kondo, A., J. Ishikawa, T. Yamasaki, and T. Konishi, Microvascular Decompression of Cranial Nerves, Particularly of the Seventh Cranial Nerve. *Neurol. Med. Chir. (Tokyo)*, 1980. **20**: pp. 739–751.

81. Kondziolka, D., L. D. Lunsford, and J. C. Flickinger, Stereotactic Radiosurgery for the Treatment of Trigeminal Neuralgia. *Clin. J. Pain*, 2002. **18**(1): pp. 42–47.

82. Kreutzberg, G. W., Neurobiology of Regeneration and Degeneration the Facial Nerve, in *The Facial Nerve*, M. May, Editor. 1986, Thieme: New York.

83. Kugelberg, E., Facial Reflexes. *Brain*, 1952. **75**: pp. 385–96.

84. Kuroki, A. and A. R. Møller, Facial Nerve Demyelination and Vascular Compression Are Both Needed to Induce Facial Hyperactivity: A Study in Rats. *Acta Neurochir. (Wien)*, 1994. **126**: pp. 149–157.

85. Laha, R. K. and P. J. Jannetta, Glossopharyngeal Neuralgia. *J. Neurosurg.*, 1977(47): pp. 316–320.

86. Lang, J., *Clinical Anatomy of the Posterior Cranial Fossa and Its Foramina.* 1981, Thieme Verlag: Stuttgart.

87. Lang, J., Facial and Vestibulocochlear Nerve, Topographic Anatomy and Variations. *The Cranial Nerves.* M. Samii and P. Jannetta, Editors. 1981, Springer-Verlag: New York. pp. 363–377.

88. Lang, J., Anatomy of the Brainstem and the Lower Cranial Nerves, Vessels, and Surrounding Structures. *Am. J. Otol.*, 1985: pp. 1–19.

89. Lovely, T. J., Efficacy and Complications of Microvascular Decompression: A Review. *Neurosurg. Quart.*, 1997.

90. Lovely, T. J. and P. J. Jannetta, Surgical Treatment of Geniculate Neuralgia. *Am. J. Otol.*, 1997. **18**(4): pp. 512–7.

91. Marion, M.-H., Hemifacial Spasm: Treatment with Botulinum Toxin (Long Term Results), in *Hemifacial Spasm. A Multidisciplinary Approach*, M. Sindou, Y. Keravel, and A. R. Møller, Editors. 1997, Springer: Wien. pp. 141–144.

92. Matsumoto, Y., J. L. Pulec, M. J. Patterson, and N. Yanagihara, Facial Nerve Biopsy for Etiologic Clarification of Bell's Palsy. *Ann. Otol. Rhinol. Laryngol. Suppl.*, 1988. **137**: pp. 22–7.

93. Matsushima, T., T. Inoue, and M. Fukui, Arteries in Contact with the Cisternal Portion of the Facial Nerve in Autopsy Cases: Microsurgical Anatomy for Neurovascular Decompression Surgery of Hemifacial Spasm. *Surg. Neurol.*, 1990. **34**: pp. 87–93.

94. McCabe, B., Management of Hyperfunction of the Facial Nerve. *Ann. Otol. Rhin. Laryng.*, 1970(79): pp. 252–258.

95. Møller, A. R., The Acoustic Reflex in Man. *J. Acoust. Soc. Am.*, 1962. **34**(2): pp. 1524–1534.

96. Møller, A. R., Pathophysiology of Tinnitus. *Ann. Otol. Rhinol. Laryngol.*, 1984. **93**: pp. 39–44.

97. Møller, A. R. and P. J. Jannetta, On the Origin of Synkinesis in Hemifacial Spasm: Results of Intracranial Recordings. *J. Neurosurg.*, 1984. **61**: pp. 569–576.

98. Møller, A. R. and P. J. Jannetta, Microvascular Decompression in Hemifacial Spasm: Intraoperative Electrophysiological Observations. *Neurosurgery*, 1985. **16**: pp. 612–618.

99. Møller, A. R. and P. J. Jannetta, Synkinesis in Hemifacial Spasm: Results of Recording Intracranially from the Facial Nerve. *Experientia*, 1985. **41**: pp. 415–17.

100. Møller, A. R. and P. J. Jannetta, Blink Reflex in Patients with Hemifacial Spasm: Observations During Microvascular Decompression Operations. *J. Neurol. Sci.*, 1986. **72**: pp. 171–182.

101. Møller, A. R. and P. J. Jannetta, Physiological Abnormalities in Hemifacial Spasm Studied During Microvascular Decompression Operations. *Exp. Neurol.*, 1986. **93**: pp. 584–600.

102. Møller, A. R., Hemifacial Spasm: Ephaptic Transmission or Hyperexcitability of the Facial Motor Nucleus? *Exp. Neurol.*, 1987. **98**: pp. 110–119.

103. Møller, A. R., Electrophysiological Monitoring of Cranial Nerves in Operations in the Skull Base, in *Tumors of the Cranial Base: Diagnosis and Treatment*, L. N. Sekhar and V. L. Schramm Jr, Editors. 1987, Futura Publishing Co: Mt. Kisco, New York. pp. 123–132.

104. Møller, A. R. and P. J. Jannetta, Monitoring Facial Emg During Microvascular Decompression Operations for Hemifacial Spasm. *J. Neurosurg.*, 1987. **66**: pp. 681–685.

105. Møller, A. R., *Intraoperative Monitoring of Evoked Potentials*. 1988, Williams and Wilkins: Baltimore.

106. Møller, A. R. and M. B. Møller, Does Intraoperative Monitoring of Auditory Evoked Potentials Reduce Incidence of Hearing Loss as a Complication of Microvascular Decompression of Cranial Nerves? *Neurosurgery*, 1989. **24**: pp. 257–263.

107. Møller, A. R., Interaction between the Blink Reflex and the Abnormal Muscle Response in Patients with Hemifacial Spasm: Results of Intraoperative Recordings. *J. Neurol. Sci.*, 1991. **101**: pp. 114–123.

108. Møller, A. R., The Cranial Nerve Vascular Compression Syndrome: I. A Review of Treatment. *Acta Neurochir. (Wien)*, 1991. **113**: pp. 18–23.

109. Møller, A. R., Cranial Nerve Dysfunction Syndromes: Pathophysiology of Microvascular Compression., in *Neurosurgical Topics Book 13, 'Surgery of Cranial Nerves of the Posterior Fossa,' Chapter 2*, D. L. Barrow, Editor. 1993, American Association of Neurological Surgeons: Park Ridge. IL. pp. 105–129.

110. Møller, A. R., *Intraoperative Neurophysiologic Monitoring*. 1995, Harwood Academic Publishers: Luxembourg.

111. Møller, A. R., Vascular Compression of Cranial Nerves. I: History of the Microvascular Decompression Operation. *Neurol. Res.*, 1998. **20**: pp. 727–731.

112. Møller, A. R., Vascular Compression of Cranial Nerves. II. Pathophysiology. *Neurol. Res.*, 1999. **21**: pp. 439–443.

113. Møller, A. R., *Hearing: Its Physiology and Pathophysiology*. 2000, Academic Press: San Diego.

114. Møller, A. R., Diagnosis of Acoustic Tumors. *Am. J. Otol.*, 2000. **21**: pp. 151–152.

115. Møller, M. B. and A. R. Møller, Audiometric Abnormalities in Hemifacial Spasm. *Audiology*, 1985. **24**: pp. 396–405.

116. Møller, M. B., A. R. Møller, P. J. Jannetta, and L. N. Sekhar, Diagnosis and Surgical Treatment of Disabling Positional Vertigo. *J Neurosurg*, 1986(64): pp. 21–28.

117. Møller, M. B., Vascular Compression of the Eighth Nerve as a Cause of Tinnitus, in *Proceedings of the Iii International Tinnitus Seminar, Munster, Western Germany, June 11–13, 1987*, H. Feldmann Editor. 1987, Harsch Verlag: Karlsruhe, West Germany. pp. 340–347.

118. Møller, M. B., Disabling Positional Vertigo, in *Advances in Otolaryngology – Head and Neck Surgery*, E. N. Myers, *et al.*, Editors. 1990, Mosby Year Book, Inc.: Chicago, Illinois,. pp. 81–106.

119. Møller, M. B., Results of Microvascular Decompression of the Eighth Nerve as Treatment for Disabling Positional Vertigo. *Ann. Otol. Rhinol. Laryngol.*, 1990. **99**: pp. 724–29.

120. Møller, M. B. and A. R. Møller, Vascular Compression Syndrome of the Eighth Nerve: Clinical Correlations and Surgical Findings, in *Neurologic Clinics: Diagnostic Neurotology and Otoneurology*, I. K. Arenberg and D. B. Smith, Editors. 1990, WB Saunders Publishing Co: Philadelphia. pp. 421–439.

121. Møller, M. B., A. R. Møller, P. J. Jannetta, and H. D. Jho, Vascular Decompression Surgery for Severe Tinnitus: Selection Criteria and Results. *Laryngoscope*, 1993. **103**: pp. 421–427.

122. Møller, M. B., A. R. Møller, P. J. Jannetta, H. D. Jho, and L. N. Sekhar, Microvascular Decompression of the Eighth Nerve in Patients with Disabling Positional Vertigo: Selection Criteria and Operative Results in 207 Patients. *Acta Neurochir. (Wien)*, 1993. **125**: pp. 75–82.

123. Møller, M. B., Audiological Evaluation. *J. Clin. Neurophysiol.*, 1994. **11**: pp. 309–318.

124. Nagata, K., T. Matsui, H. Joshita, T. Shigeno, and T. Asano, Surgical Treatment of Spasmodic Torticollis: Effectiveness of Microvascular Decompression. *Brain Nerve (Tokyo)*, 1989. **41**: pp. 97–102.

125. Nakai, O., S. Itagaki, and S. Saito, Electromyographic Analysis of Spasmodic Torticollis. *Tenth Meeting of the World Society for Stereotactic and Functional Neurosurgery. Abstract*, 1989.

126. Nakashima, K., P. D. Thompson, J. C. Rothwell, B. L. Day, R. Stall, and C. D. Marsden, An Exteroceptive Reflex in the Sternocleidomastoid Muscle Produced by Electrical Stimulation of the Supraorbital Nerve in Normal Subjects and Patients with Spasmodic Torticollis. *Neurology*, 1989. **39**: pp. 1354–1358.

127. Nielsen, V., Pathophysiological Aspects of Hemifacial Spasm. Part I. Evidence of Ectopic Excitation and Ephaptic Transmission. *Neurology*, 1984(34): pp. 418–426.

128. Nielsen, V. K., Pathophysiology of Hemifacial Spasm: II. Lateral Spread of the Supraorbital Nerve Reflex. *Neurology*, 1984. **34**: pp. 427–31.

129. Nikolopoulos, T. P., I. Johnson, and G. M. O'Donoghue, Quality of Life after Acoustic Neuroma Surgery. *Laryngoscope*, 1998. **108**(9): pp. 1382–1385.

130. Nikolopoulos, T. P. and G. M. O'Donoghue, Acoustic Neuroma Management: An Evidence-Based Medicine Approach. *Otol. Neurotol.*, 2002. **23**: pp. 534–41.

131. Odkvist, L. M., J. Thell, and C. Essen Von, Vestibulo-Oculomotor Disturbances in Trigeminal Neuralgia and Hemifacial Spasm. *Acta Otolaryngol. (Stockh)*, 1988. **105**: pp. 570–5.

132. Ollat, H., Pharmacology of Hemifacial Spasm, in *Hemifacial Spasm: A Multidisciplinary Approach*, M. Sindou, Y. Keravel, and A. Møller, Editors. 1997, Springer-Verlag: Wien.

133. Ongeboer De Visser, B. W. and C. Goor, Electromyographic and Reflex Study in Ideopathic and Symptomatic Trigeminal Neuralgias: Latency of the Jaw and Blink Reflexes. *J. Neurol. Neurosurg. Psych.*, 1974. **37**: pp. 1225–30.

134. Ouaknine, G. E., Microsurgical Anatomy of the Arterial Loops in the Ponto-Cerebellar Angle and the Internal Acoustic Meatus, in *The Cranial Nerves*, M. Samii and P. J. Jannetta, Editors. 1981, Springer-Verlag: Heidelberg. pp. 378–390.

135. Parnes, L. S. and R. G. Price-Jones, Particle Repositioning Maneuver for Benign Paroxysmal Positional Vertigo. *Ann. Otol. Rhinol. Laryngol.*, 1993. **102**: pp. 325–331.

136. Perkin, G. D. and R. D. Illingworth, The Association of Hemifacial Spasm and Facial Pain. *J. Neurol. Neurosurg. Psychiatry*, 1989. **52**: pp. 663–665.

137. Pierrot-Deseilligny, C., I. Israel, A. Berthoz, and S. Rivaud, Role of the Different Frontal Lobe Areas in the Control of the Horizontal Component of Memory-Guided Saccades in Man. *Exp. Brain Res.*, 1993. **95**(1): pp. 166–71.

138. Podivinsky, F., Torticollis, in *Handbook of Clinical Neurology, Diseases of the Basal Ganglia*, P. J. Vinken and G. W. Bruyn, Editors. 1968, North Holland Publishing Co: New York. pp. 567–603.

139. Pulec, J. L., Idiopathic Hemifacial Spasm. *Ann. Otol. Rhin. Laryng.*, 1972(81): pp. 664–676.

140. Pulec, J. L., Early Decompression of the Facial Nerve in Bell's Palsy. *Ann. Otol. Rhinol.Laryngol.*, 1981. **90**(6): pp. 570–7.

141. Pulec, J. L., Total Facial Nerve Decompression: Technique to Avoid Complications. *Ear, Nose, & Throat Journal*, 1996. **75**(7): pp. 410–415.

142. Pulec, J. L., Geniculate Neuralgia: Long Term Results of Surgical Treatment. *Ear, Nose, & Throat Journal*, 2002. **81**(1): pp. 30–3.

143. Rand, R. W. and T. L. Kurze, Facial Nerve Preservation by Posterior Fossa Transmeatal Microdissection in Total Removal of Acoustic Tumours. *J. Neurol. Neurosurg. Psychiat.*, 1965(28): pp. 311–316.

144. Rasminsky, M. Ephaptic Transmission between Single Nerve Fibers in the Spinal Nerve Roots of Dystrophic Mice. *J. Physiol. (Lond.)*, 1980. **305**: pp. 151–169.

145. Robillard, R. B., R. L. Hilsinger Jr, and K. K. Adour, Ramsay Hunt Facial Paralysis: Clinical Analyses of 185 Patients. *Otolaryngol Head Neck Surg*, 1986. **95**(3): pp. 292–7.

146. Ross, M. D. and W. Burkel, Electron Microscopic Observation of the Nucleus, Glial Dome, and Meninges of the Rat Acoustic Nerve. *Am. J. Anat.*, 1971. **130**: pp. 73–91.

147. Ruby, J. R. and P. J. Jannetta, Hemifacial Spasm: Ultrastructural Changes in the Facial Nerve Induced by Neurovascular Compression. *Surg. Neurol.*, 1975. **4**(369–370).

148. Rupa, V., R. L. Saunders, and D. J. Weider, Geniculate Neuralgia: The Surgical Management of Primary Otalgia. *J. Neurosurg.*, 1992. **75**(4): pp. 505–11.

149. Ryu, H., S. Yamamoto, K. Sugiyama, S. Nishizawa, and M. Nozue, Neurovascular Compression Syndrome of the Eighth Cranial Nerve. Can the Site of Compression Explain the Symptoms? *Acta Neurochir*, 1999. **141**: pp. 495–501.

150. Saito, S. and A. R. Møller, Chronic Electrical Stimulation of the Facial Nerve Causes Signs of Facial Nucleus Hyperactivity. *Neurol. Res.*, 1993. **15**: pp. 225–231.

151. Saito, S., A. R. Møller, P. J. Jannetta, and H. D. Jho, Abnormal Response from the Sternocleidomastoid Muscle in Patients with Spasmodic Torticollis: Observations During Microvascular Decompression Operations. *Acta Neurochir (Wien)*, 1993. **124**: pp. 92–98.

152. Sandyk, R. and M. A. Gillman, Baclofen in Hemifacial Spasm. *Int. J. Neurosci.*, 1987. **33**: pp. 261–4.

153. Schwaber, M. K., Microvascular Compression Syndromes: Clinical Features and Audiovestibular Findings. *Laryngoscope*, 1992. **102**: pp. 1020–1029.

154. Sekhar, L. N. and A. R. Møller, Operative Management of Tumors Involving the Cavernous Sinus. *J. Neurosurg.*, 1986(64): pp. 879–889.

155. Sekiya, T., T. Iwabuchi, T. Hatayama, and N. Shinozaki, Vestibular Nerve Injury as a Complication of Microvascular Decompression. *Neurosurgery*, 1991(29): pp. 773–775.

156. Selesnick, S. H. and G. Johnson, Radiologic Surveillance of Acoustic Neuromas. *Am. J. Otol.*, 1998. **19**: pp. 846–849.

157. Seltzer, Z. and M. Devor, Ephaptic Transmission in Chronically Damaged Peripheral Nerves. *Neurology*, 1979. **29**: pp. 1061–1064.

158. Sen, C. N. and A. R. Møller, Signs of Hemifacial Spasm Created by Chronic Periodic Stimulation of the Facial Nerve in the Rat. *Exp. Neurol.*, 1987. **98**: pp. 336–349.

159. Shima, F., M. Fukni, T. Matsubara, and K. Kitamura, Spasmodic Torticollis Caused by Vascular Compression of the Spinal Accessory Root. *Surg. Neurol.*, 1986. **26**: pp. 431–434.

160. Sie, K. C. Y. and E. W. Rubel, Rapid Changes in Protein Synthesis and Cell Size in the Cochlear Nucleus Following Eighth Nerve Activity Blockade and Cochlea Ablation. *J. Comp. Neurol.*, 1992. **320**: pp. 501–508.

161. Silverstein, H., A. McDaniel, H. Norrell, and J. Wazen, Conservative Management of Acoustic Neuroma in the Elderly Patients. *Laryngoscope*, 1985. **95**: pp. 766–770.

162. Sindou, M. and P. Mertens, Microvascular Decompression (MVD) in Trigeminal and Glosso-Vago-Pharyngeal Neuralgias. A Twenty Year Experience. *Acta Neurochir. (Wien)*, 1993. **58**: pp. 168–170.

163. Sindou, M., M. Chiha, and P. Mertens, Anatomical Findings Observed During Microsurgical Approaches of the Cerebellopontine Angle for Vascular Decompression in Trigeminal Neuralgia (350 Cases). *Stereotact. Funct. Neurosurg.*, 1994. **63**: pp. 203–207.

164. Sunderland, S., Microvascular Relations and Anomalies at the Base of the Brain. *J. Neurol. Neurosurg. Psychiatry*, 1948. **11**: pp. 243–257.

165. Sunderland, S., Cranial Nerve Injury. Structural and Pathophysiological Considerations and a Classification of Nerve Injury, in *The Cranial Nerves*, M. Samii and P. J. Jannetta, Editors. 1981, Springer-Verlag: Heidelberg. pp. 16–26.

166. Sweet, W. H., Percutaneous Methods for the Treatment of Trigeminal Neuralgia and Other Faciocephalic Pain: Comparison with Microvascular Decompression. *Semin. Neurol.*, 1988. **8**: pp. 272–279.

167. Taarnhøj, P., Trigeminal Neuralgia and Decompression of the Trigeminal Root. *Surg. Clin. North Am*, 1956(36): pp. 1145–1157.

168. Taarnhøj, P., Decompression of the Posterior Trigeminal Root in Trigeminal Neuralgia. A 30 Year Follow-up Review. *J. Neurosurg.*, 1982(57): pp. 14–17.

169. Tarlov, I. M., Structure of the Nerve Root. 1. Nature of the Junction between Central and Peripheral Nervous System. *Arch. Neurol. Psychiat.*, 1937. **37**: pp. 555.

170. Terrence, C., M. Sax, G. H. Fromm, C.-H. Chang, and C. S. Yoo, Effect of Baclofen Enantiomorphs on the Spinal Trigeminal Nucleus and Steric Similarities of Carbamazepine. *Pharmacology*, 1983. **27**: pp. 85–94.

171. Tetzlaff, W., M. B. Graeber, and G. W. Kreutzberg, Reaction on Motoneurons and Their Microenvironment to Axotomy. *Exp Brain Res*, 1986. **3**(Suppl,13): pp. 3–8.

172. Thompson, P. D. and W. M. Carroll, Hemimasticatory Spasm – a Peripheral Paroxysmal Cranial Neuropathy. *Neurol. Neurosurg. Psychiatry*, 1983. **46**: pp. 274–276.

173. Tolosa, E. S. and J. Pena, Involuntary Vocalizations in Movement Disorders. *Adv. Neurol.*, 1988. **49**: pp. 343–363.

174. Valls-Sole, J. and E. S. Tolosa, Blink Reflex Excitability Cycle in Hemifacial Spasm. *Neurology*, 1989. **39**: pp. 1061–6.

175. Vasama, J. P., M. B. Møller, and A. R. Møller, Microvascular Decompression of the Cochlear Nerve in Patients with Severe Tinnitus. Preoperative Findings and Operative Outcome in 22 Patients. *Neurol. Res.*, 1998. **20**: pp. 242–248.

176. Vial, C. and A. Vighetto, Hemifacial Spasm: Treatment with Botulinum Toxin (a Report of 50 Patients), in *Hemifacial Spasm. A Multidisciplinary Approach*, M. Sindou, Y. Keravel, and A. R. Møller, Editors. 1997, Springer: Wien. pp. 135–140.

177. Wada, J. A., *Kindling 2*. 1981, Raven Press: New York.

178. Wersäll, J., Studies of the Structure and Innervation of the Sensory Epithelium of the Cristae Ampularis in the Guinea Pig: A Light and Electron Microscopic Investigation. *Acta Otolaryng. Suppl*, 1956. **126**.

179. White, J. C. and W. H. Sweet, Facial and Cephalic Neuralgias: Trigeminal Neuralgia, in *Pain*. 1955, Charles C. Thomas, Springfield, Illinois. pp. 433–493.

180. Whurr, R., M. Lorch, H. Fontana, G. Brookes, A. Lees, and C. D. Marsden, The Use of Botulinum Toxin in the Treatment of Adductor Dysphonia. *J. Neurol. Neurosurg. Psych.*, 1993. **56**: pp. 526–530.

181. Williams, P. L. and R. Warwick, *Gray's Anatomy*. 1980, W. B. Saunders: Philadelphia.

182. Wilson-Pauwels, A. O., E. J. Akesson, and P. A. Stewart, *Cranial Nerves*. 1988, B. C. Decker Inc: Toronto.

183. Xenellis, J. E. and F. H. Linthicum, On the Myth of the Glial/Schwann Junction (Obersteiner-Redlich Zone): Origin of Vestibular Nerve Schwannomas. *Otol. Neurotol.*, 2003. **24**(1): pp. 1.

184. Yeh, H. S. H. and J. M. Tew, Tic Convulsif, the Combination of Geniculate Neuralgia and Hemifacial Spasm Relieved by Vascular Decompression. *Neurology*, 1984. **34**: pp. 682–683.

185. Yingling, C. and J. Gardi, Intraoperative Monitoring of Facial and Cochlear Nerves During Acoustic Neuroma Surgery. *Otolaryngol. Clin. N. Am.*, 1992(25): pp. 413–448.

186. Yingling, C., Intraoperative Monitoring in Skull Base Surgery, in *Neurotology*, R. K. Jackler and D. E. Brackmann, Editors. 1994, Mosby: St. Louis. pp. 967–1002.

187. Youngs, R., H. Ludman, and S. Smith, Transtympanic Surgery for Hemifacial Spasm. *Clin Otolaryngol*, 1988(13): pp. 331–333.

Index